CHANGING BODIES, CHANGING LIVES

CHANGING BODIES, CHANGING LIVES

A Book for Teens on
Sex and Relationships

RUTH BELL

and other co-authors of OUR BODIES, OURSELVES
and OURSELVES AND OUR CHILDREN, together with
members of the Teen-Book Project

Random House 🏠 New York

CLINIC DISCOUNT

Changing Bodies, Changing Lives is available at a discount to clinics, groups and organizations licensed by the state to operate entirely or in part as counseling services, health clinics or mental health clinics offering health education and information to teenagers, for distribution to their members or clients. The discounted price is $4.49 per copy for the hardcover and $2.39 for the softcover, plus $.35 per copy to cover shipping. The following requirements must be met:

1) A minimum of twelve (12) copies must be ordered (on a non-returnable basis).
2) A copy of the state or federal license (or other document filed with the state or federal government indicating as one of the organization's purposes the teenager education function as described above) must be included with the order.
3) Payment must be by money order or cashier's check.
4) Money orders and cashier's checks must be made out to Random House. When ordering, write to Random House, Inc. (Box 100, Department JG-1, Westminster, MD 21157). Orders that do not fulfill the above requirements will be returned.

Library of Congress Cataloging in Publication Data
Bell, Ruth.
  Changing bodies, changing lives.
  Bibliography: p.
  Includes index.
  SUMMARY: Candidly discusses teenage sexuality and the many physical and emotional changes that occur during adolescence.
  1. Sex instruction for youth. [1. Sex instruction for youth] I. Title.
HQ35.B44   306.7'088055   80-5298
ISBN 0-394-50304-X
ISBN 0-394-73632-X (pbk.)

Manufactured in the United States of America
  456789

THIS BOOK IS DEDICATED TO
ZACHARY AND DAVID
ONE WHO IS SOON TO BECOME A TEENAGER
THE OTHER WHO, IN THE BEST SENSE, WILL
ALWAYS BE ONE

PREFACE

Those of us who worked on *Changing Bodies, Changing Lives* joined together on this project because we believe that teenagers—and all of us—have a right to honest and thorough information about sex. We believe that unwanted pregnancies, epidemics of sexually transmitted diseases and exploitative sexual relationships are harmful and unnecessary, but until people are willing to talk openly with teenagers about these issues, the problems will continue to exist and increase in frequency. *Changing Bodies, Changing Lives* is our attempt to open that dialogue with teens about sex and relationships.

The inspiration for this book came from *Our Bodies, Ourselves,* a book on sexuality and health by and for women. Several of us are part of the group that wrote that book. We learned through that experience that information and facts become meaningful when we can see the connection they have to our lives. We learned to trust our own feelings and to be proud of our own bodies. The book has reached millions of people all over the world, and we know from their letters to us that they have been affected in the same way.

In that spirit we have two main goals for *Changing Bodies, Changing Lives*: (1) to give you information about sex and body development that will help you understand and trust your own feelings and so will give you more control over your own future; and (2) to give you an opportunity to hear from other teenagers who are going through some of the same changes and experiences you are.

A NOTE TO PARENTS: Many parents have an underlying feeling that sex information will shock or disturb their children, or even worse, that it will interest them too much. Some fear that if we give young people information about sex, it will make them rush out and "do it."

It's natural to think that way, but it isn't what happens. Good sex education, which means to us sex education that is about real people going through real-life situations, doesn't encourage anybody to go out and get wild. In fact, studies show that teenagers who are taught about sex, birth control, VD and body functions are *less* likely to get pregnant before they want to, *less* likely to catch VD and *less* likely to engage in thoughtless sexual activity than teens who haven't had that education. It's when we don't teach teens and preteens about sex and their bodies that they get into trouble.

Many people helped write this book. There were the hundreds of teenagers we interviewed; their contributions are the backbone of our writing. There were the parents and sex educators and junior high and high school teachers who talked to us about their experiences living and working with teens. We had teenage editors and commentators who met with us to share ideas and philosophy, and who read and criticized our work in progress. Teenage poets contributed poems, and teenage photographers offered their photographs. And finally, there were the ten of us who did the actual writing and rewriting of the pages that follow. We would like to tell you something about who we are:

Ruth Bell, Project Coordinator: As a member of the Boston Women's Health Book Collective I have worked for many years with the others in our group giving lectures and workshops and courses on health and sexuality. Much of that work has been with teenagers. I was always struck with how sophisticated many teens appear on the surface, while inside they struggle with the same questions and uncertainties and lack of information most of the rest of us worry about. The closer I became to several groups of teenagers, the more I became convinced that a book like *Our Bodies, Ourselves* was needed for them—a book that would direct itself exclusively to teenagers and not be afraid to address their real concerns. I hope *Changing Bodies, Changing Lives* does that without compromise, euphemism or moral judgment. I would like my son, who is almost a teenager, his friends, and all the preteens and teenagers I know to be able to turn to this book when they need information or support and find within it the help they need.

Sally Bowie: Currently I am the director of the Rape Crisis Intervention Program at Beth Israel Hospital in Boston. But for the previous two years I worked for the Planned Parenthood League of Massachusetts developing an exciting new model of sex education through drama—the Youth Expression Theater. In YET teenagers do the teaching.

I learned a great deal from working with the YET cast and from talking to teenagers around the country: given the opportunity, kids can really talk honestly to other kids; they can provide each other with support, information and fresh perspectives. But the opportunity is not often given. I wanted to make that opportunity more available, at least on paper, by sharing with others what I'd learned about feelings and ways of getting help. That's why I wrote the Emotional Health Care chapter.

I was born on the fourth of July. My middle name is Independence. I come from a family of six kids, and I feel as though I've lived through the teenage years six times over.

Rob Evans: I work as the clinical director of Project COPE, a drug and alcohol treatment agency for young people in Lynn, Massachusetts. I am also a doctoral student at Harvard in religion and society. In my spare time I am a storyteller, a drummer and the husband of a beautiful woman named Mary. I am glad to contribute to this book because I want to make sure that people have honest and accurate information, both positive and negative, as they decide what to do about drugs and alcohol.

Joanne Gates: Helping to write this book has been a catharsis of the last ten years of my life. It crystallized my experiences as a mother and as a psychologist working with teens around the area of sexuality. I wanted to share in writing something that would really matter to teens and touch their lives the way *Our Bodies, Ourselves* touched mine. I wanted this to be a book that I could give to my own daughter so she would know more about life, love, relationships, and about her body, her feelings and herself as a sexual person.

My work with teens includes working as a counselor in an abortion clinic, writing and teaching a course on teenage health and sexuality, making a film and a six-part cable TV program on teenage sexuality, being a counselor in a New York City alternative high school, and for the past five years, working as a sex and family planning counselor in a New York City multiservice center for adolescents.

Elizabeth A. McGee: For eleven years I have worked in family planning—as a counselor, educator, administrator or consultant. Much of this work has been with teens. I have lived on the East Coast and in Texas, and worked with a variety of groups including two Planned Parenthoods, many abortion clinics, The Door (a multiservice teen center) and the women's collective that wrote *Our Bodies, Ourselves*. Formally, I have a master's degree in public health; informally, my best training has come from friends, teens and my own memories of adolescence. I wanted to help with this book because the teens I know are still eager for more information about the changes they are experiencing. For me, one of the best parts of being a contributor has been working with people I admire.

Monica Mizrahi: I'm eighteen and I'm in my third year at Bard College in New York. I wanted to work on this book because I think it's important to have information when you're getting into sex and relationships. But more than that, I wanted people to be able to read something that would tell them: You're OK. What you're going through is OK. Don't worry about your mistakes. All of us make mistakes. Just learn from them and get stronger.

Jane Pincus: Working on *Changing Bodies, Changing Lives* was my intellectual initiation into the complexities of these teenage years. I'm the mother of a teenager and amazed by her energy and fearlessness. My very life is being changed by my changing daughter.

Wendy Sanford: I co-authored the chapters on sexuality, birth control and abortion in *Our Bodies, Ourselves,* and acted as editor-coordinator for *Ourselves and Our Children*. For four years I worked with college students as a sexuality counselor and, for ten years, have participated in an all-age religious conference called the Northfield Conference, where I've learned a tremendous amount from my teenage friends. I just received a master's degree in theological studies. I am a Quaker, feminist, writer, dancer, and mother to a twelve-year-old son named Matthew, who I hope will read this book sooner or later and be glad his mother helped to write it.

Tim Wernette: I am director of training at Planned Parenthood/Los Angeles, where I create and lead educational programs as well as provide counseling services. I am involved in a variety of personal-growth and political activities in the Los Angeles area, including membership in the Los Angeles Men's Collective, a feminist/gay rights/men's liberation organization. My interest in contributing to this book was partly the result of the difficulty and confusion I experienced, especially about sexuality, during my own adolescence. I hope this book will make that period of growth and change easier for teens and other young people.

Leni Wildflower: I live in Los Angeles with my two children, Cassie Wildflower and Jesse Potter. For the past several years I have taught workshops in sex education, women's health, and rape prevention for teenagers as well as for adults throughout Los Angeles County. I have also developed and run programs where teenagers are trained as peer counselors in sex education. Last year, as part of one project with the peer counselors, we developed a slide presentation on sexuality and media for other teenagers.

Because I have worked so much with teenagers, I wanted to help write a book that talked about health and sexuality *from a teenager's point of view.* I also wanted to express, through writing, my admiration and support and love for teenagers.

ACKNOWLEDGMENTS

During the three and a half years we've worked on this book many people have helped us and supported us. We would like to thank them here.

Above all, we thank those of you who participated in individual or group interviews. Your words may or may not appear in the following pages, but your thoughts helped us shape the content of the book.

Special thanks go to the people who went out of their way to be helpful. We owe a tremendous debt to you, for without your help this book would be less than it is:

David Alexander
Terry Beresford
Boston Women's Health Book
   Collective: Joan, Judy, Norma, Pam,
   Vilunya, and especially Nancy,
   Paula, and Esther
Paula Bowen
Cheryl Bradley, J.D.
Judy Chason

Stuart Chason
Janice Fialka
Tony Greenberg, M.D.
The Girls at Hamburger Home in Los
   Angeles, California
Susan Kandel
Charlotte Mayerson, our editor
Kemp Roelofs
Matthew Sanford

Larry Shapiro
Judith Steinbergh
Robert Takahashi
Esther Walter
The Youth Expression Theater of the
   Planned Parenthood League of
   Massachusetts

Thanks to these clinics, centers, and schools that opened their doors to us:

Alameda Senior High School in
   Denver, Colorado
Beaver Country Day School in
   Brookline, Massachusetts
The Cambridge Friends School in
   Cambridge, Massachusetts
The Committee for Gay Youth
   The Cambridge Women's Center in
   Cambridge, Massachusetts
The Commonwealth School in Boston,
   Massachusetts
Delta Women's Clinic in New Orleans,
   Louisiana
The Door: A Center of Alternatives in
   New York, New York

Feminist Women's Health Center in
   Los Angeles, California
Gay Community Services Center in
   Los Angeles, California
Hamburger Home in Los Angeles,
   California
HOY: Help Our Youth Clinic in
   Arcadia, California
Los Angeles Free Clinic in Los
   Angeles, California
Lulu Belle Stewart Center in Detroit,
   Michigan
Madison Park High School in
   Roxbury Park, Massachusetts

Oakwood School in North Hollywood,
   California
Planned Parenthood of Iowa in Des
   Moines, Iowa
Planned Parenthood of Los Angeles,
   California
Planned Parenthood League of
   Massachusetts in Cambridge,
   Massachusetts
Rocky Mountain Planned Parenthood
   in Denver, Colorado
Routh Street Clinic in Dallas, Texas
Temple Isaiah in Los Angeles,
   California
University High School in Los
   Angeles, California

These teenagers helped us by reading our work and commenting on it, by sharing ideas with us, by discussing philosophy and point of view, and by continually reminding us not to preach, lecture, or moralize:

Ronnie Allen
Darlyne Baugh
Sarah Baum
Beverly
Paula Binkley
Nadine Borofsky
Leslie Ann Campbell
Linda Carter
Stacy Chanin
Kate Chason
Liz Chason
Leah Diskin
Hannah Doress
Hilary Eustace
Bob Fehlau
Kathy Finnerty

Jose Gabilondo
Almon Grimsted
Joshua Hawley
Lynn Hudson
Cathy Jacobs
Elton Jimenez
Chris Johnson
Rebecca Katz
Lori Kleban
Sara Kontoff
Shelly Krieb
Laurel Kronsky
Kelly Mead
Jaime Michaels
Ahrin Mishan

Jessica Mizrahi
Chris Myers
Andrew Pailas
Kathi Peterson
Courtney Philbrook
Kathy Phillips
Sami Pincus
Brigitte Serville
George Smith
Janell Smith
Stuart Swerdloff
Tom Vance
Christy Wilton
Thanks also to all the teens who participated in our photo sessions.

Thanks to the following who contributed in many different ways to our project:

Gail Abarbanel
Ashana Abu-Jefferson
Edith Alexander
Stephanie Allen
Susan Allen
Myron Arnold
Polly Attwood
Denise Bisaillon
Richard Borofsky
Dennis Boyd
Marcia Bullock
Scott Burnham
Elizabeth Canfield
Ginny Cassidy
Gwindale Cassity-Miller
Jan Cobble
Bill Connet
Mary Cosey
Irene Davidson
Sam Davidson
Carol Downer
Ben Eastman
Mary Linda Eccles
Judy Favor
Aida Feria
Rabbi Robert Gan
Julie Goudy
Dinah Gilburd
Michael Gilburd
Carol Gilligan

Sharon Gillin
Fran Goldfarb
Louis Bowie Graves
Florence Hanson, R.N.
Daphne Hawkes
Dr. Jack Horowitz
Dei Iaroli
Selden Illick
Institute for the Study of Medical Ethics
Nels Israelson
Jake
Maggie Jensen
Jana Johnson
Jean Johnson
June Kailes
Antra Kalnins
David Kantor
Meredith Kantor
Temma Kaplan
Jerrold Katz
Polly Kirkpatrick
Los Angeles Regional Family Planning
Allen Loots
Peggy Lynch
Nick Masi
Ron McClain
Alice Michelson
Michael V. Miller
Kahrin Mishan
Freida Mizrahi

Dane Morgan
Pat Nichols
Mark Pecker
Ed Pincus
Cindy Orrell
Mary Owen
Randy Paulsen
Aaron Rapoport
Lin Reicher
Linda Robak
Joan Samuels
Lisa Schaeffer
Mary Scofield
Ann Smith
Anne Smith
Leslie Smith
Steve Smith
Charlotte Taft
Lisa Tackley
Lois Tandy
Sherrie Tepper
Liz Thompson
Richard Thompson
Virginia Valian
Alice Verhoeven
Barbara Waxman
Sidra Winkelman
Janet Witkins
Francie Young
Linda Young

Illustration credits:

Drawings and diagrams were done by Leslie Stone of Leslie Stone Design, Santa Monica, California.
Cartoons were drawn by Paula Maloof, New York City.

CONTENTS

PREFACE vii

CHANGES 1

I Changing Bodies 3

by Wendy Sanford, with help from Jane Pincus and Elizabeth McGee; based on work by Ruth Bell

It Happens to Everyone 5
Boys' Bodies 9
Girls' Bodies 19

II Changing Relationships 41

by Ruth Bell, with help from Elizabeth McGee; based on work by Monica Mizrahi

Parents 41
Friends 57

SEXUALITY 71

III Exploring Sex with Yourself 75

by Wendy Sanford, with help from Elizabeth McGee; based on work by Ruth Bell

IV Exploring Sex with Someone Else 84
(Heterosexuality and Homosexuality)

Heterosexual section by Wendy Sanford, with help from Elizabeth McGee; based on work by Ruth Bell

Homosexual section by Tim Wernette, with help from Wendy Sanford and Ruth Bell; special thanks to Eric Rofes and Madge Kaplan

V Sex Against Your Will 124

by Leni Wildflower, with help from Wendy Sanford

TAKING CARE OF YOURSELF 131

VI Emotional Health Care 133

Feeling Bad, Feeling Better 133
by Sally Bowie, with help from Ruth Bell and Elizabeth McGee

Drugs and Alcohol 149
by Rob Evans, with help from Ruth Bell

VII Physical Health Care 153

Going to the Doctor 153
by Ruth Bell

Birth Control 159
by Ruth Bell, with help from Joanne Gates

So You Think You Might Be Pregnant 189
by Joanne Gates, with help from Elizabeth McGee and Ruth Bell

Sexually Transmitted Diseases 216
by Ruth Bell
Original draft by Shari Reeve Schulz
Special thanks to Esther Rome

Index 235

CHANGES

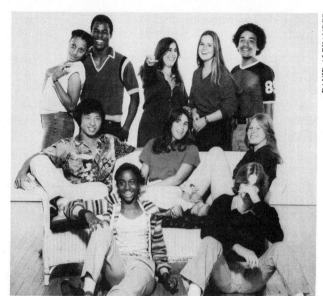

Change can take place so gradually that you don't notice it's happening until something pulls you out of the day-to-day flow of your life and makes you stand back. Sometimes when you haven't seen someone for a long time, or when you go back to an old neighborhood for a visit, you suddenly see how different things are. When it comes to yourself, one day you look in the mirror and instead of merely adjusting your clothes or combing your hair you actually see yourself. Barry, a thirteen-year-old from Texas, told us:

> One day when I was about nine I caught a look at myself in the hall mirror as I was going out to a baseball game and I saw this grown-up kid, chewing gum, wearing his baseball uniform, and I remember thinking, Hey, I'm a real kid now. In that second I remember feeling like I'd changed. I wasn't little anymore.

Just a few years later you look and see that you're not even a kid any longer. You've moved out of childhood and into the teenage years.

It's then that changes start to happen so fast it's hard not to notice them. Hair grows in places it's never been before. Breasts develop; muscles form. Voices change. Important "firsts" take place: first kiss, first date, first job, first license, first bra, first ejaculation, first menstrual period, first love. Of course, these things don't happen for everyone exactly during the eight years from twelve to twenty, but whether they happen earlier or later, they are meaningful steps. There isn't any rule book to let you know when, where or how to make the moves; you just know you're expected to come out the other end "grown up" and able to take care of yourself.

Everyone goes through these changes, but that doesn't make them any easier to handle. They involve a lot of experimenting and, usually, making a lot of mistakes. You test your abilities, make false starts, take risks, push your-self into new things, and often feel lonely and misunderstood. We all do, because that's what growth is all about.

In the middle of all this many people say they sometimes feel pretty mixed up. They feel they're in a hurry to grow up, but at the same time feel uneasy about being pushed into doing it too quickly. Fourteen-year-old Raoul, who lives in New York, told us:

> A lot of the weird things I do are just a matter of trying to prove to everybody, and I guess prove to myself, that I'm not a kid anymore. But sometimes I think to myself, Hey, wait a minute, I *am* a kid. Don't make me grow up so fast.

As your body gets bigger and develops sexually, people may *treat* you differently even before you start to feel very different inside yourself. They may expect you to act older or more grown-up in ways that don't feel comfortable to you yet. Or they may treat you like a child when you feel quite mature. All this can be confusing.

Also, as you get older you have more choices to make. When you were little, most new experiences were filtered through your parents or guardians. Now decisions come up daily, and you're the only one who can make them: Do you do what your friends want you to do? Do you take this class instead of that one? Do you ask so-and-so out for a date? Do you have sex with your boyfriend or girlfriend? Do you take this or that drug? For the most part, the decisions you are faced with are hard ones, with serious consequences. It's no wonder several teenagers we met said they feel as if they're on a seesaw—sometimes soaring gracefully, sometimes coming down with a crash. Cassie, an eighth-grader from Ohio, put it this way:

> Everyone my age is trying to grow up really quick and I can't stand it anymore. There are all these decisions to make like about drugs and sex and trying to

act older. Sometimes I get so sick of it I just want to get away from it and crawl back into my mom's lap.

Changing Bodies, Changing Lives is about the ups and downs of the teenage years. In this book teenagers talk about the changes, choices and feelings in their lives right now. We've also included a lot of information that many teens can't get very easily—information about sex, physical development, personal relationships and emotions.

We spent three years meeting and talking with several hundred teenagers all across the United States. They were different ages, from twelve through twenty. They were from different backgrounds and ethnic groups. They had different ideas and different interests. But they were all coming face-to-face with the issues that affect teens: body development, sexuality, self-esteem, changing relationships with parents and friends, and the need to establish independence.

You'll hear stories and anecdotes from many of these teenagers in the following chapters, because we've learned that listening to real people talk about their lives is usually more helpful than pages of advice written by "experts."

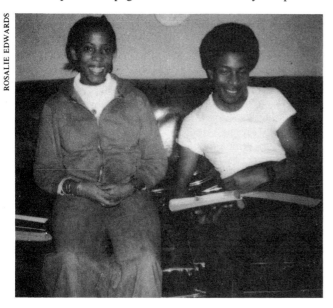

ROSALIE EDWARDS

As you read you'll probably discover that some of the problems you're dealing with are other people's problems too, and that many of the questions you have are also being asked by other teenagers.

We've changed people's names and the cities they come from to protect their privacy. Many of the quotes are very personal, telling about deep feelings and intense frustrations. Some quotes are quite frank, describing sexual activity or other intimate details. We are glad that the teenagers we met were willing to share those things with us, because their openness allowed us to discuss important issues that are often left unsaid.

Some of the quotes may sound familiar to you. Others may be very different from your experience. A number of them may surprise or even shock you. The important thing to remember is that each of these stories comes from a real teenager somewhere, and probably speaks for many other teenagers throughout the country. We hope these quotes will let you see how different people are and won't make you feel pressured to do one thing or another just because someone else is talking about it. There's no "right" way or "right" age to have life experiences.

Along with the personal anecdotes are facts and practical information about body changes and sex. You may not be at all interested in sex right now, you may already be having sexual relationships, or you may be somewhere in between. In any case, you deserve clear and accurate information to help you take care of yourself now and in the future. We think people have a right to know about how their bodies work, a right to have their questions about sexuality answered, a right to choose when and if they want to become parents, and a right to keep themselves and others safe from sexually transmitted diseases.

Some of you may not want to read this book from cover to cover. Some parts of it will be relevant to your life now, other parts you may not need for years. We hope that you and your parents will be able to use this book to open a dialogue with each other, and that groups of friends will use it as a basis for discussions about what's going on in their lives.

1 CHANGING BODIES

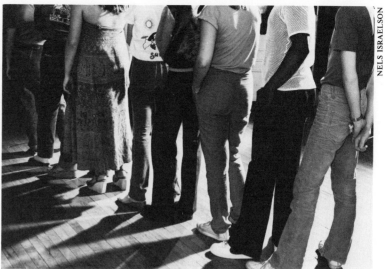

It Happens to Everyone

Sometime between the ages of nine and sixteen years, your body will start to change dramatically. As Tai, aged sixteen, said, "When I was fifteen, my body started to go crazy!"

This time of change is called puberty (*pu*-ber-tee). Everyone goes through it. It starts early for some people (around nine or ten), later for others (fifteen or sixteen). Your body may change, becoming fat, skinny or tall, hairy or smooth, big-breasted or small, pimply or not. Everyone grows and changes at different times, different rates. You may feel full of energy or lie around and sleep a lot. Your moods may shift quickly, uncontrollably, surprising you.

There are reasons for these changes. When your body reaches a certain stage of growth, a part of your brain called the pituitary (pih-*too*-it-ter-ee) gland signals your sex glands—your ovaries if you are a girl, your testicles if you are a boy—to start working. Ovaries and testicles then begin signaling certain other parts of your body, telling them to grow.

Hormones carry the signals. Hormones are chemical substances that travel in your bloodstream and reach your body organs with instructions on how to develop. There are lots of hormones in our bodies.

Testosterone (tess-*tahs*-ter-own), the main hormone special to males, is made in the testicles. Estrogen (*es*-truh-jen) and progesterone (pro-*jess*-ter-own), the hormones special to females, are made in the ovaries. These hormones cause most of the body changes of puberty—growth of body hair, pubic hair and breasts, voice deepening, pimples, menstruation and so on. Also, all of these changes, for boys who have sex with girls and girls who have sex with boys, have something to do with enabling you to reproduce—to have children. While becoming parents may be the last thing on your mind, once you go through puberty your body will be ready for it, which is why it is so important for you to get decent birth control information at this time (see section on Birth Control, p. 159).

"I feel like I'm the only one who . . ." You can fill in the blank for yourself. Maybe you feel like the only one who doesn't have her period yet. Or the only one who wakes up in the morning with come (sperm) all over his sheets. The only one with pimples at age twelve or one breast bigger than the other or one testicle hanging lower.

If you don't know anything about body changes and feelings in yourself and the other sex, you are likely to feel more different than you need to. In this chapter you'll hear from other teenagers, and see that lots of different body changes and feelings are normal.

Sexual Changes

Many of the changes of the teenage years are sexual. Your sexual organs are growing—penis, vagina, testicles, ovaries, breasts. Your sexual feelings may become more intense.

In Denver at a girls' discussion group, thirteen-year-old Roxanne said:

> I've changed in these past six months. I mean I used to be such a goody-goody and always pay attention in class and follow all the rules, and now all I can think about is my boyfriend. Actually I have a lot of boyfriends now. I'm not Miss Perfect anymore.

Darlene responded:

> I get these weird sensations in my stomach all the time. My friend read to me from this book about sex and I got this weird feeling down here, like my stomach was flipping over.

It can be hard to pay attention at school or work when all these other things are going on in your mind and body. A fifteen-year-old boy in a group at a Boston youth center said:

> I swear I woke up one day and everything changed. It was like somebody put up a big flashing neon-light sign in my head that said SEX. I was always turned on. I mean always, and all I had to do was sit across from an attractive woman in the subway and I'd feel like coming in my pants.

You may read these quotes and think, But I'm not feeling sexy all the time and *I'm* a teenager! Many times in this book people will talk about feelings you don't have right now. Or they will talk about doing things that you don't do, even though you may be their same age or older. Bodies change at different speeds. Sexual feelings are stronger or weaker at different times in our lives. Think of this book as having a conversation with lots of teenagers who are being honest about things people don't often talk about. Some will sound like you and some won't. The main point is for you to understand better what's happening with *your* body and *your* feelings.

Does Sex Have to Be a Mystery?

Since so many teenage body changes are sexual and many adults are uncomfortable about sex, teenagers don't get told much about what's going on.

Have you ever heard an older person say, "I was brought up thinking that everything below my bellybutton was off limits"? Or, "I grew up thinking I shouldn't look at anything 'down there' or touch myself or know how it all worked"? For many people in our parents' generation sexuality was a mystery, something for marriage only, and slightly shameful. As children, they were taught not to touch or explore themselves. As adults, when they did touch themselves or even look, they felt guilty about it. Generations of married couples had eight or ten children by making love under the covers with the lights off, never seeing each other's bodies.

These negative attitudes toward bodies and sex may sound strange to you. Or they may sound all too familiar. They cause many of us to be more embarrassed, shy and ignorant than we want or need to be.

If we don't learn about ourselves, do we learn much about the other sex? Here are some memories of a woman and a man now in their thirties:

> Cindy: When I was seventeen one night my girl-friends and I had a big debate about how a boy's penis worked. When it got erect, did it slip in and out of a sheath of hairy skin like a dog's penis? Some girls said yes, others argued no. Others were so embarrassed that we just got hysterics.

> Roger: One day my mother's shopping bag tore open and a box of sanitary napkins fell out on the floor. I was six. I picked it up and asked her what they were for. She blushed real red and put the box on the top shelf of her closet, saying, "This is for me to know about." Well, hell, how was I supposed to learn anything about girls' bodies?

Probably you know more about boys' bodies, if you are a girl, and girls' bodies, if you are a boy, than your parents did at your age. But the teenagers who worked on this book said there was still a lot they didn't know.

Here we're talking about what's called "sex education." Usually we learn about bodies and sex in not very illuminating ways. We hear jokes in locker rooms, on street corners, on playgrounds, at home; we hear gossip about who's doing what; we read books and see movies that make sex super-romantic or super-disgusting; we see pornographic pictures and read pornographic books and magazines, which shape our fantasies.

Some schools give sex education classes or courses. They can be good. Sometimes, unfortunately, they are not helpful: teachers themselves are embarrassed; a film on the "facts" may be dry and boring; there's no comfortable safe way or place for you to talk about your bodies and feelings.

Some parents try hard to teach their kids about sex in an open way. But many of them, like teachers, are awkward. As one girl said:

> Some parents really are not very informed. And I think that's part of the reason they're scared to talk to their kids—they really don't know all that much.

Some parents wait so long to bring it up that you've already heard it all somewhere else. ("*Mom, I know* that already!") Some parents are so private about their own bodies and their own sexuality that when they finally sit you down for "a talk" it's just plain embarrassing to have them talking about these things.

You may be lucky and find really helpful sources of information—an open-minded parent, an older brother or sister, a boyfriend or girlfriend, a well-informed friend. Yet most often we learn about sex in bits and pieces. We absorb the attitude that there is something wrong with being a sexual person, with being curious about sex. We may joke about sex, but we don't know much about it. Not knowing can make us feel bad.

We can help each other feel better by sharing information, talking honestly, not making fun of each other's differences. You may want to start a group with some friends to talk about body changes and to discover that all those things you think about and worry about are happening to others too. Margaret was in a group like this, and said, "It was so amazing to me to walk into a group of girls talking openly about sex. I didn't say a word for a couple of weeks. But I sure listened!"

Do I Like My Body?

This is a heavy question for most of us. You might say, "I better like my body, I'm not going to get another one!" But often we are pressured to dislike ourselves:

Thirteen-year-old Charlene: Sometimes when I'm all alone I stand in front of the mirror and stare at myself. I stare at all the things I can't stand about myself, like I absolutely can't stand my legs. They're so short and my thighs are huge. There's this white bump on my neck that really bothers me. It's not a pimple. It doesn't hurt. It's just there and I don't know what it is, but I can't stand it. And the worst part is my chest. I'm so flat-chested I look like a boy.

Fifteen-year-old Pablo: I've always been concerned about my body and how much I could change, in terms of manly build, broad shoulders, nice ass. How much of it can you change, through exercise, diet, et cetera? Because I can't stand what I look like right now!

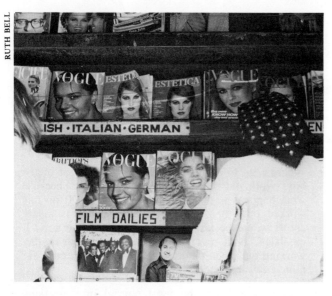

RUTH BELL

What one person suffers over *not* having may be just what another person suffers over having:

Sally: I wouldn't mind having bigger breasts.

Tai: No you wouldn't, man! Once you got there you'd want to get back down. I wish I could give you some of mine.

To change our looks we diet to lose weight, to gain weight. We lift weights, work out, use blow dryers, wear makeup, get our hair done, shave, don't shave, buy expensive clothes. We try plastic surgery, sun lamps, tanning clinics, fad diets—all of which can hurt both body and pocketbook. We buy hair spray, hair coloring, bleaches and hair-removal creams for body hair, mouthwash and acne preparations. Just think how much energy and money, at any one moment all over this country, are going into

EMERGING

The shine,
The yellow,
The golden
is rising
Can this be
the beginning?
My shining
My glow
My green
sight
so slowly
it opens
and buds into
a spotted flower.
I rise
my limbs
they open
and the dried skin peels
and reveals
the shining flesh
that will take over.

The step into
a wonderful vegetable
I hide,
and sleep,
and come out new
and blue
I step back,
one step,
but a million steps
to all
in the wooden world . . .
My old world . . .
My wooden world
seems old
seems dark
seems gruesome.
And all who live there,
without stepping
into the light
into the glow
are still speaking
the wooden language
that I have left behind
long ago.

—Lyn Bigelow

changing people's looks. It may be fun at times to play around with what we look like, but it's important to ask *who* gets the money we spend. The answer is: those companies which put unbelievable amounts of money each year into advertising their "body-beautifying" products and which do a terrific job of making us dislike our bodies as they are.

For example, deodorant companies play on your desire to be liked and admired. Their ads create worry. They make fortunes from your fear of "body odor."

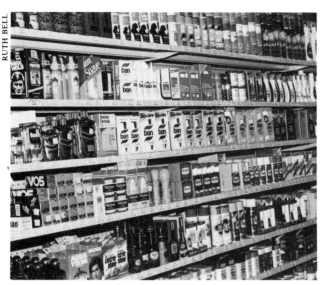

Deodorants are a big business.

When you enter puberty, new sweat glands begin to work. You sweat more. You have new smells under your arms, in your genital area. Many teenagers are sensitive about these smells. This sensitivity reflects society's belief that people should be as dry and odorless as possible. Abby remembers:

> There were some days in high school when I'd shave under my arms and then cover my armpits with adhesive tape. It wasn't much good for my skin, but on those days I knew for sure I wouldn't perspire on my blouse.

Each of you has your own particular body smells. You may like how you smell, you may just take baths and showers and not use anything. You may use deodorants sometimes or most of the time. Whatever you do, be aware of the effect that constant advertising has on you. For a start, look critically at TV ads with your friends for a laugh and an eye-opener.

Probably no one can talk us out of disliking some parts of our bodies, but it may help to look at some other reasons why we worry:

Feeling Judged by the Other Sex. Boys and girls do a lot of looking at each other, and they often judge each other harshly. Ellen complained:

> There's this kid who has a crush on me and drives me crazy wanting to sit with me at lunch and stuff. He's built like a Raggedy Andy doll—real weak and floppy.

Dan, a high school junior, said about hairy legs on girls:

> What grosses me out is the bristly part. When you think of a girl, somehow her sensuality is involved in softness, so that hard bristliness is a turn-off.

With judgments like that, can you blame boys for spending hours every day lifting weights? Can you blame girls for shaving their legs every day?

Feeling Judged by Your Friends. Chances are, if you hang around with a crowd of girls or boys or both, your crowd will have a certain idea of what looks good—and you'll feel pressured to look that way. Sandy recalls:

> I remember the first time I shaved. This girl named Janet said, "Why don't you shave your legs? You need to, you're becoming a woman now." I'm fourteen years old, right? So I went home and did this sloppy job of shaving and came back and said, "Janet, look, I shaved, I shaved!" Then she started criticizing: "You didn't do your knees! And there's a streak of hair up here . . . and you didn't do your ankles!"

Comparing Yourself with Others. Our society emphasizes competition between people, companies, countries, so it's not surprising that we feel competitive. Annie suffered from her height:

> When I was in sixth grade, I was taller than *everybody*. It was embarrassing for me. I had a really tiny friend and I used to envy her.

Bill talks about competition among his friends:

> Where I go to school, I'd say eighty percent of the boys work out with weights. It's pointless because what happens is the standards just go up. If no one worked out, then the people who had less manly chests would be just as unhappy as they are now. It escalates. Now everybody spends an hour a day working out when they could be doing something far more enjoyable and useful.

The competition may be most painful in your family. Anita remembers:

> When I was twelve or thirteen my mother told me about periods, but she said, "I don't think you'll be getting yours for a while yet." Then when my sister was eleven, she told *her* about it. She said, "You girls should be expecting periods any time now." *Then* it was really important that my sister didn't get hers before me. (*Now* I wouldn't care.) What was worse, my mother expected her to.

Feeling Judged by Your Parents. Parents may get hung up on wanting you to look a certain way. Often they feel "it's for your own good." Sometimes they're right, and sometimes they have other motives they are not aware of—they may feel they are being judged by *their* friends according to how you look, or they may remember their own adolescence. Parents often find it difficult to accept you as you are. Jeff says:

> My dad is always bugging me to go on a diet. I think it's because he was fat and unpopular as a kid. I'm heavy, but not *that* heavy. But when he looks at me with that look in his eyes, I feel like I weigh three hundred pounds.

Wendy's mother had a picture in her head of how Wendy should look:

> Every morning when I was in eighth grade my mother would meet me at the door and ask if I was going to put on lipstick that day. Couldn't she see I didn't want to? Why was she so attached to my looking a certain way?

Your Body Is OK

Next time you catch yourself saying, "I hate my legs, [or breasts, chest, face, hair]," stop for a minute and ask yourself: "*Who* hates them? *Who* says they're not good enough? Do I really agree?" Look at yourself in the mirror and name what you *do* like. Compliment yourself. Compliment your friends, help them like themselves better.

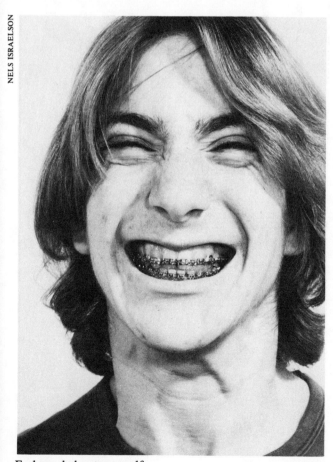

NELS ISRAELSON

Feel good about yourself.

Marge Piercy, a poet, writes: "Live as though you liked yourself, and it may happen."

Your body is OK. In fact, as one boy reading this section remarked, "Your body isn't just OK! It's great! And it does some amazing things!"

Boys' Bodies

NOTE TO GIRL READERS: When we talk to the reader of this section as "you," we mean a boy. However, when we asked a group of girls who they thought would read the different parts of this book, they said, "Girls will read the parts about boys, and the boys will read about girls!" So we figure a lot of girls will be reading this section. This is great, because girls have been ignorant about boys' bodies for too long. Just don't be surprised when we talk about "your" penis!

In a few short years a boy experiences these things:

—Your penis and testicles get bigger.
—You grow pretty close to what will be your full height.
—Your voice "changes."
—Your skin becomes oilier; you may get pimples on your face and neck and chest and back.
—Your testicles start to make semen and millions of sperm.
—Pubic hair grows around your testicles, anus and the base of your penis.
—Your body hair gets thicker, and whiskers start to grow on your face.
—You start to ejaculate ("come") when you have an orgasm—either in dreams when you are asleep, or when you are masturbating or having sex play with someone else.
—You may start having more and stronger sexual feelings.
—Your sweat glands begin working and you sweat more.
—Your muscles and strength increase.

Not all of you will go through every one of these changes. But most of them happen at some point during these years.

How you feel about yourself depends on what you know about your body's changes; what your idea of "manly," "good-looking" and "handsome" is, and how you accept the ways you *don't* match that image; whether your family and friends pressure you to grow up fast, to have a deep voice, a big penis, and a he-man body as soon as possible.*

Joe thinks competition in body development is worse among boys than girls:

> Guys notice it more than girls. Especially in the lock-

---

*We recommend the book by Sam Julty, *Men's Bodies, Men's Selves* (New York: Dial Press, 1979).

er room. Because somehow for the guy it's so much more important. He's supposed to be the virile one. He feels more inadequate if he's not as developed as his friends.

How society treats you is another big factor. Once you start growing and looking like a man, other boys and men may react to you differently than before. They may start expecting you to be tough, and pick fights with you or accuse you of doing things you never did. When girls' bodies change, they get a lot of comments on the street and sexual suggestion and harassment. Boys don't have to worry as much about being sexually abused, though they sometimes get approached. You may be treated as though all you have on your mind is fighting and sex.

Another influence on you will be the attitudes of girls and boys you know. How much do they know about boys' bodies? Is there too much mystery and embarrassment? Can you talk honestly about yourself with anyone?

There's a myth that girls are more self-conscious than boys, and that boys breeze through their teenage years never worrying what they look like or how fast they are developing. Of course this isn't true.

Steven, a seventeen-year-old from Los Angeles, speaks for many boys:

Well, for me it was weird because I didn't even start growing until last year. Everybody thought there was

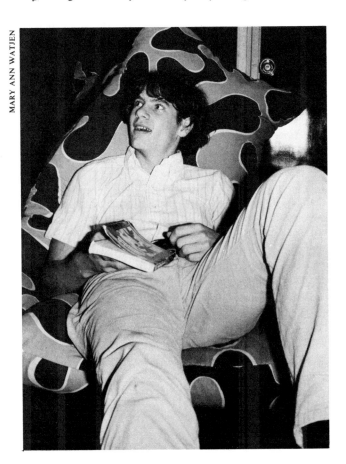
MARY ANN WATJEN

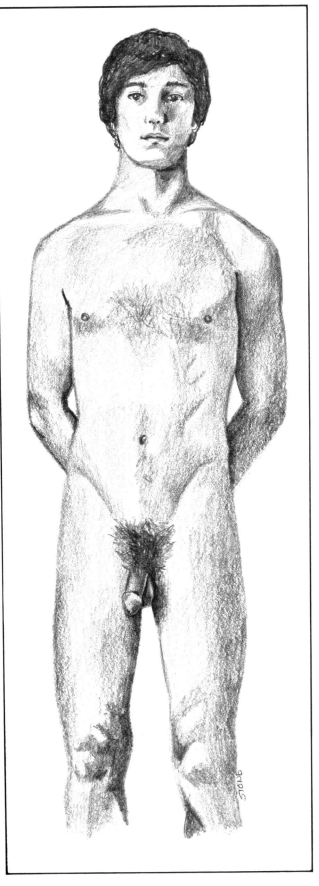

something wrong with me because I still looked like a ten-year-old up until I was fifteen or sixteen. That has been really a bad experience for me because everybody was changing around me and I was standing still. I was changing in my head but not in my body. My parents were even going to take me to the doctor to see if I was deformed or something like that, but they didn't, and finally last year I started to grow. My voice started changing and everything, so I guess I'm normal after all, but I think it's going to be a while before I stop feeling like I'm different from everybody else.

Proper Terms and Slang

Words naming sexual organs have a lot of power. While ''penis'' and ''testicles'' (so-called proper terms) are quite

sober and unemotional, they are not often used. Some families have their own private, even silly words.

Slang is especially colorful and strong:

penis		*testicles*
cock	schmuck	balls
prick	schlong	nuts
dick	pecker	jewels
stick	thing	rocks
rod	dink	cubes
gun	dinkus	nugies
wee-wee	privacy	eggs
wang	banana	
wiener	putz	
pisser	dork	
peter	meat	
hot dog	dong	

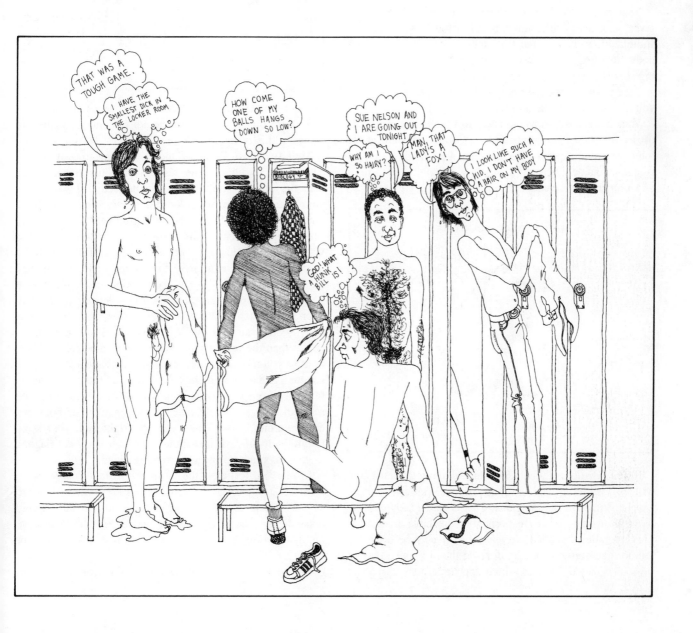

Slang is tricky because we use these words in many different ways: to express fondness and pride (then they are funny, friendly, loving, playful); to put down or to make fun of someone; or to hurt someone, to do violence to them.

Try this exercise: Say each of these words in different tones of voice, and notice how they change according to your intention. The same word can be an endearment or an insult. Some people use slang without realizing how it sounds.

You might want to know what words girls use for "penis" and "testicles." Like boys, many girls don't use any words at all. It's not that they don't know at least some words, but they are embarrassed to use them, whether they're "proper" or slang terms.

Body Parts: What Your Genitals Look Like on the Outside and Inside

Your *penis* has three functions. You urinate from it. It gives you sexual pleasure when it's touched, rubbed or stimulated, as it's the most sexually sensitive part of your body. It is the passageway through which semen containing sperm comes out of your body.

Take a careful look at your penis and testicles next time you are naked and near a mirror.

Your penis has two parts. The *glans* is the rounded head or tip, and is the most sensitive to touch. The *shaft* is the long part of the penis—the part that gets hard during an erection. Inside the shaft is spongy erectile tissue. (See p. 13 for more on erections.)

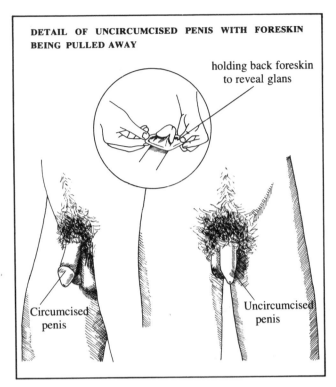

DETAIL OF UNCIRCUMCISED PENIS WITH FORESKIN BEING PULLED AWAY

holding back foreskin to reveal glans

Circumcised penis

Uncircumcised penis

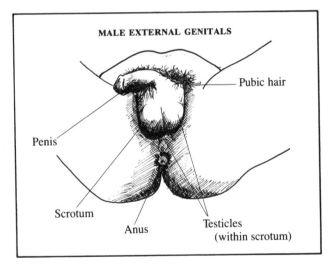

MALE EXTERNAL GENITALS

Pubic hair

Penis

Scrotum

Anus

Testicles (within scrotum)

If you have been circumcised (see diagram), your glans will be visible. If you have not been circumcised, there will be skin covering the glans. This is called the *foreskin.* Soon after some boys are born, the foreskin is removed. This operation is called *circumcision.* It may be done for religious reasons. It may be done so that a whitish cheesy substance called *smegma* which appears around the glans

will not collect under the foreskin and cause an infection. In modern times, because of the convenience of baths and showers, this is not a major problem.

Your two *testicles* are glands that hang in a skin sack called the *scrotum.* (One testicle probably hangs lower than the other.) You've probably noticed that sometimes your testicles are hanging loose and sometimes your scrotum tightens up and pulls them right up next to your body. This happens because the scrotum's function is to keep your testicles at just the right temperature for *sperm* to be made. Sperm are extremely tiny living cells. When they unite with a woman's egg, conception takes place (see p. 15). Since sperm are made at a few degrees *lower* than your body's temperature, your testicles hang from your body so that air can get in around them and keep them cooler than the rest of you. When the weather is very hot, or after you take a hot shower, or if you have a fever, your scrotum relaxes completely so that your testicles hang as far away from your body as possible. In cold weather the scrotum brings your testicles closer in to your body for more warmth. Also, when you are frightened, your scrotum tightens up. All this shows that your body is designed to give maximum protection to these glands.

Inside your testicles, the *vas deferens* tubes carry sperm from the testicles to the *seminal vesicles* where they are stored. These seminal vesicles and the *prostate gland* make *semen,* the fluid which is ejaculated when you have an orgasm (see p. 14) and which carries sperm out of your body.

The *urethra,* a tube inside your penis, brings urine out

from your bladder. It is also the passageway for semen when you ejaculate. A valve closes the urethra off from the bladder when you ejaculate so urine and semen can't mix.

Every boy knows from painful experience that his penis and testicles *hurt* when they are hit. You get pretty good at protecting them, especially in sports.

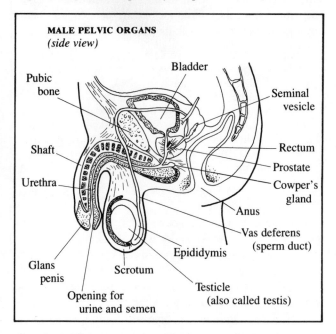

MALE PELVIC ORGANS
(side view)

Pubic bone
Bladder
Seminal vesicle
Shaft
Rectum
Urethra
Prostate
Cowper's gland
Anus
Vas deferens (sperm duct)
Glans penis
Epididymis
Scrotum
Opening for urine and semen
Testicle (also called testis)

Changes: Your Penis and Testicles Grow

At some point your penis and testicles start to grow bigger, usually when you are between the ages of eleven and fifteen, but sometimes earlier or later. Because puberty starts at different times, some boys' penises are much bigger than others' even though the boys are the same age. Since it's hard not to compare something so noticeable as a penis, many boys suffer. Roger said:

Three years ago in seventh-grade gym class, I spent a lot of time comparing myself to other guys. I felt like I was much smaller than everyone else. I started worrying if I was OK, if I had all the same things going on that everybody else did.

It's natural to compare penis size and to wonder. But sometimes there is teasing and outright cruelty:

Gym teachers in our junior high are always using sex jokes to keep everybody in line. One teacher in particular used to try to influence the guys by making jokes about them in the locker room. He was real hard on us. Like in the shower he'd go around saying, "Hey, look at that big cock over there," or to someone else he'd say, "Look at that guy, he couldn't even fill up a keyhole." I always did everything I could to avoid the shower line when that teacher was around. I mean, that was really humiliating.

Maybe one of the reasons for this teacher's cruelty was that he, too, was anxious about his penis size. In our society men are pressured to be tough and manly, to be in competition with each other. How about the disco song that goes, "He might satisfy you with his little worm, but I can bust you out with my Super Sperm!"?

The fact is that the size of your penis has *nothing* to do with how great you are, how many erections you can have, how good your orgasms will feel, or with your ability to satisfy a partner.

George and Bobby feel pretty comfortable about themselves:

I read a book on sex that said small penises could get very big when they were hard and cocks that started out big when they were soft might not grow so much when they were hard, so I didn't really ever worry about the size of my cock. I figured it would work when it had to, and that was pretty much all I cared about.

The book that George read, by the way, was right. Bobby added:

When my cock is soft it shrinks up so much you can hardly see it, and I used to look at these guys who had cocks halfway down their thighs and I'd wonder, Hey, what's my problem? But when I get excited, my cock looks like everybody else's, so I've got no complaints.

Erections

How an Erection Happens and What It Looks Like. During an erection (a "boner" or "hard-on"), your penis gets longer and harder and wider. It stands erect, away from your body. When you are sexually aroused, a nerve center at the base of your spinal cord sends messages that cause some of your blood to rush into the blood vessels and spongy tissue in your penis. The muscles inside the base of your penis tighten so that this extra blood can't easily drain out. Then your penis changes size and color—becoming larger and darker.

An erect penis looks very different from a soft one. A seventeen-year-old girl told us:

I've seen my brother naked, but I'd never seen an erect penis until the other night. When my boyfriend pulled his out of his pants, I nearly croaked. "My God, where have you been hiding that thing?!" No way it could have been in his pocket all that time!

When a penis is fully erect, it almost seems as though there were something rigid inside it, like a bone. People even call an erection a "rod" or a "boner." But in fact there's no bone inside, only blood and tissue.

When and Why You Have Erections. You have been getting erections all your life, ever since you were a

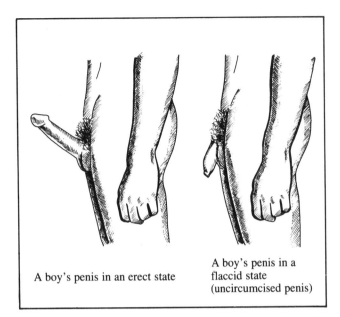

A boy's penis in an erect state

A boy's penis in a flaccid state (uncircumcised penis)

baby. Lots of boys and men wake up in the morning with hard-ons. Sometimes having to urinate will give you an erection. The friction of your pants on your penis when you are exercising can make your penis hard. Thoughts can lead to erections. One nine-year-old boy said, "Whenever I get excited about anything, my penis gets hard." Even sounds can do it!

Tony: Whenever I hear a vacuum cleaner I start getting hard. That must be because I used to love those days when I'd stay home from school, sick, and I'd be up in my room while my mother was vacuuming downstairs. That's a real good memory.

Mostly, erections come with sexual arousal. Stroking and touching your penis and testicles in a sexual way, or having them stroked by someone else, leads to an erection. Thinking sexy thoughts, reading sexy books, or daydreaming about someone can cause it. Jerry, who's twelve, was surprised at first:

When my penis first started getting hard, like at a movie during a love scene, I remember thinking, Hey, what's this? Why is this happening?

When you get an erection suddenly without planning on it and when your penis hasn't been touched, it's called a "spontaneous erection." Teenage boys have these a lot because of the high or fluctuating level of testosterone in their bodies. They can be a drag. Here's what a few boys said about spontaneous erections:

Eric (fourteen): When I get a hard-on in the subway, I think, Oh no, everybody's noticing me! I don't have any control over it, and it makes me want to slink off without even waiting for my stop.

Jim (sixteen): It's really embarrassing to have an erection just when you have to go out on to the field in a

gym class when there are girls on the field too. That's happened to me a lot.

Tom (seventeen): I get a hard-on in drama class almost every time I have to go up onstage. I can never tell if they are laughing at my performance or at my bulging cock.

Some boys worry about the number of erections they have. They may think they have too many, or compare themselves with friends and think they have too few. Joe says:

I thought I had a real problem because I would get hard-ons about fifteen or twenty times a day, for no reason at all. I'd be sitting at my desk, and maybe my mind would be wandering and all of a sudden, ZAP! there it would be. I used to put a book down in my lap and read it from there. When I asked my friend how many times he would get hard during the day, he said not so much, so I was sure there was something wrong with me.

There is in fact *nothing* wrong with Joe. There is no such thing as too many erections.

A spontaneous erection goes away by itself if you don't touch or rub your penis to add to the stimulation. An erection caused by touching can end in one of two ways. If the touching or rubbing keeps up long enough—if you are masturbating (see p. 79) or someone is fondling you—you will probably have an orgasm. After an orgasm, your penis will lose its erection and become soft again quite quickly. Or, if the touching, friction or rubbing stops without your having an orgasm, the extra blood will slowly drain out of your penis, and it will get soft again. This may take some time. You may feel frustrated or your testicles may ache slightly.

Making Semen and Ejaculating (Coming)

About a year after your penis and testicles start to grow, and just about when your pubic hair begins to come in, your testicles start to make semen.

How do you know that semen is now being made? This boy describes it:

The first time that I really came and this whitish stuff came out of my cock, I thought, Wow, this is really great, this feels great!

When fluid spurts out of your penis like that, it's called ejaculation (ee-ja-cue-*lay*-shun). Maybe you know it by another word, like coming, creaming, climaxing, juicing, milking, letting go, shooting off.

The milky whitish fluid that shoots out of your penis is called semen or ejaculate or "come." It has millions of sperm in it, as well as other fluids that help carry the sperm along. Contractions of the muscles in your penis push the semen out at the peak of your sexual excitement. This is called an orgasm. Orgasm usually feels very good.

Usually a man ejaculates when he has an orgasm, though it is possible to ejaculate without one. (It is also possible to have orgasms without ejaculating.) Some people think that because guys ejaculate when they have orgasms, women do too. They don't.

Starting to ejaculate is, for a boy, like a girl's having her period for the first time. It's a major sign that your body is growing up. Andrew said, ''I think a first wet dream is a powerful moment. It marks becoming a man. I was really excited about it.'' Another boy said:

I heard everyone talking about coming and jacking off, and at fifteen I hadn't experienced it yet. It was real mysterious to me. I would try and try, masturbating every night, and even though that felt good it didn't bring results. Finally one night, bang. It happened.

A boy's first ejaculation often happens while masturbating or sleeping. Mike, who is thirteen, told us:

I have fantasies just about every night before I go to sleep. I lie there with all these sexy things going on in my head, and of course my hand always seems to make it down to my cock. This one time I got real hard and my balls started itching like, and then there was this liquid shooting out of my cock. It felt amazing. So I went to sleep with a big smile that night.

Dennis had a wet dream:

I was about thirteen. I felt like I had this total sexual experience in my dream and I woke up and thought, Wow, did this really happen or not? It blew my mind it felt so real. After a second I realized my pajamas were wet. I sort of knew what it had to be, but still I was a little surprised.

EJACULATION, SPERM AND CONCEPTION (YOU CAN CONCEIVE A CHILD NOW)—THE NECESSITY OF BIRTH CONTROL

Once you begin making sperm and semen, you are able to conceive a child. Sperm are made inside each testicle, in tightly coiled tubes located in two hundred fifty little compartments. These tubes grow during the early stages of puberty, which is why your testicles get bigger. (If you unwound all the tubes and put them end to end, they would stretch the length of several football fields!)

Once made, the sperm move into a special compartment attached to each testicle called the epididymis (eh-pih-*dih*-dih-mis). Here they take six weeks to mature. Sperm that don't ripen or are less mature die in the epididymis. Only the healthiest sperm are ejaculated.

When the sperm mature and are ready to fertilize an egg, they go from the epididymis into a tube called the vas deferens, one for each testicle. (These are the tubes that are cut and tied when a man has the sterilization for permanent birth control called a vasectomy.) From the vas deferens sperm move to the seminal vesicles and are stored in two compartments until you ejaculate.

Your ejaculate contains both sperm and fluids made by the seminal vesicles and the prostate gland. This seminal fluid carries the sperm and protects it from the very slight acidity in a woman's vagina.

Sperm comes out through your urethra. When you are sexually aroused, a valve closes off the entry from your bladder so no urine can come out. That is why it takes a while to urinate just after you've been sexually excited.

When a man and a woman have sexual intercourse, his ejaculation puts about 400 million sperm

THE INSIDE OF A TESTICLE

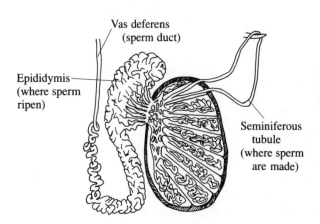

(shown outside testicle for identification)

inside her vagina. The sperm swim rapidly up through her cervix and uterus into her fallopian tubes. One of her ovaries releases an egg each month (ovulation). If she ovulates around the time she has sex with a man, her egg may meet a sperm in the tube and the two will join to start a pregnancy. There's a period of around three days when this is possible.

There are usually some live sperm in the drops of fluid that come from your penis when you get an erection and *before* you ejaculate. These drops of pre-ejaculate can cause pregnancy.

If you have sex with a girl you will have to use birth control now. (See p. 166.) *It's very important.* Just because you can conceive a child now doesn't mean you want to, or are at all ready to be a parent.

Puberty is a time to celebrate and enjoy; it is also a time to be careful, thoughtful and caring.

Wet dreams are your body's way of relieving your testicles when a lot of sperm have built up in them. (The scientific name for wet dream is "nocturnal emission.") If you have orgasms once in a while when you're awake, you may not have many wet dreams.

Many boys wonder if they will run out of semen if they come often. If you come several times in a row, there won't be as many sperm in the last ejaculation, but there will be some. You will not run out of semen.

Pubic Hair, Body Hair and Whiskers

The hormone testosterone causes boys to grow pubic hair around their genitals. Over the course of a year or two it grows over the pubic bone and covers the genital area, including the anus. Pubic hair may have been originally meant to help keep people's genitals warm and protected.

Most kids know that adults have pubic hair, and so they expect it. Dan, an eleven-year-old, said:

I keep looking for it, keep expecting to find one any day. A couple of my friends are already growing pubic hair, and I can see fuzz around my balls, but so far, only fuzz.

Pubic hair starts with just a few hairs. Gradually more hair grows, and it often gets coarser and curlier. For a while it covers a limited area and then fills out in a kind of upside-down triangle at the base of your abdomen and all around your genitals. People with naturally light hair or red hair may have pubic hair of the same color as the hair on their head, or it may be darker. Some people have a lot, and others not much at all.

· Your first pubic hair may begin to grow without your noticing. Or it may be a shock. Three boys in a discussion group in Providence found they had feelings in common:

Juan: Pubic hair scared the shit out of me. I saw all these little bumps and I didn't know what they were. I thought maybe I had VD but I hadn't even had sex.

Eric: I thought I was growing pimples.

Juan: I told my father right away, because I was terrified.

Richard: I was scared to say anything to anyone. I just waited. And then I noticed hair was growing out.

As with most of the changes in puberty, the kids who get pubic hair early usually are teased, and the ones who get it late are teased too.

You also will grow new, thicker body hair. To get an idea of how much hair you will have, look at the men in your family. If they have lots of hair, then you probably will too. How you feel about body hair is basically up to you. Some people are turned on by thick body hair, and some people like bodies with hardly any hair. It's personal, and a matter of individual taste. Having a lot of body hair doesn't mean you are more "masculine" than someone else.

Face hair usually starts to grow when a boy is between the ages of fourteen and eighteen. A sixteen-year-old said:

I had to shave a lot earlier than most of my friends. I was already shaving every day by the time I was fifteen, and even though I felt macho about it, it really was a pain in the neck. My dad's the same way—he has to shave twice a day to look good.

Shaving can be a real symbol of growing up. One man remembered:

I was late in getting a beard; it was a big deal if I had to shave once every couple of weeks in high school. I looked up to this friend who had a full growth of face hair when he was a junior. I couldn't have grown a beard if somebody paid me a million dollars.

Usually your face hair first starts coming in as sideburns and mustache. A seventeen-year-old said:

When I was fourteen I went around for about two weeks with this dirty smudge on my upper lip. I kept trying to wash it off but it wouldn't wash. Then I really looked at it and saw it was a mustache. So I shaved! For the first time.

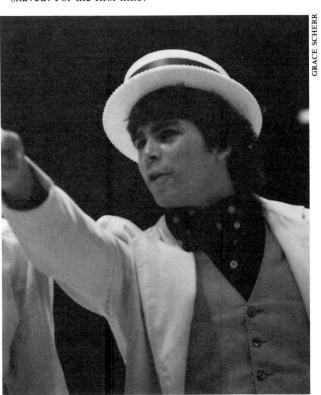

GRACE SCHERR

Voice Change

One of the cartoon stereotypes of a teenage boy is this guy who's talking along in a deep, impressive voice and all of a sudden his voice cracks and he's squeaking along like a kid. Voice change, brought on by testosterone, happens somewhere around fourteen or fifteen years.

Your voice deepening isn't necessarily any big drama. Tony said:

All of a sudden I realized my voice was low. On the telephone people started thinking I was my father, not my mother.

For George it was more noticeable but brief:

Last year it happened over two weeks. My throat was really killing me. I was feeling this scratchy thing every night when I called my friend. My voice would start cracking and he'd say, "What's the matter, you got a cold?" and I'd say "What?" because I didn't notice it. Then when I listened to myself talk, I heard my voice get heavier. In two weeks it was stronger, more mannish. It didn't bother me that much.

Some boys have a harder time. Dave reports:

I know a kid whose voice has been changing for a year. It cracks all the time and kids tease him.

Ian said:

You feel self-conscious, especially talking to a girl. I hear my brother talking on the phone with his girlfriend and he seems to be controlling his voice. He doesn't let himself sound angry or real happy or surprised. Your voice usually goes high when you get emotional or angry. So you try not to get too emotional. That way your voice will keep steady and low.

Your Breasts

Sometimes boys' breasts will ache during puberty just as girls' breasts do. They may be sensitive. Eddie said:

When I was in eighth grade my nipples felt so sore that it hurt to wear any shirt at all. For a while I was real sensitive.

Taking Care of Your Genitals

Until you start having sexual partners, the only special care you need to take of your penis and testicles is washing them with soap and warm water every day or two. Clear away any smegma (p. 12) that collects, especially if you are uncircumcised. Also, it's good to get in the habit of checking your testicles once in a while, lying down to feel for any changes or lumps, just as a girl does when she checks her breasts.

Of course, things may come up that a doctor should look at. Some of the signals that should send you to a clinic or doctor are:

—an open sore or persisting sore spot around your penis
—a burning feeling when you urinate

—an undescended testicle
—discharge (pus or whitish fluid) coming from the end of your penis.
—a pain in your testicles that doesn't go away
—a lump that wasn't there before

Many of these things are more likely to happen once you are sexually active. They may be a sign of an STD—sexually transmitted disease (the new name for VD, venereal disease). An STD is an infection you've picked up from a lover and could pass on to someone else (see p. 216).

You'll want to find a doctor you feel comfortable with. Many pediatricians are now trained in health care for teenagers (adolescent medicine). You may want a friend to go with you. You'll want to know what to expect, and what a good medical exam is like. We'll talk about all this on p. 156.

Discharge from Your Penis. This is a common problem, which may have a number of causes. Always have yourself checked by a doctor, because a discharge might be a sign of gonorrhea (if you are at all sexually active) or urethritis, which is an infection in the urethra. (See Nongonoccocal Urethritis, p. 226). Both of these diseases require antibiotic treatment.

Also, if you stop yourself regularly from ejaculating during masturbation or sex play, you may develop a condition known as retrograde ejaculation. That means that the semen has gone back down the urethra into the glands and is building up there. That buildup can cause pain and a discharge from the penis. The best way to avoid retrograde ejaculation is to let yourself come at least occasionally, when pregnancy isn't a risk.

Pain in the Genital Area. Pain in the groin or genital area can be caused by many things. It might be a swollen lymph gland or a hernia or an infection. If it lasts more than a day or two you should have it checked by a doctor. Sometimes when you stay sexually aroused for an extra long time without ejaculating, you'll feel a painful discomfort around your testicles—sometimes called "blue balls"—which can be relieved by masturbating. Or else it will go away by itself after a while. It is no cause for alarm, and certainly no reason to feel you have to talk someone into having sex with you.

Undescended Testicles. Ordinarily a boy's testicles descend shortly before or just after his birth. Sometimes, especially in the case of premature babies, the testicles do not descend for several months. When they have not descended by themselves, the condition can be corrected by surgery or hormone treatment.

When one of your testicles has descended only partway, it can become twisted and cause you a great deal of pain. An operation is called for to untwist the cord that supplies blood to the testicle. If you have pain in your testicles that hasn't been caused by an immediate injury, or if you've been hit in the testicles and the pain lasts for a very long time, see a doctor.

Testicle Cancer. It is very rare for teenagers to have a problem with cancer. But since cancer of the testicles can occur, it is a good idea for you to get into the habit of examining your testicles, just the way a girl has to learn to examine her breasts. Lie down and gently feel around the entire area to see if anything is out of the ordinary. You can also examine your testicles while you are in the shower or bath. Feel each testicle separately. If you find any lumps, have them checked by a doctor. They are probably cysts, which will go away by themselves, but they ought to be looked at by someone with experience and knowledge. When you start examining yourself regularly, you become the best expert on how your body looks and feels normally.

Doctors gave a human-made hormone called DES (diethylstilbestrol) to some women during the 1940's, 50's and 60's to help prevent miscarriage. If your mother took DES while she was pregnant with you, be sure to tell your doctor when you go for a checkup. There may be some relationship between DES and testicle cancer. (See p. 40 for more information.)

Jock Itch, or Jock Rot. If you have itching and a damp feeling in your genital area, you may have jock itch. The skin will be sore and red around your testicles and on the inside of your thighs, and it usually will itch a lot.

Jock itch can be caused by wearing clothes that are too tight or that are made of fabrics that don't let the air circulate.

Lightly rubbing cornstarch on the area will often be enough to cure it, but you may need to use a fungicide. If the condition doesn't go away, you may want to see a doctor, especially to make sure nothing more serious is involved.

Keep the area clean and dry, wash your clothes a lot, and don't wear jeans or other pants that rub or irritate you.

How to examine your testicles.

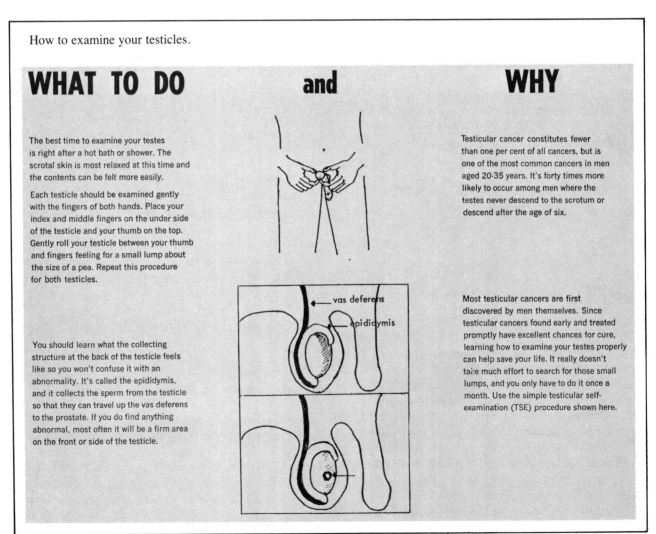

THANKS TO THE AMERICAN CANCER SOCIETY

Girls' Bodies

NOTE TO BOY READERS OF THIS SECTION: Many boys look at girls' bodies—a lot—because they are curious and fascinated, because it's a pleasure, and because they are forced to look by a culture which "sells" women's bodies along with products. Girls, too, look at girls' bodies almost as much as at boys' bodies.

There's a big difference between *looking at* and knowing about. A group of teenage boys helping us with this book were "experienced" lookers: they always knew whether a girl was wearing a bra or not; they had opinions about hairy legs and body shape. Yet they still had many questions about girls' feelings and about what goes on inside their bodies. They asked: Do you care how big your breasts are? Does getting your period change how you feel? Would you ever use pads in your bra? As the girls working with them answered these questions, you could actually see the boys moving from looking at the girls to really understanding their feelings.

Remember that the "you" from now on in this chapter is addressed to girl readers.

Girls' Changes

Somewhere between the ages of nine and eighteen, a girl will experience these changes:

—Your breasts will grow, a little or a lot, depending on the body shape you inherited from your family.
—The hair on your legs will grow thicker, maybe darker, and hair will grow under your arms.
—Pubic hair will grow around your vulva (the whole genital area, where your legs come together).
—You will get taller, growing to what will probably be your full height.
—Your hips will get bigger and your body weight may shift.
—Inside, your uterus and vagina will grow. Eggs in your ovaries will start to mature each month. You will be able to get pregnant.
—Your period will come, though it may not come regularly for a few months.
—You may get pimples, your skin may become oilier.
—Your romantic and sexual feelings may become more insistent.
—You will start to sweat more.

All these changes are caused by hormones, which become strong and active in a teenager's body.

Your Feelings about the Changes

How you feel about yourself will depend, as it does for boys, on how much you know about your body's growth, on what your idea of "beautiful" or "attractive" is and whether you accept the ways you *don't* match that image, and on the attitudes of your family and friends toward your growing up. Are they supportive? Hostile? Competitive?

Growing girls become especially vulnerable to male reactions. On the streets men who notice your growing breasts and hips make comments. Sometimes they simply compliment you, but often they call out, hoot, ogle you

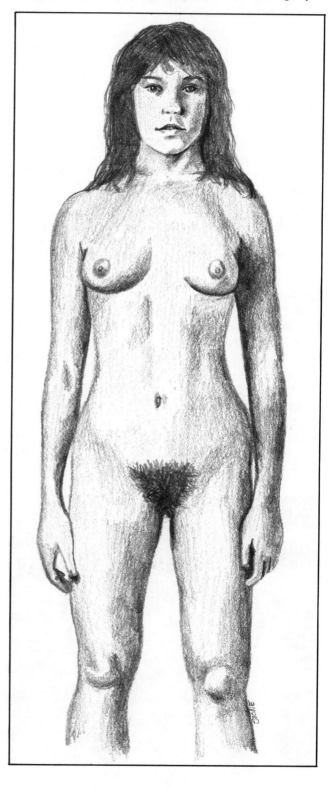

and make suggestive remarks. Girls especially are vulnerable to verbal attacks and even physical attacks by boys and men who take advantage of them (see p. 124):

> Cathy (sixteen): How about guys whistling at you and bugging you on the street? I hate that. And it's pretty scary, too, people whistling at you when you're walking home late at night.

> Denise (twelve): Since I've gotten more physically mature I get a lot of stares when I go out. Sometimes it feels nice or funny when I'm with my friends, especially when it's someone nice. But when it's some weirdo or when some older man says something like "Ooooooooh," then it's scary and I want to say, I'm only twelve, leave me alone.

In school and on the streets some boys imitate older men, or they act out their curiosity and nervousness by picking on you. Jenny, a seventeen-year-old from Washington, remembers:

> During the seventh and eighth grade I always wore a coat to school. It didn't matter what the weather was. I was embarrassed about my body because the guys at our school would always go around grabbing parts—you know, sexual parts—and I hated that.

In other situations people may react in a sexual way to your changing body. When you apply for an after-school job the boss may make sexual remarks. A neighbor who used to treat you like a kid may begin teasing you suggestively.

Girls often wonder when someone makes a sexual remark if they "asked for it"; if it's their fault. Not at all, unless you dress or act in an exaggerated obviously suggestive way. Unfortunately, even if you feel comfortable wearing a certain dress, you have to be aware that many clothing styles for girls and women are designed to be provocative. Even if you don't give a second thought to going

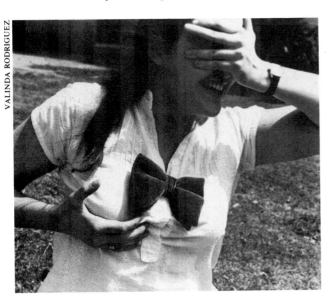

VALINDA RODRIGUEZ

bra-less, your not wearing a bra may be seen as provocative by boys and men, and they may respond to you in ways you don't expect.

You certainly have a right to grow into your woman's body, to feel good and look good without being teased or harassed. Talk with other girls about these situations if they come up. You can give each other important support in handling them and in finding other people you trust to help you.

Slang and Girls

Here are some slang words for girls' body parts:

vagina	*vulva*	*clitoris*	*hymen*	*breasts*
cunt	snatch	clit	cherry	tits
box	twat	button	maidenhead	knockers
hole	pussy	joy button		bonkers
beaver	meat	panic button		melons
honeypot	poontang	clint		boobs
muff				caldoons
				mammies
				tetons
				honkers
				jugs
				pair
				knobs

In the section on boy's slang (p. 11) we discussed how tricky slang can be, because the same words can be used in different ways. Try saying each one of these words in a loving tone, and then in a hostile tone, and notice how they differ in impact.

Even so, some of these words for parts of women's bodies have been used as insults for so long that it's almost impossible to avoid frightening a girl or hurting her just by saying them. There's really no way to make someone feel loved if you call her vulva "meat." If the word "cunt" (or "prick") is spit out in anger against someone you hate, it's hard to use those words again with affection. Think about how often our vocabulary for sex is used hatefully or—especially against women—to degrade other people.

Changes: Your Breasts Develop

Your breasts develop because estrogen, the female hormone in your body, causes the growth of mammary glands (enabling you to produce milk) and the increase of fat. Your breast, which is mostly made out of fat tissue, grows on the outside while the mammary gland grows within.

The changes in your breast come in stages. The areola (ah-*ree*-oh-la), the area around your nipple, is usually the first part to change. It gets thicker and darker. Depending on the amount of color in your skin, it can range from a light pinkish color to a very dark brown. Some hairs may grow around it.

When your breasts are cold (when swimming in cold water or taking a cold shower), when you feel sexually excited or when your breast is touched or stroked, your areola may get bumpy-looking and your nipples stand out more than usual. Otherwise the areola is usually quite smooth.

Before your breasts really start to form, your nipples will probably get larger, and they will stand out more than they did. A fourteen-year-old girl said:

One day I realized that my nipples had started growing and one was really pretty big. I thought, this is weird, everybody else has breasts and I'm going to have big nipples. I didn't really get breasts for another year, until I was about twelve.

Another girl said:

A boy came up to me at school the other day and said, "Ginny, you're totally flat!" I wanted to say, Well, you haven't seen my nipples, they're enormous! Instead I said, "Give me time, just give me time."

A sophomore from New Jersey told us:

My little sister says she feels embarrassed to wear tight shirts because her nipples are showing, but my mom says she's too young for a bra. I remember when I felt the same way—glad that I was starting to develop but embarrassed about people noticing, especially at school.

Some people have nipples that stand out a lot and other people's nipples hardly stand out at all. Some nipples sink into the areola. These are called inverted nipples (see p. 23).

Starting to develop is exciting. It's a sign of growing up, as these two girls found out:

My mom and I are really close, and when I first started getting breasts she took me out to celebrate. It was around my tenth birthday, and I remember feeling very grown-up about it.

I have three sisters who are older than me, so I was real charged up when I started popping out in front because that made me feel I was joining their club. In fact, when I got big enough, my oldest sister took me downtown to get my first bra.

Breasts: When?   Some girls begin to develop breasts at eight or nine, others not for years after that. Several girls said it was hard to be the first of all their friends to have developing breasts:

Janet: I started maturing physically when I was very young. And I never wanted to. When I was about nine I already started having breasts and I hated it. I was still a tomboy, and I used to do anything to hide my chest, like wear baggy shirts and overalls all the time. Now that I'm older I realize that I just didn't feel ready to grow up then. My body was leading the

way and my feelings about changing were about a mile behind.

Judy: When my breasts first started growing I used to wear really supertight shirts—my little sister's T-shirts. I'm serious—to flatten me. Then I'd wear another shirt over that because I was really self-conscious. I was only in third grade and every other girl in the class was flat as a board.

Sometimes breasts grow slowly:

I must have been about ten or eleven when I first started getting breasts—well, not exactly breasts but swellings on my chest. I was so proud I went around showing everybody who was interested, you know, everyone in my family and some close family friends.

The change can be more dramatic:

Ava: And my breasts, wow! Those just started going nuts. They were popping out. My sister used to call me "squished strawberries" and "busted egg yolk." Now she calls me the names I used to call her—basketball woman, grapefruit. I'm almost up to her. Another year of this kind of growing I'll be up there.

These changes may not be even. For example, one breast often starts to develop before the other one:

When I first started growing I was totally lopsided. My left side was a size-A cup and my right side was absolutely flat. It seemed to me that it was like that for a long time. I remember thinking, Uh-oh, I'm going to look very strange if this keeps up.

Usually breasts grow to be about the same size, but many women have one breast larger than the other. Ethel is twenty-two:

One of my boobs is bigger than the other one. It's not noticeable with clothes on, but when I'm naked I can really see the difference. I don't like to go around without a bra because of that—you can notice it more. It seems like my whole left side is bigger than my right side, all the way up from my foot to my hand to my boob.

Breasts: How Big?   The size and shape of your breasts depend mostly on the amount of fatty tissue they have: if there is a lot of fat in your breasts, they will be large; if there is little fat, they will be small. The major factor is heredity; that is, the body shape you have inherited from your mother or from women in your father's family. Weight has less to do with it. We've all seen thin women with large breasts and heavy women with small ones.

One group of teenagers working on this book joked about all the ways people try to develop their breasts. Exercises, they decided, just make your pectoral muscles (the muscles under your breasts) bigger. They don't really affect your breasts, but since most of the girls in the room had tried the exercises, they demonstrated a few. One of

---

THE MAMMARY GLANDS

From the time of puberty onward, your mammary glands are ready to change elements of your blood into milk if you should get pregnant and give birth.

A mammary gland is made up of areas that make milk called alveoli (al-*vee*-oh-lie), and passageways, called ducts, through which the milk travels to the nipple. You can see a few small openings in your nipple: these are the ends of the ducts. Sometimes a little bit of discharge (some liquid) will come out of these. (See p. 23.)

INTERNAL VIEW OF THE FEMALE BREAST

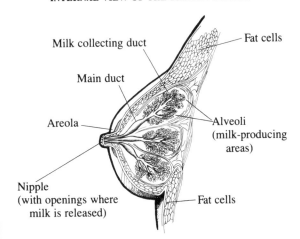

Milk collecting duct

Main duct

Areola

Nipple
(with openings where milk is released)

Fat cells

Alveoli
(milk-producing areas)

Fat cells

While a woman is pregnant her mammary glands get bigger as hormones make them ready to produce milk. Hormones released during birth trigger the milk-making a couple of days after the baby comes. When a mother holds her newborn to her breast, the baby sucks instinctively on the nipple. This sucking pulls the milk through the ducts and out. Since the baby's sucking causes more milk to be made within a few hours, there will be more milk for as long as the mother wants to keep nursing, no matter how big or small her breasts are. If she doesn't want to breast-feed her baby, the first milk will dry up and no more will be made until another birth.

the boys asked, "Is it true that if you put butter on your tits they get bigger?" Charlene had heard this too. "Last year I went to my girlfriend's house and her younger sister was in the bathroom rubbing butter and onions on her boobs because someone told her that makes them grow. It hasn't worked yet, but you never know!" Actually, there's nothing much you can do to make your breasts bigger.

Some women with very large breasts wish theirs were smaller. If you are overweight, losing weight may help. Once you are fully grown (past adolescence) you *can* have an operation to remove some breast tissue. This operation, called plastic surgery, seems like a lot of money and discomfort and risk to make yourself look different. But some

women feel it's worth it if having large breasts causes them a lot of physical and emotional suffering.

Breasts: We Care What They Look Like. Breasts come in all shapes and sizes. There's nothing much you can do about what yours look like. It would be fine if we didn't tease each other or if we liked our own and other people's bodies. It would be fine if *Playboy* magazine and Madison Avenue didn't produce·endless images of "perfect" busts. It would be fine if boys didn't grow up learning to judge a girl by her breasts or judge their friends by their girlfriends' breasts.

As women in the women's movement started to see how much they had all suffered over having the "wrong"-shape breasts, they decided that what was "wrong" was not their shape but society's attitudes. So whether your breasts are big or small, pointed or rounded, we hope this section will help you hold your own against all those voices that say they should look different. We hope that boys will begin to ask themselves where they get the message that breasts of one size or shape are best.

Taking Care of Your Breasts

Wearing a bra: If you have small breasts or very firm ones, you may not need a bra. If your breasts are large, they probably need some support; otherwise they may begin to droop. Also, during sports or dancing or any other vigorous activity, your breasts may feel much better with the support that comes from wearing a bra.

Sometimes you are given too much advice about whether or not to wear a bra. Try to make up your own mind about it. Sharon says:

I was in sixth grade and a friend told me I should wear a bra. I had never thought of it before, never thought I was big enough, and she said, "You need a bra." Who is she to be telling me I need a bra? After that, I got all self-conscious.

Mary's friends had the opposite opinion:

I had a few friends who thought it was sick to wear one. So if I ever wore one I'd wear a lot of sweaters over it. By that time I wouldn't even need to wear one.

Ellie added:

I know girls whose mothers bought them bras and said they should start wearing them. But I don't think you should start wearing a bra until you want to yourself.

Monthly Swelling. Many girls and women have swelling and tenderness in their breasts just before their period arrives. Your tissues tend to hold liquid before menstruation; this often makes your breasts feel heavier than usual. Wearing a well-fitting bra may be more comfortable. Also, since eating salt can cause tissues to hold water, cutting down on salty foods may help.

Getting Hit in the Breasts. Your breasts are sensitive. If you bump them or if they are hit, it can be painful. But your body is able to handle bruising and minor accidents, so unless your breasts are badly bruised you probably don't have cause for concern.

Some girls worry about having their breasts handled roughly during sex play. Sucking and rubbing won't cause them damage, but if it hurts or makes you feel uncomfortable, make your partner stop.

Hair. Lots of women have hair on or around their breasts. You may grow hair if you are taking the birth control pill. *Never* pluck hairs from around your breasts, for you could cause a serious infection.

Secretions. You may sometimes notice a discharge coming from your nipples. This is normal and occurs naturally as your body's way of keeping the nipple ducts open. The discharge may look like very thin milk, or it may be clear or green, gray or yellow. Women who take birth control pills may have this discharge. It can come during sexual arousal and at certain times in your menstrual cycle. Be sure to keep your nipples clean by washing with warm water and soap so the discharge won't dry and accumulate. If it has pus or blood in it, or if it is brownish in color, see a doctor, for it might be a sign of infection.

Infections. If you have an infection in or near your breasts, you will probably feel soreness and see swelling or redness. Have it checked by a doctor. Sometimes nursing mothers get infections if one of their milk ducts gets plugged up and doesn't drain properly.

Inverted Nipples. Some nipples turn in instead of sticking out. Sometimes, as your breasts continue to grow the nipples will be pushed out. If not, don't worry. It won't stop you from enjoying sex. It won't stop you from breast-feeding your baby if you have one; there are now special nipple shields made especially to help women with inverted nipples breast-feed. Lots of women have inverted nipples, so it's nothing to feel strange about. The only problem you might have is that if your breasts discharge any fluid, the secretions might get caught in the folds around the inverted nipples and dry there, possibly creating a chance for infection to develop. Be especially sure to keep your nipples clean to avoid this. *If your nipple has been normal and suddenly becomes inverted, you should see a doctor right away*. It might be because of a tumor.

Lumps. Breasts can be very lumpy. Some girls and women find changes in breast tissue throughout their monthly menstrual cycle. *If a lump stays in one place for several weeks, see a doctor*. Most lumps will be benign (noncancerous). For instance, if a lump hurts, if it is tender or sore, then it's most likely benign.

Teenagers of both sexes get a kind of lump called an adolescent nodule, a sore swollen spot right under your nipple. It will disappear by itself, but it can be scary if you don't know that. See a doctor to make sure. Teens very seldom have breast cancer. Occasionally, though, a lump can be a sign of cancer.

If you or someone you love does have a malignant or cancerous lump, be sure to learn about alternative forms of treatment.* Doctors often disagree about treatment, so remember always to get a second opinion. You'll want to choose the doctor whose approach seems most sensible to you.

Examining Your Breasts Is Important

Learn how to do a breast self-exam each month. (See diagram on p. 24.)

Many women don't examine their breasts because they haven't learned how. Others are too busy, too embarrassed, or afraid they might "find something wrong."

Take the time. You'll learn about the normal (for you) changes in your breast tissue. With practice you'll feel comfortable touching your breasts. Rarely will you find

---

BREAST SELF-EXAM

First stand in front of a mirror. Look at your breasts, with your hands at your sides; with hands raised above your head; with hands pushing firmly on your hips; or with your palms pressed together. Look for differences in shape, not size. Look for a flattening or bulging in one but not the other; for puckering of the skin; for discharge from a nipple when it is gently squeezed; for a reddening or scaly crust on a nipple; for one nipple harder than the other.

Then lie down on a bed or couch, or in a bathtub. As you examine each breast, raise the arm on that side above your head. Or bend your arm and put your hand under your head, your elbow lying flat. (A small pillow or large folded towel placed under your shoulder will distribute breast tissue more easily.) Feel your breast gently with the flat of the fingers of your opposite hand. Move them in small circles or with a slight back-and-forth motion, being sure to examine the whole breast. Pay special attention to the area between nipple and armpit, for most tumors are located there.

Breast self-exams should be done frequently at first (every few days) so that you can learn about the different ways your breasts feel during the course of a month. Later, examine them once a month at the same time each month. A few days after menstruation is good, as they will be less full then.

If you feel a definite lump that doesn't go away after a week or so, see a doctor.

---

*See pp. 128–35 in Boston Womens' Health Book Collective, *Our Bodies, Ourselves* (New York: Simon & Schuster, 1976).

something wrong. Remember, though, a breast self-exam can save your life if you find a malignant lump early enough.

Pubic Hair and Body Hair

Pubic hair grows around your genitals—over your pubic bone, around your vulva, vagina and anus. When it starts growing it covers only a small area. Then it fills out in a kind of small or large triangle or diamond shape over your pubic area. You may have just a little, or it may extend up to your navel and down the inside of your thighs.

Your first pubic hairs sometimes begin to grow without your noticing. Many people remember it as a big moment. Ann, an eleven-year-old, said:

Me and my friends go swimming at the center every week. In the shower there aren't any doors, so we kind of check each other out. Well, a couple of weeks ago Amy showed me these hairs that were starting to grow down there, and I thought, Oh my God, that isn't going to happen to me, is it? Then I examined

myself closer and I had three hairs there too. Three little dark hairs.

Also during puberty the hair on your body—in your armpits, on your legs, maybe on your forearms or upper lip and chin—gets longer, thicker and sometimes darker. Some women have very little body hair, and others have it even on their face, sometimes on their chest and back.

Boys usually welcome their thicker hair as a sign of manhood. For girls it's different. The beauty standards for women in this country right now tell us, ''Smoother is better'': smoothly shaven skin is supposed to be beautiful and body hair is supposed to be ugly. Did you ever see a magazine model with lush curly hair on her legs and tantalizing tufts under her arms? New body hair may be a sign of growing up, but for most girls *shaving* is the true sign of womanhood. Many girls are eager to start shaving:

Vicky: When I was fourteen and not even much hair had grown yet, I had a contest with my friend to see whether my mother's electric shaver or her razor could get a closer shave under our arms. I forget who

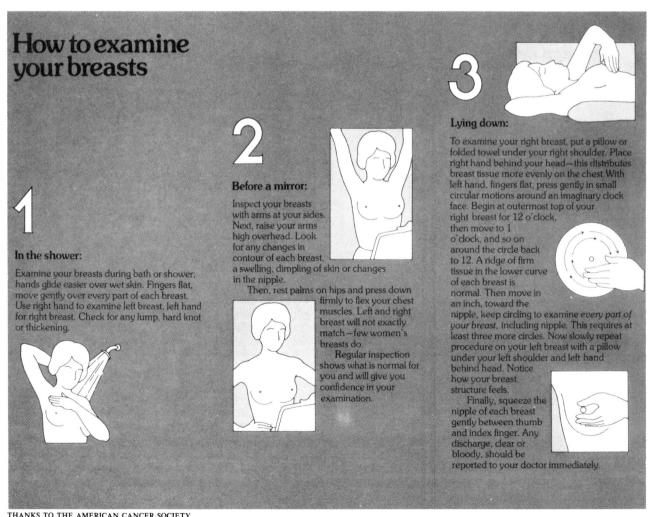

How to examine your breasts

1 In the shower:

Examine your breasts during bath or shower; hands glide easier over wet skin. Fingers flat, move gently over every part of each breast. Use right hand to examine left breast, left hand for right breast. Check for any lump, hard knot or thickening.

2 Before a mirror:

Inspect your breasts with arms at your sides. Next, raise your arms high overhead. Look for any changes in contour of each breast, a swelling, dimpling of skin or changes in the nipple.
Then, rest palms on hips and press down firmly to flex your chest muscles. Left and right breast will not exactly match—few women's breasts do.
Regular inspection shows what is normal for you and will give you confidence in your examination.

3 Lying down:

To examine your right breast, put a pillow or folded towel under your right shoulder. Place right hand behind your head—this distributes breast tissue more evenly on the chest. With left hand, fingers flat, press gently in small circular motions around an imaginary clock face. Begin at outermost top of your right breast for 12 o'clock, then move to 1 o'clock, and so on around the circle back to 12. A ridge of firm tissue in the lower curve of each breast is normal. Then move in an inch, toward the nipple, keep circling to examine *every part of your breast*, including nipple. This requires at least three more circles. Now slowly repeat procedure on your left breast with a pillow under your left shoulder and left hand behind head. Notice how your breast structure feels.
Finally, squeeze the nipple of each breast gently between thumb and index finger. Any discharge, clear or bloody, should be reported to your doctor immediately.

THANKS TO THE AMERICAN CANCER SOCIETY

won, but, boy, do I remember how sore and raw my armpits were.

Cindy: When I started getting hair under my arms it was in the spring. People were starting to wear bathing suits and I had these hairy underarms. I wanted to shave, but I was afraid to because my mother never talked to me about it. So finally I said, ''Ma, is it OK if I shave?'' She said, ''Oh, yes. I just thought you were liberated.'' Because I always talk about women's rights and stuff she thought that meant I wouldn't want to shave my underarms.

Many girls shave so as not to look different from everyone else. Three girls in Boston discuss shaving:

Eileen: I shave in the winter when it's time for gymnastics because you don't want to be the only one on the gym team with hairy legs.

Iris: Yeah, you're under a lot of pressure to shave your legs.

Liz: There's a difference between what you want and what you think other people want. I don't think hairy legs are that bad. It doesn't bother me on me, and it doesn't bother me on other girls. But still I do it at times.

Many girls who have dark hair on their arms or thighs, or on their faces, wish they didn't have it and dream of ways of getting rid of it. They tweeze it out or remove it with wax. They use chemical bleaches and hair removers sold commercially; they go to the expense of electrolysis. Sometimes they feel fine about having hair but are pressured to use one of these methods by parents or older women in their families. The idea ''No hair is beautiful'' goes deep. It's up to each of us to decide how *we* want to look, and how much body hair we are comfortable with.

Your Genitals and Reproductive Organs

Your genitals are easy to see: Take a hand mirror and squat over it or hold it between your legs as you sit on the edge of a chair. Be sure you have plenty of light. Make sure you have enough time, too, and enough privacy so you can feel relaxed.

You may be surprised when someone first says, ''Take a mirror and flashlight and look at your genitals,'' or ''If you reach your finger up inside your vagina you can touch your cervix.'' You may feel shocked. Doreen said:

I know a lot of girls who think they're dirty down there and are taught not to touch themselves.

Becky, a sixteen-year-old helping with this book, said:

I absolutely can't stand to think about doing that. It gives me the shivers. Even when I have to wash myself, I can barely do it.

She had been taught that it was wrong, dirty and shameful to touch herself. When she was a child her parents punished her when they found her masturbating (see p. 79). She learned that ''nice'' girls don't have anything to do with that part of their bodies.

The funny thing is that Becky didn't mind when her boyfriend touched her down there or even when he looked. Her genitals were off limits only to herself. The other girls in the group she belonged to tried to help her feel that it was her right to get to know her body. They explained that the more she knew about her body, the better care she'd be able to take of herself. As Doreen said to her:

I figure it's a part of my body, just like any other part, except it's not right out there like your boobs are. Anyway, I sure as hell don't want someone else playing with it if I don't know what it is myself.

Lots of girls start out feeling like Becky. One of the best lessons to come out of the women's movement has been that we owe it to ourselves to know what our bodies look, feel and taste like.

Your Genitals: What You Can See on the Outside. Starting from the front, you'll first see a soft, fatty mound called the *mons*. It's sometimes called mound of Venus or mons veneris: Venus was the goddess of love. The mons is the pad of fatty layers that covers your pubic bone. If you press it, you can feel the bone right above where your legs join. If you have pubic hair already, this mound will be covered with hair.

Next you'll see the *outer lips* or *major lips* (labia), two pads or flaps of skin. Unless you spread your legs apart, these lips fall together, protecting the rest of your genitals as they were meant to do.

If you gently separate these lips, you'll see the *inner lips* or *minor lips,* another set of folds of skin with no hair on them. These give more protection. They may hang below the major lips. They are sexually sensitive.

As you carefully spread open the inner lips, you see that where they come together at the front they form a hood over a small, sensitive pea-shaped bump, which is the top of the *clitoris* (*klit*-or-iss). The clitoris is densely packed with nerves, extremely sensitive to touch, and the center of sexual sensation for a woman. This sixteen-year-old said:

It's not hard to find your clit. Just put your hand down there and feel around. When you get to the place that feels great and turns you on, that's your clit.

Your clitoris, like a penis, has a *glans,* or head, which is the most sensitive part, and a *shaft* under the skin which is the main part of the clitoris. Glans and shaft contain the same spongy tissue that makes a penis erect. When you are sexually turned on, extra blood rushes into the spongy areas (erectile tissue) and causes your clitoris to get a little bigger. The whole area around it swells too, and becomes sensitive to touch. Rubbing the area can feel very good and may make you have an orgasm—a climax of sexual

FEMALE EXTERNAL GENITALS

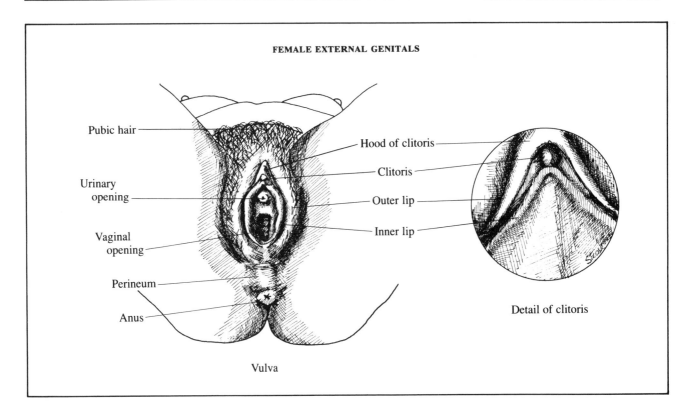

Pubic hair

Urinary opening

Vaginal opening

Perineum

Anus

Hood of clitoris

Clitoris

Outer lip

Inner lip

Detail of clitoris

Vulva

excitement. Your clitoris is so sensitive that rubbing or touching the glans directly often hurts.

Your clitoris is special, its only purpose sexual arousal—it's just for pleasure. It's amazing to realize that for centuries most women didn't know about the clitoris. Many still don't. Women have had sex not knowing about the important role of the clitoris. Their partners share this ignorance. Imagine not knowing about such a source of feeling good!

Next in line from your clitoris, also inside the inner lips, you'll find your urethra, a small dot or slit. You urinate through this little round opening. The urethra is the opening of the tube that carries your urine from your bladder (which holds the urine). The urethra is about 1½ inches long.

Next you will see your *vaginal opening,* which is larger than the urethral opening. It leads to your vagina. Menstrual blood, vaginal discharges and babies come out through the vaginal opening.

Look around the opening. You might see your *hymen,* a membrane (a special kind of tissue) that covers the vaginal opening partway. It almost never blocks the opening all the way, since there must be a way for menstrual blood to leave your body once your period begins. The hymen gives your body extra protection. It becomes stretched if you are very active or if you have had intercourse.

You can stretch your hymen open by yourself by putting one or two fingers into your vagina and moving them gently from side to side every day until it stretches. You may

want to use a tampon. Be gentle. Even after stretching, you can see little folds of hymen tissue around the opening.

A big deal has been made of the hymen over the centuries. For many people it's the symbol of a young woman's purity, the sign that she is still a ''virgin''; that is, that she hasn't had sexual intercourse with a man. The sexy parts of lots of books have dramatic scenes where the hymen (the ''cherry'' or ''maidenhead'') is torn during first intercourse, with lots of blood and anguish and passion. These accounts are pretty exaggerated! (See the section on virginity, p. 99). Some girls are born with no hymen at all;

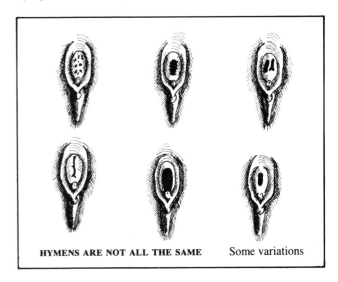

HYMENS ARE NOT ALL THE SAME   Some variations

some have a naturally large hymen opening; some stretch their hymen open during the normal play of childhood, including masturbation. Having a hymen or not is no sign of "virginity." Also, first intercourse isn't necessarily bloody.

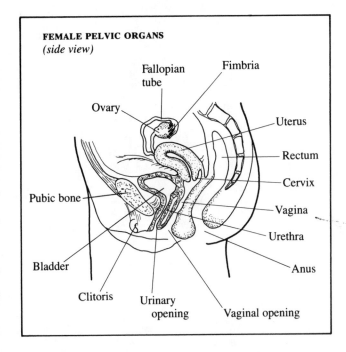

FEMALE PELVIC ORGANS
(side view)

Fallopian tube — Fimbria — Ovary — Uterus — Rectum — Cervix — Vagina — Urethra — Anus — Pubic bone — Bladder — Clitoris — Urinary opening — Vaginal opening

Now put a finger into your *vagina*, which is the passageway from your uterus to the outside of your body. A moment before, the vaginal walls were touching each other, but now they are spreading around your fingers. The walls seem to hug them. Feel the soft folds of skin. The stretchy walls allow the vagina to change shape, to fit whatever is inside. This may be a tampon or fingers; it could be a penis or a baby.

Maggie was surprised to find these walls touching each other:

> I always pictured my vagina as open, like a box or something, a hole I carried around between my legs. It's nice to realize I'm not so wide open.

Now move your finger. Notice how it slides around. Sometimes the walls of the vagina are almost dry, sometimes they feel moist. The degree of moistness depends on your age, on where you are in your monthly cycle, or on whether you are sexually excited.

The walls of your vagina give off a liquid, called *mucus*, most of the time. Mucus is your vagina's natural way of cleaning itself—which means that you don't have to douche. The mucus is slightly acid, keeps many infections from starting, and tastes salty. You may find signs of this mucus discharge on your underpants at times, which is normal. It may, though, be a sign of a vaginal infection (see p. 230).

Do you notice that when you are turned on sexually, even by a picture or a fantasy, the lips of your vagina get wet? The vagina's natural mucus increases when you are sexually excited (see p. 81).

Push gently against the vaginal walls. Try it all the way around. The outer third of the vagina, closest to the entrance, is very sensitive because it contains many nerve endings. This sensitivity is important in lovemaking.

If you squeeze in the entrance to your vagina and then relax, you'll feel the muscles called *pelvic floor muscles*. These muscles hold your pelvic organs—your uterus, bladder and ovaries—in place. When these muscles are weak you may have trouble holding your urine or having orgasms. Pregnant women do an exercise to make these muscles stronger. We can all do these exercises (Kegel exercises) to keep in shape. The pelvic floor muscles, like mucus and nerve endings, play a role in lovemaking.

To locate these muscles, spread your legs apart while urinating and try to start and stop the flow of urine. Exercise these muscles by contracting (squeezing) hard for a second and then releasing completely. Repeat ten times in a row (which takes about twenty seconds) to make up a group of exercises. Try to work up to several groups a day. You can do these exercises anytime—while you are sitting, talking, walking, reading.

You may be feeling with your finger or noticing from the diagram that your vagina doesn't go straight up into your body. It goes back at an angle toward the small of your back. When you are trying to put in tampons for the first time this is a good thing to know. Your vagina ends after a few inches. Nothing that goes into your vagina can get lost in the rest of your body.

If you reach your middle finger as far up as you can, you should get to a lump that feels like the tip of a nose or (if you've had a baby) a chin. This is your *cervix*, the lower part of your uterus, or womb. (If you have trouble reaching it, bring your knees and chest closer together.) Marie said:

> I had always thought my womb was so far up in there that I could never touch any part of it. The first time I touched my cervix you could have knocked me over with a feather. Amazing!

You may not always feel your cervix in exactly the same place every day because your uterus moves slightly during your monthly cycle. Some days you can barely reach it. It also shifts when you are sexually excited.

In the center of your cervix you should be able to feel a small dimple, called the *os*. About as wide as a straw, it is the opening to your uterus. Blood comes out through your os when you have your period. Believe it or not, when a pregnant woman goes into labor the os opens up wide enough to let a baby through. Most of the time it is very tiny. No tampon or finger can go through it. No penis can, either. But germs can, so to avoid infections make sure that everything you put into your vagina is clean. And sperm can go through it, too, so always use birth control if you have sexual intercourse with a boy or a man and don't want to get pregnant.

When an instrument called a speculum is put into your vagina to hold the walls apart, your cervix can be clearly seen. (It looks like a small pink doughnut.) A doctor or practitioner does this in a gynecological exam (see p. 157), but you can do it, too, with a speculum, flashlight and mirror. Feminist health centers and self-help groups often sell inexpensive clear-plastic speculums for girls and women who want to examine their vaginal walls and cervix.

Your *anus* is the third opening in your vulva. It is where your bowel movements leave your body. It leads from the rectum, where wastes are stored. In fact, since only a thin wall of skin separates the vagina from the rectum on the inside, if you have your finger in your vagina you can sometimes feel the feces in your rectum right through the wall. They will feel like a lump in the bottom or back side of the vaginal wall. By the time your pubic hair is fully grown, you will also have hair around your anus.

Your bowel movements have germs in them that can give you serious infections if they reach your vagina and urethra. It is important to wipe yourself off from front to back after urinating or defecating so that the bacteria do not get into the vagina. Also, in sex play be careful: if a penis or finger has been on or in the anus, don't put it in your vagina without cleaning it with soap.

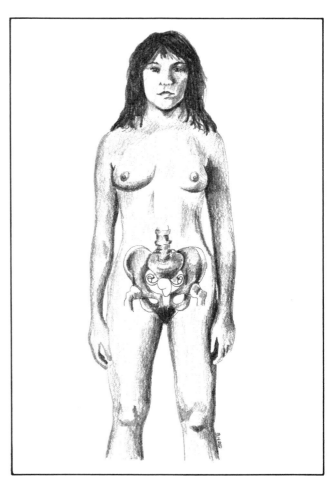

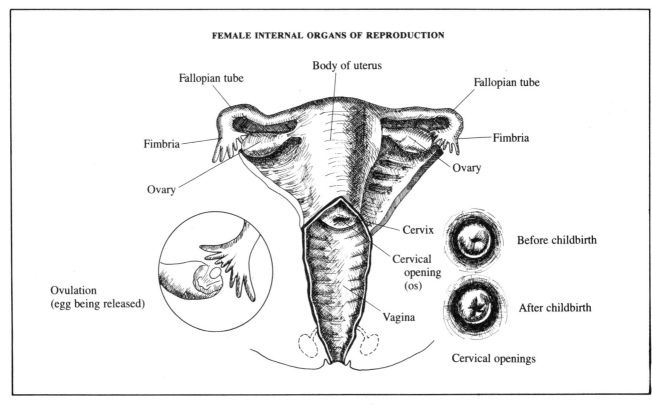

FEMALE INTERNAL ORGANS OF REPRODUCTION

Fallopian tube

Body of uterus

Fallopian tube

Fimbria

Fimbria

Ovary

Ovary

Cervix

Cervical opening (os)

Before childbirth

Ovulation (egg being released)

Vagina

After childbirth

Cervical openings

Further Inside: Your Internal Reproductive Organs. Except for your cervix (the lower part of your uterus), your internal organs are too far up inside your body for you to see or feel them.

Your *uterus* (*you*-ter-russ) or *womb* (woom) is an organ about the size of your fist and the shape of an upside-down pear. It has thick walls of strong, stretchy muscles.

Two tubes, called the *fallopian* (fell-*low*-pee-yan) *tubes,* lead out from the top of your uterus, one on each side. They are about four inches long, and narrow, about the width of a fine needle. The outer end of each tube has fingerlike fringy ends (*fimbriae*—*fim*-bree-ay) that wrap around your ovary but do not touch it.

You have two *ovaries* (*oh*-vah-rees), one on each side. An ovary is the size and shape of an unshelled almond. Your ovaries make the important female hormones estrogen and progesterone. These hormones are chemicals that travel through your bloodstream when triggered by certain glands and processes. They cause most of the changes of puberty.

Both ovaries contain eggs. These eggs, stored in little pockets called *follicles,* are in a girl's ovaries from the day she is born. When you reach puberty, one egg matures each month and leaves the ovary. The fimbriae guide the egg into the fallopian tube.

Menstruation, or Getting Your Period*

All women menstruate unless they are pregnant, nursing a baby, very underweight, ill, or have some problem with their reproductive system). A woman usually begins her period between the ages of nine and eighteen (this is called *menarche*—muh-*nar*-key). She continues to have it for the next forty years or so. A menstrual period comes about every 21 to 40 days. Some women are very regular; they have their periods at the same time each month. Others are not. Most women are irregular sometimes. Though there are negative words (like the "curse") for a menstrual pe-

*A great book for girls (and boys), ages eight to fourteen, is *Period,* by Jo Ann Gardner-Loulan, Bonnie Lopez and Marcia Quackenbush (My Mama's Press, P.O. Box 2086, Burlingame, CA 94010).

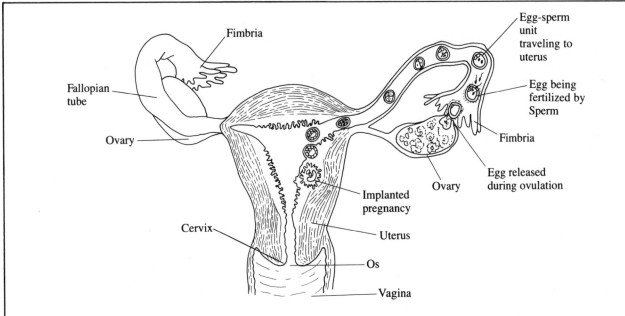

Fimbria
Fallopian tube
Ovary
Cervix
Implanted pregnancy
Uterus
Os
Vagina
Egg-sperm unit traveling to uterus
Egg being fertilized by Sperm
Fimbria
Egg released during ovulation
Ovary

CONCEPTION: HOW YOU BECOME PREGNANT

If you have had sexual intercourse with a man and used no birth control, if your birth control method hasn't worked, or if some semen from a man's penis has gotten close to the lips of your vagina and sperm have swum in, then the sperm will swim up the vagina through the cervical os into the uterus and then into the fallopian tube. The egg just released by the ovary may be penetrated by sperm. This can happen during two or three days a month. This is called *fer-*

tilization or *conception.* Fertilization most often takes place in the fallopian tube. From there the fertilized egg takes about six days to move through the tube to the uterus, where it attaches itself to the inner uterine *wall,* or *lining,* and grows for about nine months.

While you are *pregnant,* hormonal signals sent to the uterine lining keep it thick and nourishing for the developing fetus. Because the lining is in use, you don't get your period. Not getting your period is one of the signs of pregnancy (see p. 190).

I AM WOMAN

As time goes by,
the memories remain, the laughter, the joys,
even the great depth of pain.

Remembering when you started to walk,
remembering when you fell—that first fall was
  great.
Knowing someone was there.
I wonder what it would have been like
if no one was there,
  that first step may have been the last.
The first day of school and you couldn't reach the
  water fountain,
  tried to get up to your chair—it was too tall.
When you had to go to the bathroom and couldn't
  undo your clothes.

As time goes by
the memories remain,
that first pain and discomfort of being a woman
not knowing who to tell—or what to do.
Your body flows of red rivers and your mind races
  in time,
remembering your mother walking in your room
  saying,
"You're a young lady now, and ladies don't run
  around
with a lot of little boys playing boyish games.
You should sit properly and dress neatly."
Never did she tell me that it was okay that I am
  Woman.

—Annette Barnes

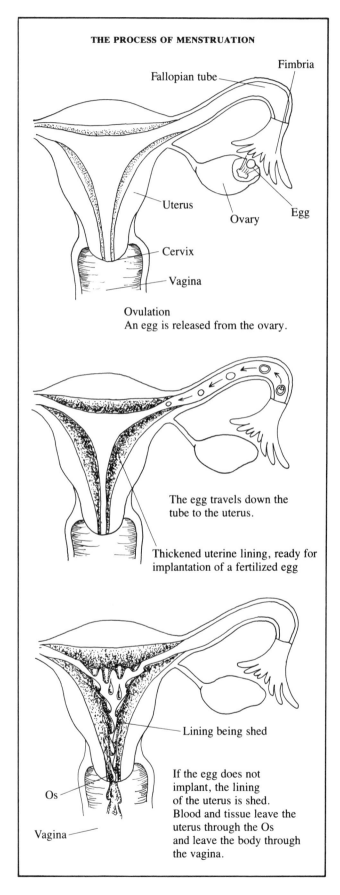

THE PROCESS OF MENSTRUATION

Fallopian tube — Fimbria

Uterus

Ovary — Egg

Cervix

Vagina

Ovulation
An egg is released from the ovary.

The egg travels down the
tube to the uterus.

Thickened uterine lining, ready for
implantation of a fertilized egg

Lining being shed

Os

Vagina

If the egg does not
implant, the lining
of the uterus is shed.
Blood and tissue leave the
uterus through the Os
and leave the body through
the vagina.

riod, getting your period is normal, healthy and very positive.

Your Menstrual Cycle. Medical people count your menstrual cycle from *the first day your period comes*. This is called Day 1. They talk in terms of a 28-day cycle, just for simplicity. We will, too, to help you understand what goes on. Very few women in fact have a 28-day cycle.

Look at the cycle at Day 5—that is, five days after your period begins. At this point the pituitary gland near your brain sends a signal to several of the thousands of eggs in your ovaries. Some eggs begin to ripen, but usually only one egg will mature. Meanwhile the ovary sends out the hormone estrogen, and signals your uterine lining to become thicker with blood and tissue.

About Day 14 the ripened egg breaks out of its follicle and rises to the surface of your ovary. This is called ovulation (ah-vue-*lay*-shun). You may feel a cramp or twinge when you ovulate. The egg is then swept into the fallopian tube. Meanwhile the ruptured follicle produces the hormone progesterone and causes the uterine lining to continue its buildup. If the egg has *not* been fertilized (if you have not conceived), it breaks apart and disintegrates. Then the estrogen and progesterone signals to your uterus get weaker. By Day 24 they have stopped. The uterine lining starts to break up. By Day 28 it has loosened so much that bits of it start to break off and come out of your cervix and vagina as menstruation begins. This is Day 1. Five days later the cycle starts all over again. This is called your *menstrual cycle*.

As you can see, ovulation occurs *before* menstruation. That is why it is possible to get pregnant before your first period comes. Many girls get their period a few times before ovulation starts, but some ovulate right from the beginning. If they are having unprotected intercourse, they can get pregnant even before they begin menstruating.

What comes out of your vagina is usually called "blood" because the blood in it makes it red, but it's really a mixture of tissue, mucus and blood. So when a clump of it comes out all at once we may call it a clot but it is not a blood clot. You do lose *some* blood during your period, but not as much as it looks like.

You have *cramps* when the muscles of your uterus tighten up to push the menstrual fluid out, and when the muscles of your cervix open the os a little bit to let it out.

When Will Your First Period Come? You have no definite way of knowing when you will menstruate for the first time. Usually you start about two years after your breasts begin to develop and one year after your pubic hair begins to grow. When you begin will depend on your health and on when the women in your mother's or father's family began their periods. There's no time when you "should" start. Menstruation comes according to your body's own time.

Two girls talk about waiting for their first period:

Lisa (eleven): I'm glad I haven't gotten my period yet. I'm still a kid. No way do I want to worry about that every month.

Toni (sixteen): I wish I would get it already. Just about everyone I know has it and I feel like a freak not having it yet. Like friends come up to me and say, "Oh, do you have a Tampax I could borrow?" and then they'll say, "Oh, sorry, I forgot you don't have it yet."

When your period comes for the first time, it can be a big event. Sally, a twelve-year-old from Buffalo, described her first time:

The whole weekend I had this terrible stomachache, but I just thought it was a stomachache. Then on Saturday night while I was in the bathroom, I saw this brownish stuff in my pants and I thought, No, it couldn't be . . . because it was brown and I thought a period was red. So I didn't put a sanitary napkin on or anything. Then in the morning I had this big mess in my pajamas and that's when I knew for sure. I was really excited. I was sort of waiting for it to come,

because I have an older sister who got her period around her twelfth birthday.

Not Feeling Ready. Some girls are not ready for their periods. Either they haven't been told it will come, or they don't feel grown-up enough:

Crystal: I didn't know what was happening. I had these cramps and a headache, so I went to the bathroom, but it wasn't like I had the flu or anything. I didn't know what I had. When I got up from the toilet I noticed this blood in there and then I saw some blood on my thigh, so I started to scream. I thought I was bleeding to death. Nobody told me about periods, nobody told me about anything. I was in the fifth grade and I still thought babies grew in your stomach and came out your bellybutton. I can't believe how scared I was.

Holly: When I got my period, it wasn't OK with me and I cried and cried because I never thought I'd ever actually get my period. I was eleven and I remember crying and thinking, Oh, now I'm a woman and I'm too young to be a woman. I was such a kid. I was so upset I didn't want to tell my mom at first. I had this crazy idea that she was going to be mad at me for getting it, but when she saw how upset I was, she asked

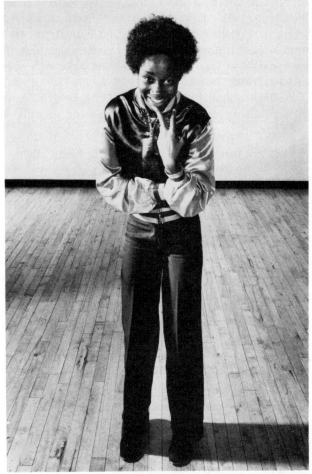

me what was wrong. I finally told her. She turned out to be wonderful about it and really made me feel better.

Being Ready. Being ready for your period makes a difference. It helps a lot if someone—a parent, aunt, sister, friend, teacher—has told you ahead of time what to expect. Most schools try to teach the girls (rarely the boys!) something, but often those classes start after half the girls already have their periods. Most of the time you don't feel comfortable talking about your own feelings and questions. You and some friends could help your school start a good discussion group for both sexes so that more of you will be prepared.

Darlene is luckier than some girls. At twelve, she said:

I'm ready for it when it comes. I sent away for that Kotex kit, you know, where they send you this book about it and some napkins and stuff. And my mom showed me how to put on a napkin, so when it comes I'll be prepared.

There are a lot of mothers like Darlene's, who give their daughters the help they need in getting ready for their period. If your mother hasn't been much help, remember that *her* mother may not have told her anything. She may have no practice in talking about these things. Maybe reading this chapter with you would give her a chance to talk with you in a way she'd really like to. But even if you can't learn what you need to know from your mother, you do have a right to know. Try to find some older woman or man you trust to talk to.

Feelings about Menstruating. Girls have a lot of feelings about menstruating. Some are proud, like Karen and Ginny:

I got my period early, when I was in fourth grade, and all my friends were jealous. They wanted to get theirs too.

I told everybody when I got my period. Everybody! I celebrated and went out and bought myself a present.

Some, as we have seen, are embarrassed about being the first one of their friends to get their period, embarrassed to be so young, shy to tell their mothers and their friends. This embarrassment is a sign that menstruation makes a big change in your life. You are becoming a woman. What's happening to your body is new. It's natural to feel strange at first, full of mixed emotions.

Some girls have more negative feelings:

Alice: My friends sort of teased me when I got my period—like something was wrong with me for developing faster than them. I think I was a little ashamed of myself for getting it. No one told me it was something to be proud of.

Charlotte: When my best friend moved away, we swore to each other that we would tell the other one

when one of us got our period. Well, she got it and she didn't tell me, and I had a funny feeling about that. She sort of got shyer. It was like she was ashamed she got it.

Ruth: I didn't want to tell my mother when I got it because I thought she would be mad at me for knowing what it was. I thought she was going to think I was dirty for having it so young.

We believe that girls feel such embarrassment and shame because our society (like many others) has a negative attitude toward menstruation. Often we are taught that it is dirty or ugly, or to be kept secret. These things are not true, but many people are uncomfortable about bodies, and women's bodies in particular. Too many girls and women suffer needlessly because of these attitudes.

Brief History of Attitudes Toward Menstruation. Attitudes toward menstruation are very old. All through history, and in the Bible, women were said to be "unclean" when they had their periods. Many times menstruating women weren't allowed to take part in festivals or religious ceremonies. In primitive cultures women were sent away from the settlement on those days. They weren't supposed to touch or go near certain objects for fear the objects would be ruined. To this day, in certain religions and cultures men aren't supposed to have sex with their menstruating wives.

Those taboos around menstruation were based not on fact but on fear. Women's blood was a special kind of blood. It didn't come from sickness or injury. It was related to a woman's ability to give birth, and that ability was and still is a power that only women have. You can imagine that before much was known about periods and childbirth, some people thought these events were caused by magic. Primitive men may have been jealous of that "magical" power. Both women and men may have made up stories about it and been afraid of it.

Now we know that menstruation and childbirth are not caused by magic. We know there is nothing to be scared of. But the same kinds of attitudes persist.

Here are some modern ways they are expressed: "A woman wouldn't make a good President because she'd be too emotionally unstable during her menstrual cycle." "Women can't be priests because what if they were menstruating when they were at the altar?" Menstruating women are warned that exercise is bad during menstruation. (In fact exercise helps lessen cramps and keeps your spirits up.) You may have been told that you shouldn't take a bath or wash your hair or feed your dog or cook or water the plants or have sex or go swimming when you have your period. Actually, none of this is true. But such beliefs act like the ancient taboos, restricting a woman and making her think she is more helpless at this time.

Women today are questioning myths like these. You and your friends can too. If you ever find yourself or a friend feeling ashamed or bad about having a period, remember that it's a normal event, even an event to celebrate. You and your friends can learn about women through the ages who have menstruated, borne children, made history, healed each other, been strong. Maybe there *is* a special power in menstruating women, after all—but it's a power for creating and healing, not for destroying.

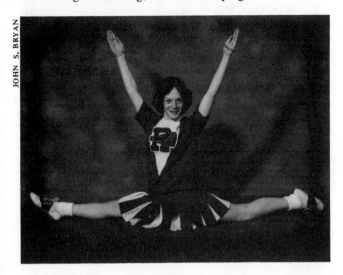

Some Difficult Moments. Attitudes about menstruation won't change overnight, and even if they did, people will still get embarrassed at times, for hundreds of reasons. Many girls (and older women too) talked about their fear of getting caught without a pad or tampon, or of getting blood on their clothes. Nancy remembers:

This didn't happen to me, it happened to my friend Paula, but I've always prayed it wouldn't happen to me! She went to the movies with a bunch of kids. She sat on her legs for some of the movie. Her period came right in the middle and she didn't know it. When the lights came on there was blood all over her white knee socks. She was so mortified!

We feel so vulnerable when something like this happens. Though menstrual bleeding is natural, many of us still have "learned" that this evidence of our periods should be secret; when it stains our clothes we are ashamed. Your period won't necessarily start when you're at home. Some months it comes when you're in school, on a date or at work.

When our periods become "public" we find it difficult. Debby, a thirteen-year-old from Denver, said:

I almost died when I had to go to the store to buy pads for my period. My mom and I were out shopping and I got my period right then and we didn't have anything with us, so we had to go to the drugstore to get some pads and a belt. Just as we were going up to the counter I saw a boy I knew from school. He didn't see me, but my heart started beating like mad and I turned bright red. As soon as the lady at

the counter put my stuff in a bag I felt so much better, but then as we were walking out, we ran into him and I could hardly even say "Hello" to him, I was so nervous thinking, Oh my God, what am I going to do if this bag rips!

A fifteen-year-old from Los Angeles said:

That was the most embarrassing thing I've ever done in my whole life, buying my first box of tampons. I'll never forget. I was in the store and I kept waiting until the guy at the register went into the back. I waited and waited until there was a lady there, and then I bought something else that I absolutely did not need just so I could hide the box of Tampax behind it. I really needed a big box, but I only bought a small one so I wouldn't be so conspicuous.

Doris's embarrassing-moments story is one of the most dramatic:

My mother always told me, when you have your period you take off the used pad and wrap it up in toilet paper and throw it in the wastebasket right away. Well, I was at my girlfriend's house and I was in the bathroom and I had my period, so I took off the old pad and put it up on the top of the toilet while I was putting the new one on. For some reason I totally forgot about the old pad sitting up there on the toilet and I walked out of the bathroom and left it there. Well— here's the most embarrassing part—her brother went into the bathroom a few minutes later and found it. Can you believe it? I really wanted to die. He was older and he knew about girls getting their periods— plus he had three sisters, so that had probably happened to him before anyway—so he was pretty understanding. He made a little joke about it and made me laugh, but still I was dying inside. I made some excuse and went home real soon after that and I went into my room and started crying. My girlfriend was really nice about it the next day in school, and she didn't tell anybody, but I waited a long time before I went over to her house again.

Those kinds of experiences are so common. When Doris was telling her story, one of the other girls in the room said, "Oh my God, the same thing happened to me once, but it was my cousin who saw it and he teased me about it for weeks."

Lots of girls are teased by boys about having their period. Most boys can't be blamed—probably no one has told them what is going on, and they are nervous. Some girls find that if someone takes the time to talk to boys about menstruation, they are interested in a serious way.

Predicting Your Menstrual Cycle. Some women have regular menstrual cycles; others have irregular cycles. Many teenagers have irregular cycles for a while. In a discussion group, Carrie said, "My sister went for almost a year with only one period. When I first got mine, six months passed without another one." Mark commented,

"It must be scary if you sleep with a guy because you never know if you are pregnant or not." He's right: girls who skip periods, who make love with boys and don't use birth control, often can't tell if they are pregnant. Sometimes just worrying about being pregnant can make your period come late.

Even if you don't have sex, it can be puzzling and frustrating to be irregular. You may be regular for a while but then skip a month, or be late because of events and pressures in your life: you may lose or gain a lot of weight, go on a trip, get sick, or worry a lot about something. It's amazing how connected our minds and bodies are. Usually your menstrual cycle settles into its own pattern. As you grow older it may change again.

There are ways of knowing when your period is due:

(1) Find out the average length of your cycle. You have your own rhythm. Even if your periods seem to come in no regular pattern, try keeping track of them on a calendar for several months. Each month mark an X on Day 1. After six months count the number of days from Day 1 of one cycle to Day 1 of the next. Add the number of days in all the cycles together and divide by 6 to find out your average cycle length. If the length of your cycle varies greatly from month to month, the calendar method won't be helpful.

(2) You may notice some body signs. For instance, when you ovulate you may get a pain or cramp in your back or abdomen. Two weeks after ovulation your period should start.

(3) Often your breasts feel bigger, heavier and lumpier after ovulation and before menstruation. Familiarize yourself with how your breasts feel. If they change, mark it down and notice when your period comes.

(4) You may get headaches or backaches just before your period. You may not sleep well. Your face may break out in pimples, or you may feel depressed or cranky. Some or all of these signs can mean that your period is about to begin.

(5) Another way of figuring out your cycle seems too complicated at first but in fact is pretty accurate. It's called the mucus method. At the time of ovulation your vaginal mucus is runny and wet. Closer to your period it gets thicker and dryer. You can learn to tell the difference simply by how wet or dry the lips of your vagina feel, or by

---

HELPING YOURSELF FEEL BETTER

If you have painful periods and/or depressing premenstrual moods, here are some things that women have discovered help to make them feel better. You and your friends may also discover some of your own remedies. Since each woman's body is unique, some of the remedies will work for you and some won't. Pay attention to how the remedy you choose affects you.

1. Watch your own body signs so you can begin to notice when your period is due. Then you'll be able to plan your schedule around whichever days are hardest for you. You'll be able to take steps like watching your diet or getting exercise or getting enough sleep when you know you'll need it. (See the section "Predicting Your Menstrual Cycle," p. 33.)

2. Watch what you eat. If you know when your period is due, cut down on salty foods before and during. Salt makes your body retain water. Water retention can add to your feeling of heaviness and swelling during your period, as well as to tension and depression beforehand. Salt—in chips, pretzels, nuts, spicy foods, soy sauce—can make you more uncomfortable than you need to be. For about ten days before your period, also cut down on sugar, white flour and caffeine. This list covers a whole lot of what you eat and you may not be able to cut down on them all at once. But try to avoid cola drinks, chocolate, coffee, soft drinks, junk foods, and most cakes, pies and breads.

Alcohol, too—especially wine and beer—may increase cramping and headaches. Drink natural fruit juices. Some herbal teas—raspberry-leaf tea, for instance—are soothing and may help relieve cramps.

If you have very painful periods, you might ask a nutritionist to recommend a special diet with vitamin and mineral supplements. Experiment to see what works well for you. Eat well-balanced meals. You might find that when you change your diet you'll feel better in general.

3. Some women find that taking several dolomite calcium tablets and vitamin C supplements each day for a week before their period helps to relieve tension and depression. You can buy these tablets in a drugstore or health-food store.

4. If you have heavy menstrual flows, iron supplements are recommended to help you avoid anemia. Blackstrap molasses contains B vitamins, which help you absorb iron, and calcium, which reduces cramping.

5. If your cramps are severe, you may feel better if you lie down and relax your whole body. That's easier said than done, because when you are in pain your body almost automatically tenses up. Tenseness often comes from a fear that there's something wrong because you're hurting so much. Tell yourself there's nothing wrong. Remind yourself that your body is just working to let out the old uterine lining. Many women have learned to keep themselves from tensing up by breathing deeply and slowly, and by keeping their bodies as relaxed as possible.

putting your finger into your vagina to test the mucus closer to your cervix. About fourteen days after the day of runniest mucus you'll get your period. (This method is used by some women as a form of birth control. See p. 188).

Knowing about Side Effects. Menstruation brings a number of side effects. Some women experience none of them; others experience just a few. Some of these side effects are headaches, backaches, skin problems, mood changes, depression, cramps, nausea and water retention (when the liquids you drink tend to stay in your body and you feel puffy and heavy). Many women find that as they grow older some of the painful symptoms become less severe or go away.

You may not even notice that your period is coming and not feel any different at all. You may feel heavy or extra tired before your period but be fine once the flow starts. Gini, at sixteen, is a swimmer and a lacrosse player:

My period is no problem and it never really was. When I first got it, I got it when I woke up one morning, and even now, four years later, it still usually comes in the morning, so I almost always know I have it before I go to school. I also had no trouble learning how to use tampons—I used them right from the beginning. And I hardly ever get cramps. I mean, I feel so lucky about that. Some of my friends really get pretty bad cramps, they even have to miss classes sometimes, but for me my period doesn't affect my life at all.

For other people, it's not so easy. Ruth is sixteen, too, and has the opposite experience from Gini:

I hate my period. I almost always get really bad cramps, and for about a week before it comes I am the biggest bitch and I cry at the drop of a hat. I hate it. I never know when it's coming, and even now, after I've had it for three years, it's so irregular that sometimes I skip a whole month. I know a lot of people who don't have any problems with their period at all, but for me it's the biggest problem of my life.

Connie is a senior from Los Angeles who is on the drill team and exercises all the time. She said:

You know, I thought that I was going to die the first few times I got my period, the cramps were so bad. Even now, even with all the exercise I get, I still have at least a day with such bad cramps that I can't even

Childbirth breathing techniques are very helpful. Lie on your side or sit up with your back supported by pillows. Get as comfortable as you can. Then take a full breath in and blow it all out. Repeat that deep breath. Then begin breathing deeply so that you can see your stomach rise with each breath in and fall as you breathe out. Make sure you blow out all the air very slowly. Keep up that deep stomach breathing for as long as you feel cramps.

You may notice that your cramps come in waves. Their strength rises and falls. Try breathing with the waves.

6. Gently massaging your stomach or your back may help. In childbirth this gentle rubbing is called *effleurage*. It is very relaxing. Someone else can do it for you, or you can do it yourself while you are breathing deeply.

A back rub or whole-body massage will often relieve cramps caused by tension. Apply pressure on your tailbone (coccyx) by hitting or pounding it with your fists or pressing into it with your knuckles or fingers. Work only as hard as is comfortable. You can do this yourself or ask someone else to do it. You can find other kinds of menstrual and general massages in books on yoga, shiatsu, polarity therapy, etc.

7. A hot-water bottle or a heating pad on your stomach or back may help. Also a warm washcloth on your forehead may make you feel better. Some people prefer a cold washcloth. That's up to you.

8. Sometimes curling up in a knee-to-chest posi-tion with a hot-water bottle or heating pad on your back helps. Try to keep yourself relaxed, though.

9. For some women, having an orgasm or being sexually aroused helps to ease the pain and tension and also helps to start the flow of your period.

10. Many women find that aspirin brings fast and complete relief from cramping. Unless you are allergic to aspirin—which is rare—small doses should not cause any serious side effects.

11. Exercising throughout the month and getting enough sleep in the week before your period can relieve your symptoms and will make you feel better in general.

12. Some doctors prescribe the birth control pill to help ease the side effects of menstruation. The birth control pill causes you to stop ovulating, which means your hormone balance of estrogen and progesterone will be more steady. Consequently, some women feel less tension and pain during their periods when they are taking the birth control pill. Also, women on the pill tend to have shorter periods.

We do not recommend the birth control pill for young teenage women, and many doctors don't, either. Since it takes your body about a year, and sometimes more than a year, to get used to the cycle of ovulation and menstruation, it doesn't seem like a good idea to tamper with that process—at least not until it is firmly established. Also, introducing human-made hormones into your system has its own dangers (see pp. 177–82 for a complete discussion of the birth control pill).

go to school. The only thing that helps is if I stay in bed with a heating pad. And I bleed so much I always have to bring another pair of pants with me to change into. I go through everything, even when I wear a Tampax and a napkin both.

Some people, like Connie, suffer from bad cramps and heavy bleeding. Usually the worst cramps last only a day or two, but for these girls these are days each month when their lives are disrupted.

For other women, the week or few days before their period arrives is the most difficult time. They feel tense and depressed. They are even more likely to fall or hurt themselves accidentally. Molly keeps being surprised:

This month it happened again! I was feeling real depressed. I had this terrible fight with my best friend and it looked like we'd never talk to each other again. When I woke up the next morning I just wanted to crawl back down under the covers and never go to school or see anyone. Then the next day I got my period. You'd think I'd remember when I'm feeling bad that my period's due soon. When it comes it doesn't change my situation, but it changes how I'm looking at it. I'd save myself some grief by remembering.

(For Molly, keeping a calendar would help. See p. 33.)

Some people say they appreciate the changes in their moods. "Usually I try to act happy a lot even when things are troubling me," said one woman in her thirties. "So when I get real moody and vulnerable for a few days before my period, it gives me a chance to know the darker part of my feelings."

Sometimes people feel extra good around the time of their period, especially when they are feeling good about themselves that month. There are many different ways you can feel.

Why Side Effects? We don't know as much as we'd like about the side effects of menstruation and why some women seem to suffer more than others.

Not enough medical research has been done on menstruation. You would think something as common as this—something half the world experiences—would have been studied very well. But not much research money is spent on learning about "women's problems." These days more women want to know about their bodies. Since more women are entering the sciences and medical professions, we hope they will look for ways to relieve menstrual problems.

People may try to tell you that your menstrual side effects are "all in your head." For years, for instance, no one knew exactly what caused cramps. Girls would be told they had cramps because they were tense or nervous or because they were thinking about it too hard, or because they didn't "accept their womanhood"—whatever that meant. The girl herself was blamed for having cramps! Those of us who get bad cramps *know* that they are real. It makes

us angry to think of all the girls who curled up in their rooms or stood at their jobs with terrible cramps and thought somehow it was their fault.

What causes cramps and premenstrual tension? While today people agree that there are real physical causes, they don't agree on what the causes are. Three theories have been suggested: 1) Muscle contractions in your uterus and cervix may cause pain and cramping. Your uterus contracts to push out the old lining. It clenches like a fist, especially when there are clots to expel. At the same time, your cervix pulls itself open a tiny bit to let the blood and tissue out. 2) The low level of estrogen and progesterone in your body just before your period causes many of the side effects, including depression. 3) It is possible that hormone-like substances called *prostaglandins,* made by the lining of your uterus, cause your uterus to contract.

Taking Care of Yourself. If you suffer from cramps or weight gain or depression, you can do certain things to make yourself feel better. Women have been passing these hints along and making up new ones for generations. In the box below you'll find a list of ideas, some old as the centuries and some new.

It's important for all of us to remember that we deserve to go through menstrual periods as comfortably as possible. Some of the negative attitudes toward women and women's bodies can subtly make us believe that we deserve to suffer. Nonsense!

Dorie, a twenty-five-year-old woman from Massachusetts, described how she learned to take care of herself:

When I first got my period I was twelve and a half and for the next two or even three years I had very painful periods. I used to get so tense when I felt the cramps that I'd just curl up in a tight ball or run around the room or just cry because I couldn't stand it and I didn't know what else to do. My mother and I found some things that seemed to work to make me feel better. Like first of all, when I learned to stop fighting the cramps and just go with them, just relax and breathe with them, I found they were really not constant pain, but just kind of short waves of pain. When the wave would come, my mother or I would rub my stomach and I'd try to relax. I liked using a hot-water bottle or a heating pad, the heat always made me feel more comfortable. And my mother—she really was pretty terrific—would make me some tea and I'd sip that hot tea and something about that ritual made me feel so much better. Even now when I'm feeling tense or sick, I like to crawl into bed and have a cup of hot tea. It makes me feel taken care of.

What to Use for the Flow. Women in different cultures have used many different ways of soaking up the menstrual flow. Since earliest times, women have made tampons and pads using natural materials like sponges, grasses or bits of cloth. Your great-grandmother may have used rags, which she washed out in cold water each night.

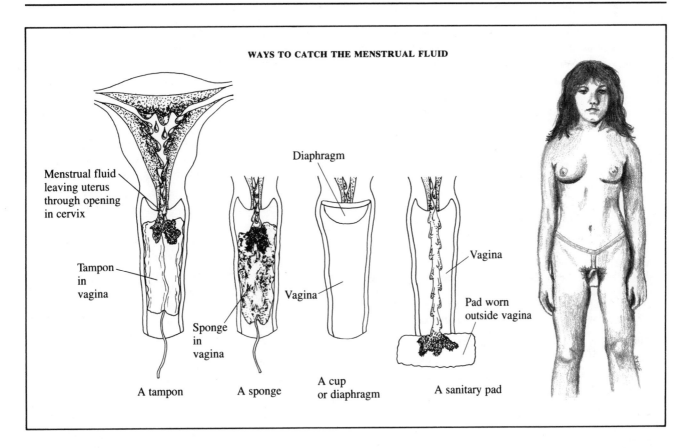

WAYS TO CATCH THE MENSTRUAL FLUID

Menstrual fluid leaving uterus through opening in cervix

Tampon in vagina

Sponge in vagina

Diaphragm

Vagina

A tampon

A sponge

A cup or diaphragm

Vagina

Pad worn outside vagina

A sanitary pad

A woman today in this country has a choice among commercial sanitary napkins and tampons, natural sponges and cups. You might end up trying all of them before you find the one you like using best.

Sanitary napkins. Although you don't have to, most girls start out using *sanitary napkins*. These are rectangular pads of cotton, usually with a plastic lining either between the cotton layers or on the outside. You wear one in your underpants until it is nearly soaked with menstrual flow, then change it for a fresh one.

Sanitary napkins seem bulky at first. Alice said:

When I tried on a pad for the first time I felt like a cowboy—like I was walking bowlegged. I always felt like the pad was slipping out of place and I'd have to slide up against a desk to push it back. I was so self-conscious all day long. I was sure that everybody could tell by the way I walked that I was wearing one.

Actually, no one can tell you have one on—it just feels that way.

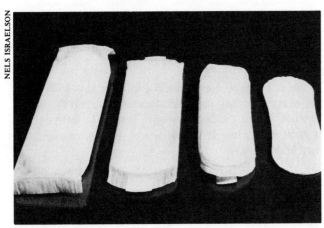

Sanitary napkins come in different sizes and thicknesses.

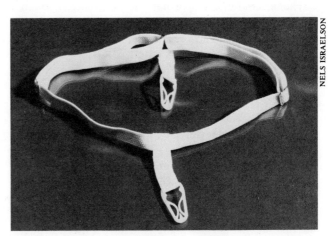

A sanitary belt is worn with some napkins.

When menstrual fluid hits the air outside your body, it dries and can develop a stale odor, so you'll probably want to change your pad several times a day. Some girls feel embarrassed at first when they buy pads or carry around a purse just for their extra pads. A sixth-grader from San Francisco devised a very imaginative way to handle her embarrassment:

What do you do when you have to change your pad at school? That really worried me when I first got my period because nobody at my school carries purses and I always felt kind of obvious carrying a purse around on the days when I had my period. Also it was creepy for me to have to buy pads in the machine in the girls' room, so I worked out this solution. I always wear knee socks under my pants when I have my period. I stick an extra napkin in each sock and then I always have them with me when I go to the bathroom and have to change my pad. It works fine except when the weather gets really hot. Then I swelter. I can't wait until my mom lets me use Tampax.

Tampons. A *tampon* is made of soft cotton pressed together. It fits into your vagina, where it expands as it soaks up the menstrual fluid. You push a tampon in with your fingers or with the applicator that comes with some brands. It has a string that hangs from it outside your vagina; to take it out, you pull the string.

> **As of the day this book went to press, there were reports that using tampons—especially superabsorbent brands—had caused a disease called toxic shock syndrome. The problem seemed particularly to affect women under thirty. While there were few cases, some of them *were fatal*. To be safe, it may be better to use sanitary napkins until more is learned about the situation. Watch for newspaper and TV reports. If you do use tampons, be sure to change them every few hours.**

The material in a tampon holds lots of fluid, so you may not have to change it as often as you would change a pad. On the other hand, if you are flowing heavily, you still may have to change the tampon often or use a pad for extra protection.

Since the tampon sits inside your vagina, it can't be seen, so you don't have to worry about it showing through your clothes. And since no air gets at it, it doesn't have any odor. You can swim more comfortably with a tampon than with a pad.

Each package of tampons comes with directions explaining how to insert them. But even with written directions it's sometimes hard to do it the first few times. Many girls have spent hot, sweaty hours in the bathroom trying to get the first one in. The best thing is to have a friend or mother or sister show you how to put the tampon in. It helps to remember that your vagina angles back and doesn't go straight up.

Some girls worry that the tampon will get lost. But except for the tiny hole in the cervix leading up to your uterus, your vagina doesn't open into the rest of your body. There is *no way* you can push the tampon up too far or lose it in there.

Avoid deodorized tampons and pads. They have chemicals in them that may irritate your tissues. Even with pads, odor can be avoided by changing your pad and by bathing. *We don't need deodorants in our vaginas at any time.* Manufacturers make money by making us think we smell bad.

When you remove a tampon or a sanitary napkin, wrap it up with tissue or toilet paper or newspaper and throw it away in a wastebasket. Do *not* throw it in the toilet. Napkins will definitely clog plumbing, and tampons often do, too.

Sponges. Recently women have rediscovered using natural sponges to absorb menstrual flow. They are cheaper than tampons or pads in the long run, more ecological and less bulky to carry around. Worn inside your vagina like a tampon, the sponge is soft and comfortable and, when damp, takes the shape of your vagina.

Get a piece of natural sponge, and divide it into pieces about the size of a regular tampon. You can also buy sponges ready-made at some health-food stores or feminist stores. Sponges with small holes absorb more than those with large holes.

To use a sponge, tie a piece of strong string or dental floss around it or through one end. Dampen it with water and wring it out, then push it gently into your vagina just as you would a tampon. A sponge holds about as much as a tampon or napkin. When you think the sponge is full, pull the string to remove it. Wash it well in cool water and soap. Before reinserting it, squeeze it in a towel to remove excess water.

When you are finished with your sponges for the month, wash them well and let them dry completely before you wrap them to store them for the next period. When the sponge starts to fall apart, throw it away and get a new one. Don't boil the sponges because that makes them disintegrate faster.

Recent reports have raised questions about the safety of using internal methods to catch menstrual blood. Probably, until more is known, it may be better to use sanitary napkins. If you do use a sponge, change it every few hours.

Menstrual Extraction. Some women involved in a women's self-help health project in this country have designed a way to remove the entire old lining of the uterus in five minutes. The method is called menstrual extraction. The menstrual blood and tissue are pulled out of the uterus by

Many of the premenstrual and menstrual symptoms we've discussed happen to most of us at one time or another. When we lose or gain a lot of weight, when we travel or get sick or worry a lot, our period might be affected. Sometimes it just doesn't come at all, or sometimes it comes early or late. There may be times when we have a very heavy flow and other times when our flow is really light. Our mind and our body work together, so whenever we experience problems or changes, we might also experience irregular menstrual symptoms.

Sometimes, however, our body is signaling us that something is not working right. In that case it is important to have a medical checkup to find out what's going on. Some signs that mean a checkup is in order are:

—a very heavy menstrual flow that lasts more than four or five days;
—severe menstrual cramping or pain that lasts more than three days each month;
—a sudden irregularity in your cycle that isn't due to sickness, travel or weight gain or loss—if suddenly your period doesn't come one month and there's no reasonable explanation;
—bleeding in the middle of your cycle or at any time other than during your period;
—severe cramps at times *other* than when your period is due.

These five symptoms are warning signs that something might be interfering with the normal functioning of your body, and they mean you should see a doctor.

suction. A special flexible tube called a cannula (the same kind of tube used in some abortions) is inserted through the cervix into the uterus. The tube is connected to a bottle and a syringe, and the woman's period is sucked out, all at once, into the bottle. This may cause some cramps, but they are over soon.

Although some women in self-help groups are using this method regularly, it is still only in the experimental stages and its long-range effects are not known. Even if it is not something you would choose to do, we're glad to know that women are exploring new frontiers of relief from menstrual pain.

Some Problems Related to Unusual Symptoms

Pregnancy. If you have been having intercourse or petting heavily (so a boy ejaculates near your vagina) and you miss a period, the first thing to consider is pregnancy. Go to the local clinic or a doctor's office and have a pregnancy test as soon as possible. (See p. 192 for more information.)

Ectopic Pregnancy. If a fertilized egg doesn't implant in your uterus but gets stuck in your fallopian tube and starts growing there, you have a tubal or ectopic pregnancy. When the fetus grows too big, the tube usually bursts. You will probably miss your period as you would with a normal pregnancy, but before the tube bursts you will feel very severe sharp pains in your abdomen, chest or shoulder. Go to a doctor immediately because a burst tube brings internal bleeding and other serious symptoms that can lead to death.

Ectopic pregnancies are not common, but if you have had an infection in your fallopian tubes your chances of having one are greater. Scar tissue may have formed in the tube after the infection, which sometimes blocks the sperm-egg unit from reaching the uterus.

Endometriosis (en-doh-*mee*-tree-o-sis). When the tissue that usually grows in the lining of the uterus begins to grow in other places, such as your vagina, urinary tract or bowel, you have endometriosis. Its symptoms are very painful periods that may last a long time and be quite heavy. Your period may also come more frequently than usual—for example, every twenty-four days or less. Endometriosis is more common among twenty-, thirty- and forty-year-olds than it is among teenagers. Treatment for this disorder varies according to the particular case. If your doctor advises surgery to remove the extra tissue, you may want to check the diagnosis with another physician.

Pelvic Inflammatory Disease (PID). PID is a general name for different infections in the pelvic area, the area around your uterus and vagina. Symptoms of PID are extreme cramping with periods, irregular bleeding, cramps even when you're not having your period, general pelvic pain and sometimes chills and fever. Gonorrhea is a major cause of PID, but other infections cause it as well. Sometimes a PID is a problematic side effect if you use an IUD for birth control. Treatment for PID is a heavy dose of antibiotics, lots of rest, and no sexual intercourse for at least two weeks after you begin treatment. PID can cause scar tissue to form in your fallopian tubes which may result in ectopic pregnancy or infertility (inability to get pregnant). If you develop PID, seek medical help at once.

Fibroids and Other Cysts. Fibroids are growths in the uterus. Cysts and tumors can develop in the ovaries, too. These growths can affect your period by either blocking the flow altogether or causing extra bleeding during your period or at some other time during the month. Usually fibroids don't occur in teenagers, but if they do they are almost always benign (not caused by cancer). However, they should be regularly checked by a doctor. He or she can usually tell if you have fibroids by feeling them in your uterus. Since fibroids usually stay rather small, they don't always cause problems, and some women live with them for years. They usually disappear during menopause. If they get large enough to create pain or heavy or irregular bleeding, they can almost always be removed by surgery without removing your uterus.

Cancer. Cancer is probably the scariest word in the English language. Teenagers get cancer very rarely. Most important, the best chance of cure is early discovery of the disease. So it is crucial to have your symptoms checked out by a medical person as soon as you suspect something may be wrong. (For example, symptoms may be irregular bleeding during the month from your vagina or a breast lump that doesn't go away.) Some cancers affect a small percentage of teens. One type is vaginal cancer, which has been appearing recently in some teenage women whose mothers took a drug called DES (diethylstilbestrol) while they were pregnant with these daughters. DES is a human-made estrogenic hormone now known to be linked to cancer. Doctors gave it to women in the 1940's, 50's and 60's to prevent miscarriage during pregnancy.

If your mother took DES when she was pregnant with you, write to the DES Action Group in New York to get more information about what to do. Their address is: DES Action National, Long Island Jewish-Hillside Medical Center, New Hyde Park, NY 11040.

Be sure to see a doctor for a complete checkup if your mother took DES. Tell the doctor why you're there. Say that your mother may have taken DES and you want to check to make sure everything's all right. The doctor should give you a Pap smear and a thorough pelvic exam, including a close look at your vaginal walls and your cervix, as well as a general checkup.

Also, if you are a DES daughter, both the birth control pill and the "morning after" pill are very risky for you to use because they contain chemicals (estrogen and diethyl-stilbestrol) that increase the risk of cancer.

You may feel nervous or worried when you go to the doctor, so be sure to bring along someone you like and trust. (See p. 156 for a description of the exam you will get, called a pelvic exam.)

II CHANGING RELATIONSHIPS

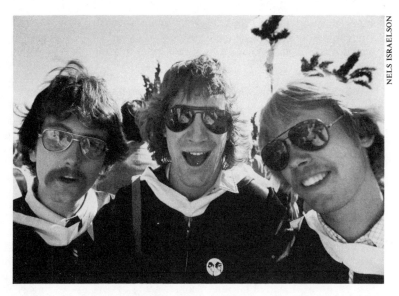

NELS ISRAELSON

It's not just how people look that changes during the teenage years. How we see also changes. It's as if we're wearing a pair of "life" glasses, and as we go through each new stage of growth we change the lenses. What used to look really big suddenly looks a lot smaller. What used to seem like the whole picture now becomes only a part.

Most of the teenagers we interviewed said that one of the biggest changes they notice is in the way they feel about their parents and their friends. In this chapter we'll be talking about those changing relationships.

Parents

The teenage years can be pretty hard on the way parents and children get along together. Although your feelings about your parents and their feelings about you will probably remain strong throughout, they are usually not *only* positive feelings. In fact, there may be times when you feel very definitely unloving toward each other, times when you each feel completely misunderstood or unappreciated, times when you can't even believe how much anger there is between you.

The reason for all these intense feelings is not so hard to understand. It comes from what your relationship is all about in the first place. Parents try to raise children who'll be able to leave them and live independently when they get old enough. But they feel it's their responsibility to take care of and protect their children until they *are* able to live on their own. Children need their parents but they also want to grow up, have more independence, live on their own. The problem for both sides is: when to hold on to each other and how much and when to let go.

During the teen years, the holding-on/letting-go conflict can get so bad that it feels like a game of tug-of-war, with each side pulling harder in response to the other's strength.

As you read this chapter, try to keep in mind the larger picture: that you and your parents are saying good-bye to one sort of relationship with each other—a relationship based on the child's dependence—and you're trying to find a new way of relating that is based on independence. If there is stress between you now, it's probably directly connected to that change. *It's not easy to let go of a familiar routine.*

Separating

By the end of the teenage years lots of teens have moved out of their parents' home, made plans for their own future, and started to earn some or all of their own money—a big change from how they were at the *beginning* of the teen years, not too long before. Steve, a sixteen-year-old from Denver, has mixed feelings about that change. He said:

Some of my friends say that once you're eighteen you're *free* and you can do anything you want. You're out from under your parents' control. But for me . . . I'm going to get out in that world and I'm going to say, "Uh-oh—now what do I do?"

Like Steve, you may not think you're completely ready to go "out in that world yet." Maybe you realize how much you still depend on your parents or the other adults in your life.

If you have doubts or anxieties connected to your increasing independence, you're not alone. Most of the teens we interviewed said they aren't sure they feel equipped yet to take on the full responsibility of adulthood. At the same time they are pretty glad to be making more choices by and for themselves now. Most teens we met said they spend much less time at home now than they did when they were younger. Alexandra, a seventh-grader from Seattle, said:

You start doing more stuff. You're out of the house

more, meeting more people, getting more friends. You can get around by yourself now, so you want to be out more. You don't want to always be with your family.

Some parents of teens wish their children weren't gone so much. Fifteen-year-old Joe, one of the people in a group we interviewed in Los Angeles, told us:

> With me, every time I'm with my friends my mother tells me, "You're never home. You don't care about your family anymore." And it's sort of true, because these days I don't really enjoy doing that much stuff with them. I have other things I want to do.

And Stephanie, a ninth-grader whom we met in Washington, D.C., said:

> Last year I started doing more things on my own. It was exciting—I started meeting people, going to parties, sleeping over at friends' houses, and my mother felt that I wasn't spending enough time with her anymore. She's divorced and I guess she feels lonely, but she makes me feel guilty.

Joe's mother and Stephanie's mother feel neglected. Other parents said they feel that way too. All of a sudden their kids, who were always home before, can hardly be counted on to show up for dinner. Many parents are glad to have a bit more time to themselves or at least one less person around to relate to all the time, but pretty soon they start missing you. They may begin to feel left out of your life.

Barbara, age thirty-nine, a mother of two from Boston, said:

> Suddenly in the last six months I look at my two teenage sons and they're like strangers living in my house. I don't know them at all. I don't even know what they like to eat anymore. One week they're off eggs altogether, the next week one of them's a vegetarian. You could go crazy. And it was just last year we could say, "Oh, let's all do this," or "Let's all go here." And we'd do it and we'd have a wonderful time. But now no one's ever home anymore. I don't know if we'll ever be able to collect the whole family together at the same time in the same place again. There's been a real breaking away and it's sad. It's sad for us as parents anyway.

This mother told us she really is glad to see her children growing up and pleased that her kids are so independent. But it's happening too fast for her. She doesn't feel prepared to let go yet, and many other parents we interviewed feel the same way. George, forty-three, a father of three teenagers, said it this way:

> You make a plan: "OK, two weeks from today we're all going over to Uncle Jerry's for a barbecue. Can everybody come?" And everyone says they can. Then two days before, there's grumbling and bad moods and one of them says, "Oh, but I want to go to the show with Peter," and another says, "Well, I can't go because Sally got me a ticket to the concert," and then even my thirteen-year-old says he can't go because he has a term paper to do. So that's when I put my foot down and say, "No excuses. Everybody's going to the barbecue." And then they all go moping around the house for two days and act like we never let them do anything on their own. Just because we ask them to be a family with us *one* day. One day in maybe a month. Is that asking too much?

Thirteen-year-old Maddy talked about what this feels like from a teenager's point of view:

> My family is *always* doing something together, and they always want me to be with them. It used to be a lot of fun, but now it seems like the only time I'm away from them is when I'm at school. Sometimes I can't stand it anymore, so I'll say to my mom, "I'm going out for a walk." She always wants to know where I'm going, but I'm not going anywhere. I go just to be alone for a while. Or I'll lock myself in my closet with the light on and read or think in the quiet. Nobody knows I'm there, so nobody bugs me.

Most people we met agreed that they have to be able to get away at times. A few said they were beginning to feel they didn't really belong at home anymore at all, but others just wanted some privacy and a feeling of their own separateness.

Your parents may consider you selfish for wanting to be on your own so much, and you may feel guilty about that if you are still living at home and you count on them for support and love. Actually, rather than being selfish, you may have a real need to experience a life of your own, as one boy from New York said:

> When I'm home I'm still my parents' kid. When I'm out in the world, I'm a person.

So if it seems to you that your parents are holding on too tightly, you may feel you have to push them away, shouting "You *never* let me do anything." A lot of the most frustrating arguments that happen during this period have to do with the clash between what teenagers want to do and what their parents want them to do.

A few parents do have a particularly hard time letting go. They want to keep on watching over you, and they want you to continue participating in the family as if nothing were changing in your life. If your parents are like that, try to talk with them about your need to be with friends or alone more. But when you talk to them, don't expect to get anywhere if you do it five minutes before you have to run out the door. Talk to them when you're relaxed and when they're not busy. You'll need time to really listen to each other.

Moods

Many teenagers find themselves going through wild mood swings, from high to low and back again. We discuss this in more detail in the section "Feeling Bad, Feeling Better." Some discussion of it belongs here, too, because your moods usually affect the way you get along with your family.

Since most teenagers live at home, the folks there are usually the ones who catch the worst of the bad moods. If it happens that way at your house, it's actually a funny kind of compliment because it means you feel comfortable enough at home to let out feelings you may have been carrying around all day. Dwayne, a fifteen-year-old from the Midwest, described the scene with his mother when he comes home from school sometimes:

Let's say I have a tough day at school and I walk in and first thing she'll say to me is, "Go walk the dog" or "Take out the garbage." When that's the first thing someone says to you when you walk through the door, you get mad. So I throw my books down, go to my room and slam the door. Then I'll come out and we'll have a big argument over nothing. If my father's there he'll laugh at how stupid it is. If we would just stop for a second and think how stupid it was, we would never have the fight in the first place. It was just that we didn't click when I first walked in.

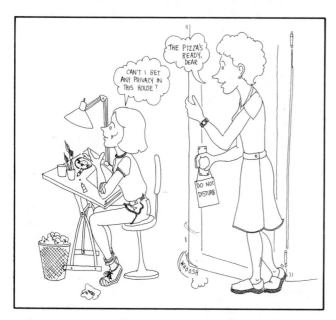

Some people get into a kind of habit, knowing that they can let out their anger at home. It's important to be able to have a release for pent-up emotions, but it isn't fair to let parents—usually mothers—be the object of all the attacks. One mother of a fifteen-year-old girl told us:

I don't know what's going on with Lori these days, but she hasn't said a nice word to me in at least a month. However much I try to understand, still it makes me feel bad. We used to have such an open relationship, and now I feel like I'm her enemy.

Lori's mother doesn't care if Lori's anger is really a compliment in disguise. She wants to feel appreciated again.

In some families, though, everyone seems to understand that blowing off steam at home can be useful, as long as people make up afterward. Cheryl is fourteen. She said:

It's fun to scream and yell at home, like if you've had a really hard day. It's really great to be able to yell at someone and take out your aggressions on them and to know that they won't be hurt because they know you love them.

And thirteen-year-old Jordy had a similar attitude:

Me and my brother got into a really heavy fistfight the other day. We swore at each other too. Then he went outside and I went outside to cool off. And when we looked at each other, we were laughing. We couldn't believe how stupid we were. But the feelings had been bottled up all week because my mom was away on a business trip and usually I fight with her.

Sometimes, just the fact that your family is in a good mood can put you in a bad one. They're being friendly and happy when you may feel grouchy and miserable. Leslie, a sophomore from Ohio, said:

I find it hardest to get along with my parents when they're cheerful. I see my mother at five-thirty when she comes home from work and she's like, "Oh hello, how was your day?" with a big smile. Then she thinks I don't like her if I don't want to talk. But it's not that, it's just that by that point in the day, I've just had it. I just have to be alone.

Since parents are only human, they may not always respond the way you'd like them to when you're in one kind of mood or another. If you are taking out your bad moods on your family day after day, someone is bound to want to know why you're acting that way. They may do it by yelling at you to stop looking as if you hate the world, or they may be very kind and understanding and ask you if something's wrong. Either way, some teenagers take offense and feel that it's none of their family's business, but in the long run it usually does help to talk about what's bothering you.

Your Own Style

During the teenage years your looks change, your interests change, and your image of yourself changes too. You have a chance to start shaping a style that will be yours in the years to come. You may try out many different roles, costumes, accents, attitudes before you settle on what expresses the *you* you like best and are most comfortable with.

Lots of people use their appearance to make a statement about themselves. Whether you spend hours in front of the mirror adjusting and studying how you look, whether you dye your hair fuchsia, go barefoot to your brother's wedding or polish your shoes every day, your appearance says something about you to other people.

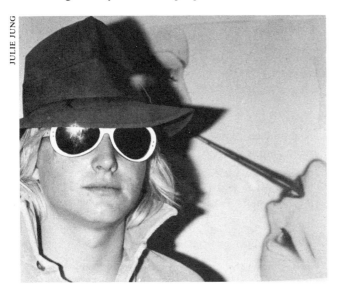

JULIE JUNG

Often *your* idea of who you are and how you want to look is quite different from your parents' idea of who their child is and how he or she *should* look. Simple things, like whether you've taken a bath or worn a bra or changed your shirt can take on huge significance now. You and your parents may end up battling with each other over things like the rip in your jeans, the length of your hair, the amount of makeup you have on. Allen, a fifteen-year-old from Denver, told us:

My parents are always bugging me that my hair's too long. Every time I walk into the house my mom tells me I need a haircut. And if we go anywhere, they're always complaining about how I look—my pants are too sloppy, my hands aren't clean, my face is breaking out. I swear they spend every minute telling me what's wrong with me. So I just say, ''Sure, Mom, right, Mom,'' and go up to my room and close the door.

Allen closes out his parents' comments because he doesn't want to change his appearance—which is his statement about who he is—and the criticism makes him feel bad. Other teens said the same thing. Cheryl-Ann, a fourteen-year-old from Connecticut:

My little sister needs a bra, but my mom keeps saying, ''You don't need a bra yet.'' It embarrasses Amy—like she's not old enough to wear a bra. It wouldn't hurt my mom to let her get one. And I want to grow my nails long, but my mom makes me cut them. She makes me cut them even though I say, ''It's not fair, they're *my* nails.'' It's like her saying

I'm into my urban existential cowboy act tonight. I'd donned my denims, boots and leather-collar up, of course. I'm the fucking Marlboro man. I take the steps two at a time, clicking my heels on the last step. Dancing my way through life? Naw, not enough tension there: you can't be too slick, and I ain't flashing. I stop, reach down under my coat into my sweatshirt pocket, snag the open flip top of my Kools—''The Kool Box. Flip open extra coolness''—and pull out a smoke. Sweatshirts are handy things. So are turtlenecks, it's on account of ''the feel like.'' You say something, no response and everyone looks around checking out the reception and then the eyes once again focus on you. Another few seconds go by till someone lifts their forefinger to their forehead (pointing up), lowers their head and looks for redemption. You do as instructed, if you got a turtleneck and I don't. I stopped playing Iliya Kuriackin long ago, you buried your head in it. If you got a sweatshirt, you flip the hood around and stick your face in it. If you have neither, you can improvise. Jimbo did a doubleflip and tuck and roll into a coffee pot at I.H.O.P., once. I don't worry. I feel like the cock of the walk taking my cock for a walk. It ain't strapped to my ankle tonight. Back at the ranch . . . I take out two Ohio blue-tip matches: one I light my cigarette with, the other I jam between my jaws, flipping it up and down between hauls. I step out into the street (sidewalks are for old ladies and their dogs). Full moon out—getting all disturbed tonight, as Cuckoo Caruso would say. Walking uptown down Beacon, I'm a panoramic anti-hero. Walking slowly, strutting strong—shit, I'm so slick I slide when I walk. It's early, around seven, no one's at the 825 so I go in Brighams. Looking around, I don't see anyone I know: eyes bold, I look from person to person, checking them out and then discarding them. They look in turn, maybe I'm not subtle enough but would they rather have me clog in, with an expectant look on my face that turns to a frown accompanied by raised eyebrows, my look saying ''Duh, which way did he go, which way did he go?'' I walk back down to the sub shop. A lady, sitting in the passenger seat of a Cadillac locks her door. I go up to the window and say ''Don't worry, lady, we only come out at night.'' I laugh and trip into the sub shop. Dickie says, ''Hey, whaz happenin? You want anything, or you killing time?'' ''Killing time,'' I answer over my shoulder as I stroll over to the jukebox, slap a dime in to play ''Born to Run.'' I'm in the mood for a horror show—maybe I can get my hands on Ed's madman machine and go a little dovial.

—Jamie MacDonald
Age 16

to me, "I'm going to cut your hair whether you like it or not." It's my hair and I should be able to wear it any way I want to. And they're my nails. I want long nails to make my hands look better, not to look hotsy-totsy. I wish she would let me grow them, but if I go against her she punishes me.

Cheryl-Ann said she doesn't think her mother is willing to let her or her sister grow up. Seventeen-year-old Susan remembered:

When I started junior high my mom always wanted me to wear these little Alice-in-Wonderland dresses to school. I couldn't believe it. Everyone is wearing jeans and I'm supposed to wear little dresses.

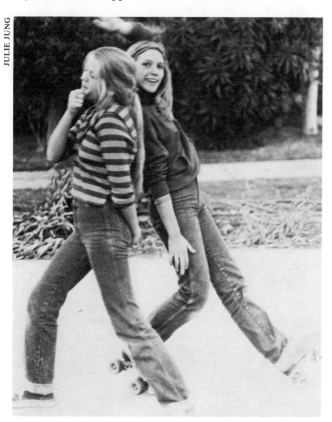

Sisters and brothers may get into the act too. Eighteen-year-old Carolyn told us what happened when she came back home after her first semester at college:

I'm not in the house more than a half hour and my sister says, "How come you're talking so funny? What are you trying to prove?" I didn't know what she was talking about. I didn't think I was talking funny at all. "That's how I always talk," I told her. Then she starts laughing at me. And my father looks at me and says, "Don't *you* look like Miss Collegiate." I had these special kind of socks on and tennis shoes and I was wearing a college sweatshirt. So big deal. I couldn't understand why they all had to start picking on me. It was like I was a stranger in my own house.

Being "examined" this way can be annoying, but it may be a sign that your changing style means something important to your family. They may see it as an indication that you aren't a little child anymore, and that can be a worry to them because it means the family's changing.

Some parents may have a hard time adjusting to the fact that they are no longer in charge of how you look. When you were little they probably dressed you and picked out your clothes. Now they have no say over what you wear except in the comments and/or criticisms they make. Suddenly, the way you look is not their responsibility anymore, and although they may welcome not having to take you for a haircut or to buy shoes now, it is a change they have to get used to.

A mother we talked with in a suburb outside Boston had a different reason. She said:

When we go somewhere with Richie, I think it's rude if he doesn't wear clean pants or comb his hair. I know he doesn't care about those things, but *I* do. It's showing he doesn't respect me or my friends when he goes out looking like a slob.

Richie's mother considers a neat appearance a sign of respect, and she consequently feels ashamed when he shows up looking messy by her standards. She cares about her own appearance and she wants him to care about his, since as far as she's concerned, he's almost a *part* of her.

LEMON

They try to tell me I'm not what I think.
They dye me and feed me full of their things.
Conform me.

I am myself.
I am fresh and sunny.
Me.

They take me and reap me. Stamp me.

Sun Kissed.

They use my juice. Squeeze my life out of me.
They take my scent to clean dishes and make hands softer.
They use my seeds to grow more.
They throw away my skin, my shell. Nothing left.

I want to peel my skin off and show you the sun!

Well damn you. Yes you
I want you to see me.
You don't know me.
Don't say I'm fake.
I'm not unreal.
I am me!

—Amy C. Rosen

Like many parents, she sees her child as a reflection of herself. When you stop to think about it, Richie's appearance may be his way of telling his mother, "Look, I'm me. I'm not part of you."

Of course, not all parents make an issue of what their children wear. Many parents seem perfectly satisfied if you're warm enough and wearing something on your feet—"It's cold tonight, shouldn't you bring a sweater along?" or "Put some shoes on your feet, do you want to catch pneumonia?"

He told me that I was pretty
　　My mother told me I smell like some chemical.
He told me that we will run away together
　　My mother told me I better clean up my room.
He told me, "You are my ultimate friend."
　　My mother told me, "Get off the phone."
Then he suddenly disappeared
　　And that's when my mother, smelling of warm milk, told me that I was beautiful.

　　　　　　　　　　　　　　　　　　　　—Anonymous

But if your parents really do care about your appearance, and you and they are always getting into arguments over it, you might try asking yourself why it's important to *you* to keep irking them that way. Like Richie, you may be telling your folks something about how your values are different from theirs. Perhaps you feel totally misunderstood when they criticize your hairstyle or choice of clothes. You may take it as a sign that they don't respect *you*. Here your parents are saying that you ought to show more respect for them by dressing in what they consider an appropriate manner, and you're feeling that they're not respecting you by asking you to do that. These are the kinds of missed communications that seem to happen a lot during the teen years and usually leave everyone upset. If you and your folks can talk about what's happening, that might clear the air of some of the bad feelings.

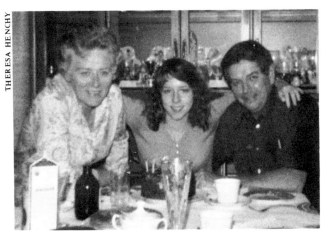

THERESA HENCHY

Looking Older

Once your body develops and you get bigger and more grown-up-looking, your parents can't help realizing that you're not a child anymore. One father of two teenage daughters said:

I watch my daughters grow and I think, This is beautiful. It's exciting to see children turn into adults. That's when I see it objectively. But when I look at them and see *my little girls,* when I say to myself, "Those are my children and they're becoming adults and they're going to have to deal with that outside world without me along to protect them," *that's* when I get emotional. They're beautiful and they're sexy. My daughters are sexy young women and I worry for them. This world is rough and they could get hurt and I know there's nothing I can do about it except teach them good values and hope they make good choices.

You're not just getting bigger, you're also getting "sexier." Can you imagine how complicated it is for your parents to watch that happening?

It is pretty common for parents to have mixed feelings about their children's sexuality. After all, in our society sex is a complicated subject. It's considered part of the "adult" world. In some ways, because your body is becoming sexual, you are stepping into your parents' world—whether you want to or not, and whether they're ready to let you or not. They can see, and you can probably sense, that you *are* a sexual person. And that means they have to think of you in a new way.

This mother of four said:

With my son it affected me very strongly. I think when he became really physically grown it made me feel strange to think that he would be going out with girls and sleeping with girls someday. With my daughters it didn't affect me so much, maybe because I'm a woman.

Another mother said:

My daughter's body changes were more obvious. We could watch her developing gradually. But a male changes in subtle ways and you don't always get to see the gradual development. I remember the first time we saw our son with pubic hair. My husband's reaction was, "Oh my God, when did that happen?" You see that and you feel it's not your little boy any longer.

Around this time even families who used to walk around naked in front of each other may start covering up. If there is a kind of shyness between you and your parents now, it's very understandable. Your body is different and you need a chance to get comfortable with it.

As you become more sexual, you may see your parents in a new way too. Some teens feel funny about that. They think they shouldn't notice their parents' sexuality. But remember, adults *are* sexual, and it's perfectly natural to notice that about each other.

A few preteens and teens, who see that their parents are having an especially difficult time accepting their children's body changes, try to protect their parents and themselves by attempting to hide their development. Some teenagers will start overeating to the point where the extra fat on their body covers up any sexual growth. Other teens will stop eating almost completely. They lose so much weight that normal body functions—such as menstrual periods in girls—cease, and their bodies look small again, like little children's bodies. Often these reactions occur without anyone, including the teenager, understanding what's causing them. Some of the teens who stop eating think they are just going on a diet because they feel "too fat."

If you or your parents are having a hard time accepting your body changes, help yourselves by talking over your concerns with a competent person who has experience dealing with this kind of issue. If you can put your feelings into words, it may be easier on your body. Remember, our bodies were intended to change and become sexual. It happens to everyone, and it can bring you a lot of pleasure.

Unfortunately, you can't control how other people react to your changing body. If your parents or other members of your family seem to be taking more notice of your sexuality than you'd like, or if they are acting sexual with you in ways that make you uncomfortable or just plain scared, find someone to help you. There may be another family member you can talk to.

Mentioning this will undoubtedly be shocking to some of you, but sexual abuse in families does exist, and it is far more common than people in our society have been willing to admit. There's more on this in Chapter V. Also, look in the "Emotional Health Care" chapter for suggestions on how to find a counselor or therapist for professional help.

Parents' Concern: Is My Child Normal?

There's a very wide range to what's "normal," so in fact the word doesn't mean much. What most parents are concerned about is whether or not their child's development is happening the way they think it should be happening. That's because most parents don't want their kids to have a hard time growing up.

Unfortunately, some parents go overboard, worrying about your size, your shape, your maturity or lack of same. If your folks are like that, it may seem to you that they aren't aware that there's no such thing as a perfect human being. Their concern about you may make you feel that you *should* be different from the way you are—in other words, perfect.

Most parents try to keep their worry about your development to themselves, but very often you can sense it in something they say or the way they look at you. Some people learn to laugh at it. Others let it get to them, and that usually makes them anxious too. Liz, an eighteen-year-old from Oregon, found that she was able to laugh at her father's anxiety:

I developed physically kind of slow. I looked about two years younger than I was up until I was about sixteen. And my dad kept worrying that I was worried that something was wrong. He would say, "Now, if you want to go to the doctor to see if everything is all right, I'll take you." Finally I brought him this book that said what the normal ages for a girl's development are, and it said that if you were a little slower in growing it didn't mean anything was wrong. So he read it, and after he read it we both started cracking up because we both knew it was *him* who had been worrying all along.

But Lewis, a sixteen-year-old from Los Angeles, said his parents are making him upset:

My dad and my brother are both over six feet tall and I'm only five-five at age sixteen. They keep telling me, "Oh, don't worry, there's still plenty of time for you to grow," but the more they talk about it, the more it feels like they couldn't stand it if I didn't grow. I'm getting pretty disgusted with the whole thing. I mean I am who I am, and if I take after my mother's family, maybe I won't grow much more. They make me feel like there's something wrong with being short.

Comments on your development or comparisons with your sisters and brothers can be very hurtful. Tell your parents they're making you feel bad by saying things like that if they are. They may not be aware of how insensitive they're being.

Some of the teenagers we interviewed have special problems that affect their lives. They have physical disabilities, and they told us how important it is to them to be accepted for who they are. Lois, a sixteen-year-old from New York, was born with a spine problem. She said:

My mother and I have such a hard time communicating. She's not affectionate with me at all—I guess because I'm disabled. She makes me feel like there's really something wrong with me. Like she says I shouldn't be interested in sex because I'm handicapped and will probably never get married. That drives me crazy. I say, "Well, how do you know? You don't know *me*. You're not inside *me*. You don't know what I feel." I keep saying to her, "Don't put me down. I'm just like everyone else. I have the same feelings as everyone else. The only difference is I have to walk with leg braces."

And fifteen-year-old Paul, who's spent most of his life in a wheelchair, told us:

> My mom just can't deal with my handicap because she blames herself for it. But I don't think she should. I don't blame anybody for it. It was something that happened. I just want her to be able to accept me as a person. I mean, I do have limitations and I can't do certain things, but disabled people always try to find a way to get around those things. I would rather that she treat me the same way she treats my brother than to keep treating me like there's something wrong with me.

We all want to feel we're OK, especially in our parents' eyes. But some parental concern is justified. A mother from New York told us:

> A kid I know had a degenerative spine problem that only turned up in his teenage years. At first his parents kept nagging him to stand up straight, but pretty soon they began to realize that their son needed medical attention. Without their concern, the boy would never have gotten himself to the doctor.

Parents worry about your social life too. They have their own ideas about what's OK for a person your age to be doing. Their expectations come from their own upbringing, the values they hold, the opinions of the community, and their concern for your health and emotional well-being.

Many of the teens we interviewed said they feel their parents are *expecting* them to be different from the way they are. A thirteen-year-old boy from New England said:

> Every time I get off the phone my mom wants to know if I was talking to a girl. Or if a girl calls, my mom says, "Peter, it's a girrrrrrrrl for you. Anything serious?" She makes me feel like I'm not normal if I'm not always wanting to go out with girls.

And Patty, who just turned fifteen, said:

> My parents are worried because I don't go out yet. I mean I go places with my friends, but I don't date or go to parties. And I don't have a boy that I like. They make me feel like there's something wrong with me, like I'm turning into this prize wallflower or something.

These teenagers are saying they want their parents to be able to love them and feel good about them no matter what's going on in their lives. When you stop to think about it, that's what we *all* want: to be accepted for who we are without anxiety or disappointment.

Seeing Your Parents as People

We've talked so far about how your parents are seeing you differently, but during these years most teenagers start seeing their parents differently too. Many of the people we interviewed said they've begun to realize that their parents

are people: ordinary people with faults and weaknesses and insecurities and problems just like everyone else. Some children learn this about their parents early on—especially children who've been mistreated or abused. Some of these children grow up knowing that they can't always count on their parents.

But if you've grown up thinking of your folks as shining examples of perfection—or at least the ultimate authorities on most of the world's problems—seeing them as regular people can come as a shock or a disappointment. In Ohio, Melissa, a sixteen-year-old who was working in one of the clinics we visited, told us:

> You know, I've been noticing lately that when my mom and my grandmother fight with each other they sound like a bunch of babies. I can't understand why they can't just talk about what's on their mind. My sister and I act more mature than they do most of the time.

Fifteen-year-old Bernie said:

> My parents are always picking on each other. Always arguing. It seems so stupid. I don't see how they can stand it.

As little children you may have accepted the fights between your parents or their funny habits or their style of doing things as just the way life was. As you get older you have more exposure to the world. You meet other people who do things differently and begin to have a broader picture from which to develop your values.

Once you start forming your own values you may find yourself criticizing your parents all the time for the things about them that aren't up to *your* standards. Several teens we interviewed told us they get embarrassed by the way their parents talk or dress or act. Fourteen-year-old Geri was part of a group we met in Denver. She said:

> My mother doesn't know how to act. She came to this meeting at my school, and she was bossier and talked louder than everyone else there. It embarrassed me so much I tried to pretend she wasn't my mother.

Everyone is tempted in one situation or another to pretend that their parents aren't really their parents. It's a hard feeling to live with while it's happening. Your own parents may have felt that way about their parents when they were your age. Ask them.

Maurice, a sixteen-year-old from Los Angeles, brought up another area of conflict that can occur as you begin to look at your parents as people:

> I like going to church every week and I get so mad at my parents for not going. They're such hypocrites. They're always talking about people who don't have a religion, but then they only go to church on the big holidays and that's all. My dad has his golf game on Sunday morning and nothing can interfere with that!

You too may feel your parents aren't giving an all-out effort to support the values they say they believe in—whether it's religion, politics, honesty or simple human kindness. Like Maurice, you may think they're acting like hypocrites, and you may feel like telling them they're setting a bad example.

On the other hand, you may think your parents are devoting themselves to the *wrong* values altogether. If you try to convince them of that, and lots of teens do, you and your parents may end up fighting over whose ideas are right. Huge political arguments take place in some families. Violent disagreements occur over whether there should or shouldn't be a draft, whether we should or shouldn't go to war, whether the Equal Rights Amendment should be passed, whether homosexuals should be discriminated against.

Occasionally you may find that you disagree so strongly with your parents' views that you go against their wishes openly. Fifteen-year-old Barry did that. We met him during the summer when he was staying with his grandparents on Cape Cod, in Massachusetts. He said:

I'm having a really hard time with my parents. I even had to leave this summer to get away from them, because we keep having these fights over whether I should be allowed to visit my mother's parents. My folks don't talk to them, and they want to keep us kids from seeing them because I think my folks want to punish her parents for something that happened before I was even born. Well, I think that stinks. I think it's really childish and selfish on my parents' part to do that, and now I feel like I'm old enough to do something about it. That's why I decided to come here this summer to be with my grandparents even though my parents were dead set against it. I worked during the year to save the money for this trip.

Sixteen-year-old Ruthie gave us another example:

My parents are so conservative it drives me crazy. They believe that everything the government does and says is right, like they think the oil companies have a right to their profits, and they're in favor of nuclear power. I can't even talk to them without screaming. But our worst fight was last summer when I was part of this demonstration at this nuclear energy plant and I got arrested, and they wouldn't even post bail for me. I had to stay in jail until strangers gave enough money to bail us all out. And then when I got home they wouldn't talk to me for about a week.

Ruthie and her parents may never work through their political differences, but in the years to come they may choose to relate in other areas and just leave politics alone. In a few families disagreements over values and beliefs lead to permanent splits between parents and children. In other families parents and teenagers learn to respect each other's views and accept the fact that each of them is entitled to have differing stands.

Some parents have serious problems. People don't automatically become grown-up just because they turn thirty or forty or fifty. They don't lose their selfishness or childishness or fear of the world just because the size and shape of their body has changed. You may find that your parents are acting in ways that you just can't accept. For example, if they have a drinking problem or a drug problem, it can cause you a lot of pain and heartache. If your parents mistreat you or someone else in the family, you may even feel like standing up to them physically and defending yourself or the abused person. Several teens we interviewed said that they've felt like hitting their parents at times, and a few have in fact gotten into fistfights with their mom or dad. But there are *always* better ways to let people know what you're feeling than by hitting them. While physical violence may give some immediate relief to tension, it does nothing actually to solve the problem that caused the fight in the first place. Yet nineteen-year-old Phillip told us he didn't know what else to do:

When my dad gets drunk he gets out of hand. He starts beating us up or pushing my mom around and I can't stand it. I caught him punching my little brother a couple of weeks ago, and I broke it up by giving him some of his own medicine. I had to move out of the house for a while, until he settled down again.

It is a terrible situation when it comes to violence like this between parents and children. If it does exist in your family, it is not a violation of family privacy to seek help. You can comfort your parents by giving them as much love as you can, but you must realize that *you can't solve their problems, nor are you the cause of their problems*. The seeds of their personal conflicts were probably planted during their own childhood and they need professional or peer-group help now to change their behavior. Some services that are available are Alcoholics Anonymous (in the phone book) and Parents Anonymous. Parents Anonymous is a self-help group for parents who abuse their children. There are chapters in many of the larger cities. Look in the phone book.

As a teenager, seeing your parents' imperfections can be a shaky experience. If you have always depended on them for your security, when you see that they have some problems it may make you feel insecure. If you've always based your view of the world on their model, seeing that they aren't always right may make you start questioning everything. For a while you may feel that the rug's been pulled out from under you. Rosie is a sixteen-year-old from Detroit who said:

When your parents are having problems you just have to learn to depend on yourself. Like my mom and dad are always fighting and sometimes I think they take it out on me. So I don't go by what they say anymore. They each say something totally different, and if I listened it would drive me crazy. You just have to go by what you feel down deep inside yourself. When you don't have anybody to turn to, you just have to depend on yourself.

Many people feel the way Rosie does, that when you're going through a hard time you can only depend on yourself. But at those times, most of us benefit from sharing some of our troubles with a friend or relative, someone who really cares about how we're feeling.

Parents Go Through Changes Too

In many families, parents see their teenagers becoming young adults and they start worrying that *their* life is slipping away from them. They watch you growing and it makes them feel *old*. They see your strong young body and suddenly their wrinkles look wrinklier and their sags look saggier.

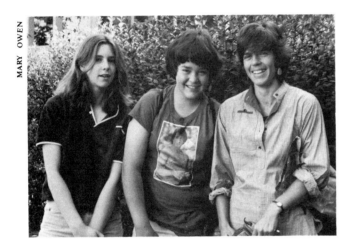

MARY OWEN

When people become parents they don't stop growing and developing. They go through changes over the years just the way children do. One of the stages many adults experience is called a mid-life crisis. It's a time when many adults look at themselves and their lives and say, "I'd better start doing some of the things I've always wanted to do before it's too late."

One thirty-nine-year-old mother of three told us:

I'm ready for a giant change because a little change just won't do it for me. My kids are getting ready to leave home soon and I want to sell the house and do something crazy, like go around Europe for a year, or move back into the city and get a job or go back to school. I'm not willing to wait till I get cancer or until somebody dies, or until Peter and I get divorced. I know those kinds of tragedies make people change their lives, but I want to do the things I want to do *now*. Not wait until something forces me into it. At least now we still can enjoy ourselves.

Some people change careers at this time. Others get separated or divorced. Most people don't go to such extremes,

but they may start reexamining things they've taken for granted up till now. Some married couples begin to argue more about issues that may seem silly to their children. Men and women both may start dieting or exercising or redoing their wardrobes. A few couples decide to have another baby.

This crisis often happens between the late thirties and early fifties—just the time when many people's children are in the teen years. So while you're off experimenting and having adventures, your parents may decide it's time for them to do the same. Some parents take a second honeymoon and feel satisfied with that. Other parents start acting very differently from the way they used to act, and that can be upsetting to the family.

We met seventeen-year-old Gordon in Wisconsin. He told us:

Everything was going along like usual and then all of a sudden my dad started doing crazy things—like staying out real late, not telling my mom where he was, showing up late for work or not showing up at all. My parents were arguing a lot and he would get real defensive, so it just kept building up and up. I could see it but I didn't want to say anything. I knew something was going on. I was expecting something. And pretty soon my dad came to me and said, "Well you know me and your mom are having problems and I think I'm going to have to leave." And we both started crying. It was a heavy scene. My little sister, who's only eight, didn't really know what was going on. I didn't want to cry, I was trying not to cry, but I couldn't help it. Finally after a couple of months my mom and dad started talking about it and they went to see a man who helped them sort it out. And it seems like it helped them because they're back together now and my dad's living at home again. It's not exactly the same as it was before, but they both seem OK.

And in San Francisco, seventeen-year-old Wendy said:

My mom's just starting her career now. She's going to become a legal assistant and she's going back to school and all, but she's saying "Now I'm first, you kids come second now." She says, "All these years you kids have been able to do what you've wanted—well, now I'm coming first for a while. Now I need you to watch the little ones while I go back to school. Now I need you to take care of the house." And I say, "Gee, Mom, that's great for you, but where am I supposed to come from now? I mean, what about the job I wanted to get and the money I wanted to save for college?" She really came on strong and I could understand, but I thought, This isn't fair. This isn't like my mom.

If your family is going through serious changes—for example, if your parents are getting separated or divorced, if a parent loses his or her job or changes careers, or if someone gets very sick—the children who are still living at home may feel disoriented, as if there's nowhere for them to turn. That's the time when talking to a school counselor, a favorite teacher, a person at church or temple, or a close friend of the family can really help.

Often people feel that no one will understand or that others will judge or criticize their families, so they keep their personal problems to themselves. One thing to remember is that whatever is happening in your family has probably happened in many other families too. You're not alone.

Discipline

With all the changes that take place during the teenage years, the old rules about discipline may no longer apply. You're older and more capable than you were a few years ago, and your parents can't watch you twenty-four hours a day even if they wanted to. You have to be responsible for yourself a lot of the time.

You may even be bigger and stronger than your parents now. Imagine how it feels trying to discipline someone who's six feet tall if you're a mother who's only five-foot three. Fifteen-year-old Jeffrey said he and his mother ended up laughing over that one day:

You know, when your parents get mad at you now it's different. I'm about five inches taller than my mom now, so it's a joke when she yells at me. Once she got real mad and tried to hit me, but I blocked her hand and we both looked at each other and cracked up because it was so weird.

Even if you don't tower over your parents you are still beginning to look more like an adult than a child, so discipline almost necessarily has to be approached in a new way. It's pretty likely you aren't going to be spanked anymore.

In most families teens get grounded or lose some privileges when discipline is called for. And many teenagers pointed out to us, if you're still living under your parents' roof, you have to follow their rules or expect to pay the consequences.

Todd, a seventeen-year-old senior from Rhode Island, said:

I'm independent and I like to come and go as I please but it's hard because you got to listen to what your parents say and even though they're pretty lenient— like they tell me I can come home around one or two in the morning sometimes—I still have to be home when they say. They have certain rules for the younger kids, and when I'm home I have to go by the rules too, whether I think they're right or not. And also I have to set an example for the younger ones.

Now that you're older and have opinions of your own, you may not always agree with your parents' rules. When that happens, if you and your parents can talk openly with each other, you may be able to figure out ways to compromise and redesign the rules.

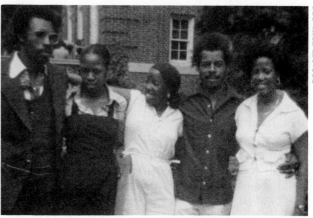

ROSALIE EDWARDS

Jane is an eighth-grader from Boston who has been helping us work on this book for the past two years. She said:

I'm beginning to see that I think differently than my parents do sometimes. I was talking to my mom and I told her about this party that was either going to be at this boy's house or at a teenage night club in the city. I asked my mom if she'd let me go if it was at the club and she said no, because she knew that club had a pretty bad reputation with drugs and make-out rooms and stuff like that. Well, I had sort of heard those things too, so I wasn't too interested in going there anyway, but I told her that if I knew that it was a safe place to go, I would want to go anyway because now I feel like I'm old enough to have good judgment about things like that.

Fifteen-year-old Patrick, of Philadelphia, told us:

When I turned fourteen my parents seemed to start to trust me more. They started letting me make some of my own decisions, have my own opinions about things. I was undecided about whether to go to a particular school or stay at my old one, and my mother said, ''Well, that's up to you, you have to make your own decisions about those things because it's your life.'' In the past she and my father probably would have told me what to do.

Darlene, a sophomore from Chicago, said:

My mother told me I couldn't go with a guy in a car until I was in my senior year of high school. I argued with her about that, but in a nice way. We ended up compromising and she said I could ride with someone as long as she knew who the person was. So now whenever I go out on a date my mother invites the guy in and sits and talks to him for a while. At first it embarrassed me, but then I started liking it because it calmed a couple of those guys down and we ended up having a nice time together instead of just being wild.

When parents are willing to bend a little to accept some parts of your life that they may not completely approve of, and when you're willing to bend enough to listen to their reasons for wanting to restrict you from doing certain things, then there's a chance to grow and separate without feeling that you have to lie or sneak out or rebel against them just for the sake of it.

Yet no matter how well you and your parents are able to work things out between you, there are bound to be some points on which you can't reach a compromise. You are probably ready to think of yourself as grown-up and capable of handling yourself in the world before your parents think you are ready. There's often a long period of time during which you struggle with each other about who knows best. You may feel that your parents aren't giving you enough credit. Elizabeth said:

> One minute my mother treats me like I'm old enough to do this, this, and this—like help her out at home by doing the marketing or making dinner or baby-sitting for my brother. And she's always telling me, "You're thirteen years old now, you should know better than that!" But then the next minute, when there's something I really want to do, like there's a party that everyone's going to, she'll say, "You're too young to do that."

And fourteen-year-old Timothy said:

> Physically I matured much faster than my friends— and emotionally I feel older too, and that causes a lot of problems between me and my parents. They're always saying to me, "Stop going out with people so much older than you. Why don't you hang around some kids your own age?" They still see me and treat me as if I were a child and I resent that because it's not who I am.

If you think of yourself as more mature than your parents do, they may worry a great deal about whether you'll be able to take care of yourself and make decisions that protect your health and your future. Maybe because of their concern they are very strict about some things.

Betsey lives in Miami, where she said lots of kids go to parties on the weekends. She said:

> When I got into eighth grade I started going out to parties with my friends and that's when my parents started setting curfews for me. I felt that was really unfair because I was always the one who had to come home first. My parents are European and they have strict rules. They just couldn't understand that it would be OK for me to stay out past midnight. That was embarrassing for me and it made me really mad at my parents.

Parents feel it is their responsibility to you to set some limits for you. When we interviewed Betsey's parents they said they wanted to make sure that she was home safe before they went to bed at night. They said when she gets older they will relax the curfew, but they think midnight is late enough for a fourteen-year-old. Betsey thinks it's unfair; her parents think it's just showing that they care about her.

Sex

Many parents feel they have to take a firm stand on the subject of sex. Fourteen-year-old Rebecca, an eighth-grader from Massachusetts, told us that once her parents found out she had a steady boyfriend, they became very strict. She said:

> I can't talk to them anymore. If I told them what me and my boyfriend do they'd tell me I couldn't see him anymore. I know my parents. My mom says to me, "You're too young to have a boyfriend." She treats me like I'm so young. She thinks I'm so innocent.

Parents are concerned about sex for many reasons. In the first place, most parents want to protect their children from the traumatic experience of an unwanted pregnancy or the dangerous complications that can come from sexually transmitted diseases. These are serious issues that many teens don't think about when they start having sexual relations. Parents would do their children a favor by telling

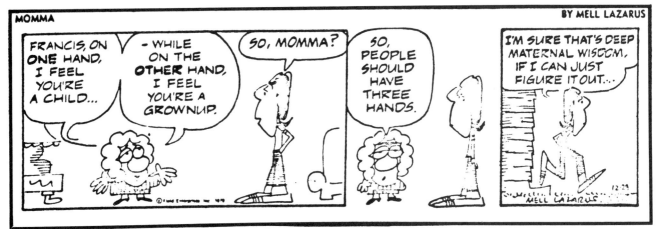

Thanks to Mell Lazarus and the Field Newspaper Syndicate

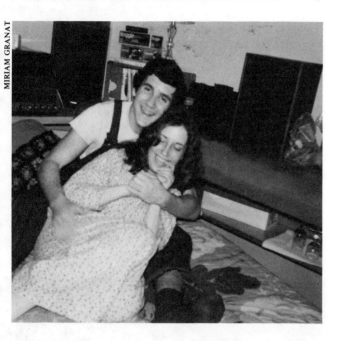

MIRIAM GRANAT

them about birth control methods and teaching them how to prevent VD. The information starting on p. 216 may help open that dialogue between parents and teenagers.

Parents also know that sexual relationships can have emotional as well as physical consequences. They don't want you getting hurt before you have enough self-confidence to be able to handle it. Corrine, a fifteen-year-old from Minnesota, told us:

> My mom will say, "Well, I don't expect you to be a virgin till you get married," since she knows I don't expect to get married until I'm in my late twenties. But she also says, "I do expect you to wait until you feel that you can handle it, until you feel responsible, until you're on your own, taking care of yourself." She doesn't think I could handle it until I'm out of school, and she's probably right.

Corinne and her mother have talked about sex openly with each other. Corinne thinks that's helped her to have a more responsible attitude about what she wants for herself. Sixteen-year-old Tom said the same about his parents:

> If I was going with someone for a long time and we were getting into some heavy sex, I'd want to talk to my folks about that. They're very understanding. After all, they went through the same thing. They wouldn't try to tell me what to do. But they also wouldn't say, "Hey, man, go ahead and do what you want." They would probably tell me to think about the consequences. They trust me.

Fourteen-year-old Brenda told us she wishes her parents *would* talk to her about sex, but instead they just tell her not to do it. She said:

> The most important thing to me is that I know my parents love me and respect me. But they just can't

accept the fact that I'm growing up and I have a boyfriend. Now I never, or rarely ever, lie to my parents, but when they asked me if I ever made out with my boyfriend, I said no. I felt I had to say no because if I told the truth they'd say, "No more Brian. No more seeing him, no more phone calls, no more parties." I'd like it so much more if they were just a little more realistic. Like if they said, "Just don't have intercourse, but you can make out. We know that's normal." I mean I don't want them to get mad at me for kissing Brian for more than two seconds. If they could only understand that I have my limits, that they can trust me.

Parents of girls may be very concerned about their daughters' reputation. They don't want them to get the label "loose" or "cheap" or "easy." Unfortunately, those kind of labels are still around. That's why many parents, like Brenda's, seem to be stricter about sex than you may think is necessary. That's also why some parents seem to be much more lenient with their sons than with their daughters, as David, a sixteen-year-old Kansas boy, told us:

> There's definitely a double standard at my house. My fifteen-year-old sister will talk about bringing her boyfriend home and it will be a tense subject, and my parents let her know that it's really not OK with them. But with me, my dad's always joking around asking me how things are going with my girlfriend and stuff like that. Whenever I go out on a date he says, "Well, I'll see you in the morning." Like whatever I do or whenever I come home is OK with him.

David feels the inequality of how he and his sister are treated. (We talk more about the "double standard" on p. 67.)

But don't get the idea that all parents of teenage boys encourage their sons' sexual activity. Many worry just as much about their sons as they do about their daughters. A mother of two teenage boys who worked on this book told us:

> When Gregg was fifteen and sixteen he was pretty wild. I used to worry about him getting into real trouble. Whenever he went out I'd wonder, Will he pick people up or get picked up in dangerous situations? Will he get mugged while looking for adventure? Is he going to get my best friend's daughter pregnant? Is he going to "corrupt" her!!

We talked with several parents who have strong feelings about their sons' sexual involvements. One mother said:

> You know, I think mothers and fathers of boys have a real responsibility to make sure their kids don't grow up to be that "love 'em and leave 'em" type of man. It's up to us to teach our boys about consideration in sexual relationships, because if we don't teach them I don't know where else they're going to get that message.

Many parents of both boys and girls worry about sex and cars—whether their teens will get picked up by the police while making out, whether drugs or alcohol will be involved. The funny thing is, if and when you become a parent of a teenager, you may find yourself worrying about the same things. That's what one of the fathers who helped us with the interviews was laughing about. He said:

> You know this is ridiculous because when I was a teenager I used to get furious with my parents for restricting me and putting the fear of God into me about VD and pregnancy. And for so many years I've advocated sex education in the schools and I've counseled teens on birth control and everything. But now that my daughter is fourteen, I'm starting to feel just like my parents. I mean I don't want her staying out late and I don't like the looks of some of the kids she goes out with. And whenever there's an article in the paper about teenage pregnancy I always manage to leave it on her desk.

Parents feel this way because they want to protect you. They don't want you getting hurt, emotionally or physically, by having sex before you're ready. The problem is, *you* may feel ready before *they're* ready to think you are. (Chapter IV, p. 99, says more about this.)

Finally, there is another very important reason why some parents are opposed to teenagers' sexual activity. They have deep-felt religious and moral beliefs that say premarital sex is wrong. Their values will not allow them to sanction your sexual behavior. Many teenagers feel the same way, and they have told us they don't want to have a sexual relationship with anyone but their wife or husband.

The "Double Life"

Many teenagers said they had things going on in their life that they just couldn't talk to their parents about.

The most common areas for secrecy were sex and drugs and drinking, but people also mentioned things like staying out late, picking up strangers, skipping school, fighting, and going around with friends their parents didn't like. Anything you are doing that you don't tell your parents about comes under this category. Some of the activities are things you know you probably shouldn't be doing because they could hurt you or get you in serious trouble. Others are just things that you're pretty sure your particular parents won't be able to accept, so you don't tell them. Lou, a sophomore from Arizona, said:

> I'm doing things that my mom wouldn't want me to be doing. I know that. But I'm level-headed, I can say no when I want to. The thing is, sometimes I want to smoke pot or stay out to see the sun rise, or do other things that would worry her, and I don't think she'd understand that I know what I'm doing. I think she'd get mad, so I don't tell her.

Cassie, a fourteen-year-old from San Francisco, is more hostile toward her parents. She feels they put too many restrictions on her:

> In seventh grade I started getting drunk, going out with friends to parties and stuff. I stopped talking to my parents except for little bullshit things. I would tell them I was sleeping at a girlfriend's house, and they wouldn't ask what we were going to do. In a way I feel good doing things they don't know I'm doing because it makes me feel important. I have a separate life from them and I don't think they're on to it at all. Like I'm sure they feel, Oh my daughter wouldn't do anything like that. They wouldn't believe half of what I'm doing, and they want reassurance that I'm not doing that stuff, so I can't tell them the truth even if I wanted to.

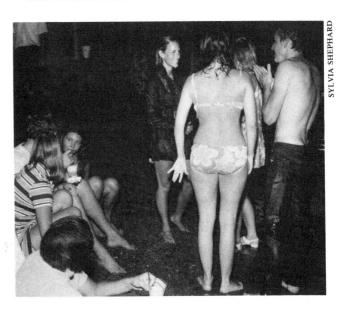

SYLVIA SHEPHARD

Like Cassie, several people said that their parents think, Oh, my child wouldn't do anything like that. Fifteen-year-old Suzanne told us:

> My parents think I'm so much more innocent than I am. That makes me feel bad, like they'd be disappointed in me if they knew the things I do. Even I think I'm too young to be doing some of the things I'm doing, but it just happens. You can't stop the way you feel at the time, and sometimes you just feel like doing that stuff.

Most people do feel "guilty" for doing things their parents think are wrong. If they've raised you to obey them and respect their rules, and then you find yourself sneaking out and lying to them, you're probably going to feel guilty. One of the women who worked on this book is a counselor who has met with thousands of teenagers. She said:

> Guilt may be a stage that people have to go through as they stretch themselves past their parents' rules

into their own new rules for themselves. Guilt comes when you're doing something (or thinking something) that you feel you shouldn't be doing or thinking. As a person gets older and starts acting according to his or her own ideas of what's right and wrong, guilt doesn't have to play a big role. You might feel sad then that your ideas are so different from your parents', and it may take a long time for you to be able to accept that it's OK to have different opinions, but you don't have to feel guilty as long as *you* think you're doing the right thing.

Everyone has at least some ideas that are different from his or her parents'. Still, you may wish you could share more of your separateness with them. You may wish that they could accept you, even if you have a different way of acting and thinking from them. Sixteen-year-old Gil said:

If I could let my parents know what's going on with me, that would help so much. If I could let them know and not get judged by them, that would be such a relief. If only they could understand that parties and staying out late and pot—and sex—are part of growing up for me.

Some parents would actually prefer not to know the details of your outside life, just as you probably don't want to know all the details of their personal life. That kind of arrangement is very healthy sometimes, but many times it makes a distance between you that can increase your anxiety and make you feel very alone. It can deprive you of guidance you need.

Fifteen-year-old Ellen told us:

I started smoking pot the summer before my ninth-grade year. And I was getting into it pretty heavy because my brother used to kind of deal in pot and he always had a lot. He even grew it out in the backyard and my folks didn't know what it was. They were just glad to see him doing something useful, like gardening! Meanwhile I'm getting to the point where I can't do without it.

And eighteen-year-old Brandon said:

One night when I was fifteen I got totally wasted and I got sick all over myself, and about one in the morning I came tripping into the house and my mom was waiting up for me. So she looked at me and said, "You've been drinking, haven't you?" and so I said, "Well, I only had a couple." And then she said, "You've been sick too." So I said, "No, I haven't. I just spilled my food all over me at dinner by accident. Somebody bumped into me." Well, I got away with it. I didn't get busted. I didn't get grounded. Nothing. I was just *asking* for her to notice that I'd been coming in drunk a lot, that I needed some help, but she preferred to overlook it. I guess she didn't want to admit she had a lush for a son. I think her philosophy is, If you don't notice, it isn't really there. She was really blind to what I was doing. She just didn't want to see it.

Brandon eventually went to Alcoholics Anonymous for help. He told us his mother still won't talk to him about his alcoholism.

It's part of the teenage experience to do things without being too cautious. But sometimes you end up getting yourself in trouble, and that's when you might want your parents to come through for you. Like Brandon, you may be asking them in your own way to notice and help you. It's hard for parents to know just when to interfere and when not to. It would benefit both you and your folks if you could somehow find a way to ask them for help *directly,* if you think you need it.

MY OLD MAN

My father,
Boy can he drive you crazy!
He sits down after dinner
With his head buried into the world's
gossip which he calls a newspaper.
    Dad I gotta talk to you.
        Silence
Ya see dad I've got this problem.
        Silence
    Dad I'm PREGNANT!!
Did you say something honey?
    No dad go back to sleep.

              —Andrea Mintz

Sometimes it takes a crisis for parents to learn what their children are doing. Eighteen-year-old Phyllis was in a group we interviewed in Iowa. She said:

I finally broke down and told my mom that I needed an abortion and she just about got hysterical. She started shouting, "My baby, my baby," like I was a three-year-old. But when she calmed down, we had the first good talk we've ever had. And after the abortion she helped me decide what kind of birth control to use and she was much more open with me about her life.

Several teens we met insisted they'd *never* be able to talk to their parents. In Washington, D.C., sixteen-year-old Freddie said:

My father's so strict that if I even look at him funny he knocks me under the table. That's the way he was raised and that's the way he treats me.

Bobbi-Jo, a sixteen-year-old from Memphis, said:

My father never talked to me at all about sex. Never one word. But one night we were out to dinner and my boyfriend was with us. As we were walking into the restaurant I put my arm around my boyfriend and my Dad gave me the dirtiest, angriest look and said to me sort of under his breath, *"You don't do that!"* I was really shocked by how angry he looked. I felt like saying to him, "Well, if you think that's bad, you should see what we do when you're not around." But I didn't say anything.

We've learned from the teens we've interviewed that most want their parents to accept them as they are—people who are growing up and experimenting with life. They are in need of support. When their parents can't give them that support, they look elsewhere. Carl, a seventeen-year-old from Los Angeles, moved out of his house temporarily, to stay with his friend's family:

As I got older I realized that I couldn't depend on my parents—being open just didn't work in my family. The few times I tried it, it was disastrous. They just couldn't understand and they would yell at me and punish me without even the tiniest bit of understanding. So finally I ran away from home and my best friend's family took me in and I lived with them for about six months. His parents became my second parents, and to this day they still are. Because they weren't my real parents I felt like I could talk to them about anything, like sex and drugs and going out to the beach and this and that. I could tell them stuff because they didn't get threatened by it. They didn't have a lot of negative feelings around it like, "Oh, we're failures. Our son's doing this, this, and this." They didn't expect me to be perfect the way my real parents did. Plus they showed me a lot of love, and I really needed that.

Some people, like seventeen-year-old Karen, find a way to support themselves and go live on their own:

My parents didn't let me do anything. They always had to know exactly where I was going and exactly who'd be there and exactly what time I'd be home, or they wouldn't let me go anywhere. And they never let me go on a single date, only on double dates, so we had to pretend we were doubling just to please them. We had to go through this whole thing of getting two other people to act like they were going with us, when they really weren't. I felt like I was too old for my parents to still be treating me like a baby. I wanted to talk to them and be friends with them, but they just couldn't handle that. I love my parents, but I just couldn't talk to them because they have a thing: what they think is right goes and that's it. They wouldn't let me express my feelings about anything, so I just closed them out of my life.

Try to open the lines of communication. You may be surprised to find your parents really do come through. Since you're getting older, they may want to talk to you, too, about things that are going on in their lives. You probably won't always be able to talk calmly. You probably won't agree with each other about everything. In fact, at times it may take a lot of strength and self-control just to listen to each other. But the alternative, which is cutting yourself off from your parents altogether, is painful for everyone. Gretchen, a seventeen-year-old senior from Milwaukee, told us she's really glad she finally opened up to her mother:

I never was very close to my parents, but when my first boyfriend broke up with me last year, I was really depressed, and he kept saying I should talk to my mom. So I did. And she made me feel a lot better. Now I talk with her about a lot of things—anything, really. I still can't talk to my dad. I know I can't because my mom tells him everything and he never responds to me, so I know he doesn't want to talk about that stuff. It's OK though. We love each other. But my mom and I are really close now. I feel like she's a friend, not just my mother.

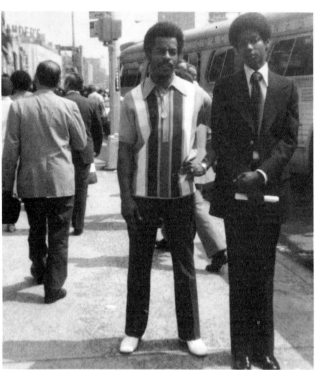

And one of the fathers we interviewed had this suggestion:

You know, almost everybody has trouble with their parents when they're teenagers. But let's say you've got really rotten parents. Well, you've got to approach them very positively. If your parents are hardnosed, you as the child have to be very diplomatic. You have to find some way to have a conversation with them about things they're interested in or things that won't threaten them. Think about them as people, not as enemies. And you can't just go to them when you need something or you want something. You have to talk to them just for the sake of talking. Find wherever you can connect up with them and try it. Start out with something simple. I think most parents would respond positively to that. After all, they want to get along with their kids; they want to have a good relationship; they want you to love them.

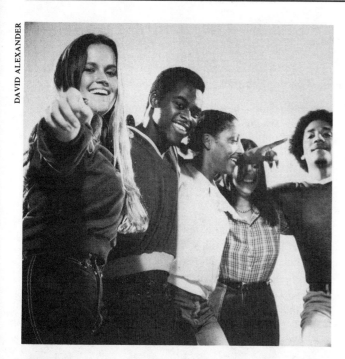

DAVID ALEXANDER

Friends

Friendships, too, go through a lot of changes during the teenage years. Most people make new friends, stop seeing some old friends, and spend more of their time with groups of friends both in and out of school. Some of the teenagers we interviewed said they're with their girlfriend or boyfriend a lot now, and that's a change from when they were younger. Many teens told us that these days their friends are even more important and closer to them than their families.

Groups

Everyone we met said that groups are part of his or her life. There are family groups, school groups, religious groups, teams, political groups, social clubs, hobby clubs and more. It's almost impossible to avoid being in some group, and most people are part of many.

A number of teens we interieved told us it's important to them to be part of a group at school. Vicki, a tenth-grader in one of the largest high schools in New York City, said:

> Some people I know think it's cool to say that groups are the pits. They say they want to be an individual. But I mean, what fun is it to be an individual if you don't have a group of friends too? What are you going to do? Be an individual with yourself? Sit at home and say, "Oh, I'm an individual." Sure.

Being part of a group can make things more fun. Something that you might not want to do alone, like going to a movie or a party, can be really enjoyable when you do it with others. And things you might feel embarrassed to do alone are usually easier to do when there are other people with you. Louisa, a fifteen-year-old we met in the South, told us:

> You know sometimes you feel scared to do stuff, but because everybody's doing it, you do it too. Like dancing. For me, dancing was really hard. To get out there and dance with everybody watching was so embarrassing for me I never could do it. But when I started going to dances with my friends it wasn't so bad. Everybody I knew was out there, so I forced myself to get out there too. I figured, If they can do it, so can I.

But not everyone we talked with was satisfied with the group scene. In fact, many people had pretty nasty comments to make about the groups at their schools. Anthony, a tenth-grade Los Angeles student, said:

> In our school it's disgusting the way everyone's in these groups trying to outdo each other in the way they dress or who's the most popular. A lot of the people on the outside sit back and watch what's going on and laugh.

Lynn, an eighth-grader from Virginia, told us:

> Usually there's one group that's called the popular group, and everyone outside it is down on the people in that group. You know, they think those people are stuck-up. Sometimes I think it's because everyone else is jealous of them.

A few people said it was different in their schools. Janie, a fourteen-year-old from New England, goes to a small school where, she said, people try to be accepting of each other. She didn't feel there was much competition there at all. And Zack, a fifteen-year-old from Colorado, agreed. He said:

> Last year I started going to this school where it's really incredible. It's like a family. You get to know everybody, even the teachers. Of course you don't have to like everybody, but it's not like you feel like you have to stick with just one group of friends to be popular. Everybody's accepted as an individual. It's like people appreciate each other for just being who they are.

Zack and Janie and several other teens we met think that it makes school life a lot easier when there's less concern about who's popular and who isn't. Several other teenagers said that even though there are definite groups at their school, they've somehow been able to stay friends with lots of different people from lots of different groups.

Some people said they enjoy being part of a crowd of friends, but the trouble comes when you get swallowed up in it. They told us that in their schools people who are in groups get labeled, and they said they don't like being categorized that way—put in a little box that says: you're a jock; you're a brain; you're a druggie; you're social;

you're a troublemaker. Those categories may say something about your group's activities or interests, but they certainly don't describe anybody as a whole person. No individual can be explained away so easily—we're too complicated for that.

David, a senior from Denver, said he's angry about the way the people in his school label him and his group. He said:

I guess in all schools there's a problem with reputations. I mean, my pet peeve has to do with that. I've done my share of screwing around and you know that it gets back to people after a while. I'm not the best-loved person in my school and neither are my friends. Not that we'd ever hurt anybody, but we do like to have our fun, if you know what I mean. But like when something happens, they just blame us.

About a month ago there was some trashing at school and I got blamed. I didn't have anything to do with it. I wasn't even there and I got blamed. They said, "Oh, it must have been Dave and the boys who did it," not because they knew we did it, but because of our reputation. You just get labeled. People don't look at you as a person anymore.

Dave's friend Gina said the same thing happens to her because she's a cheerleader and on Student Council. She told us:

I'm labeled as one of the rah-rah girls. I'm just put in this box and people think they know me. So when I overhear somebody saying something about the rah-rah's, as if we're not people, I go up to them and say, "Is it really *me* you're talking about? Or are you just making a big generalization?" Then they always say, "Oh, we didn't mean *you*." But they don't get that they're being so stupid to label people just because they go out for something like sports or cheerleading or student government. Everybody's not the same who does those things. It's like saying that everybody who likes to swim is the same.

Fitting In

Part of the identity confusion comes from a real pressure that exists in many groups for members to be like one another. The fact that your friends are doing something can give you courage to try it, but that can also limit you.

Some people get so used to doing things with the crowd that they feel funny doing anything their friends aren't doing. George, a sixteen-year-old from the Southwest, told us that's the worst part of groups as far as he's concerned:

I hate school because I have to stifle a lot of myself and I can't say a lot of the things I feel because I'd just be made an outcast. Like in English class, if you're reading poetry or something and if you have an opinion on it that's different from the rest of the class, you can very rarely express it without them all jumping on your back. You have to do and say what

everybody else is doing and saying. I don't like it at all.

Tyrone, a fifteen-year-old we interviewed in Chicago, said that things are like that in his school too:

In my school there's the "in" group and the "out" group, which is everyone else. And whatever the "in" group does, that's the thing to do. They can go out and stand in the middle of the street and get run over by trucks and, sure enough, the next day everyone will be standing out in the middle of the street getting run over by trucks. You know what I mean? It's pretty bad.

Tyrone laughed while he told us about the pressure to be like the "in" group. But it's an important issue that affects every one of us, no matter what age we are: the difference between doing and saying what we want because that's what we believe, and doing things or saying things because that's what we think everyone else believes.

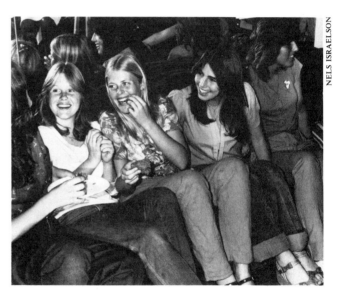

Many people feel the pressure to be accepted and to conform to group standards especially when they are in a new situation—a new school, a new neighborhood—when they don't have old friends around who know them and appreciate them for who they are. Fourteen-year-old Rachel told us about what happened when she moved from New York to her new school in California:

Last year I was new and I was beginning to make a few friends with some of the kids in my classes. Well, I had this new purse that was made of leather and I really liked it. But then this girl in the popular crowd who I was sort of becoming friends with told me that she thought the purse was weird-looking. She said it looked like saddlebags and that no one had a purse like that. I think she was really trying to be friendly, telling me how to make myself more stylish, but it really hurt my feelings. I went home and cried about it for a long time. I felt lonely and embarrassed and out of place.

The desire to be accepted by a particular group of friends pushes a lot of people into doing things they don't really want to do. Fourteen-year-old Lionel, who lives in New Jersey, gave an example. He told us about the group of boys he plays basketball with:

Friends can push you into doing stuff you know you shouldn't be doing. You try and say no and they'll probably end up beating you up or something. They tell me to do something and I do it. They're a lot older than me. Like they tell me we're going to play basketball, so they come by and pick me up and we end up going to the liquor store. And I say, "Hey, man, what's in the bag?" And they say, "Gin. Now shut up and take a drink."

That's a no-win situation. Lionel said he didn't want to drink, but he felt he had to or else it wouldn't have been cool, since he was younger than most of them anyway. He liked playing basketball with them because they were good, and he was glad they accepted him on their team, but it put a lot of pressure on him to do the things they told him to do. At least Lionel *felt* pressured.

Ben, a fourteen-year-old from Boston, explained that the pressure isn't always as obvious as it was in Lionel's experience:

I'm part of the crowd who are considered the "cool" kids at school, and it always gets into who's the coolest in the crowd. Like who's done the most or who knows the most stuff. There's this competition around who's going to lead the group—who everybody else will follow. Sometimes the so-called leaders do a drug and don't let me or some of the others do it because that makes them more experienced than us, and we sort of end up feeling less mature than them. It makes doing that stuff very appealing because you start thinking, Oh, yeah, that looks like fun. I want to do it too. It's not that anyone's telling you to do it. In fact, they may be telling you *not* to do it, but since they're doing it, and since they make it seem so great, you naturally want to do it too.

We don't mean to be saying that teenagers only do things because of the pressure from their friends. Most of the teens we interviewed told us they do what they do because they *want* to, not because other people are doing it. But even so, everyone agreed that there are times when they personally feel a little scared to do something, or maybe feel that they're not quite ready to experience something, and they end up doing it anyway because their friends are. Inside they're unsure or they're worried about getting caught or having their parents find out, but they go along. It's that way for everyone, not only teens.

The choice to go along with the crowd can sometimes get in the way of what you really want for yourself, or

what you know is right. When other people are doing something that is dangerous or destructive or humiliating or illegal, you're faced with the decision: Do I do it too because they're doing it, or do I say no?

Those kinds of decisions come up all the time throughout a person's life. Situations come up that test your values—whether to cheat on a test, drive without a license, fight with someone who provokes you, try an unfamiliar drug, go to bed with someone you hardly know, or, for that matter, with someone you know very well. No one is standing over you at those times helping you decide. It's up to you alone. And if you do take a stand that is different from the others', you risk having to put up with their teasing or their anger. That takes courage and self-confidence.

In the long run, the question is whether *you* want to be responsible for making your own choices, or whether you're willing to let others make choices for you.

There's always been and there probably always will be a certain amount of tension between what the group wants and what the individual members of the group want. If you're in a crowd which values individuals, that makes it easier to say no if you want to say no. In Connecticut, fourteen-year-old Betty said:

If the kids in my group are smoking marijuana they say, "You want to try it?" If you say no, they say "Fine." That's all there is to it. No one forces you. And no one puts you down.

If you're in a crowd of friends who take care of each other, that also helps. Georgia, a seventeen-year-old from Detroit, said her crowd is like that:

Usually the kind of drinking or smoking that goes on with us is just social. People just sitting around and smoking a little weed or having a little wine. But if you see your friends getting wasted or messing up, if you're a good friend you'll say something to them. Like if somebody's totally bombed and they want to drive home, you tell them, "Oh no, I'll drive tonight." We watch out for each other.

Some people we met are admired by their friends for doing things that can hurt them or get them into trouble. Seventeen-year-old Annie told us about her experience when she first entered high school:

Big, bad and bitching was the thing in my school—at least with my crowd. If you cut school and got away with it, that meant you were all right. You had a scam on those teachers. If you could still pass, you had an in. Everyone thought that was great. You'd be stoned in class and sit back and make a fool of yourself and everybody would laugh and you'd be considered fun. Like you'd be entertaining everyone. And if you didn't get caught, you were cool, you were OK. The thing was—just don't get caught.

Fifteen-year-old Josie told us that she couldn't count on her friends for anything but trouble:

When I was twelve I started hanging out with this crowd at school and they really had an influence on me. I always looked up to this one guy who was like the leader of the crowd. He was a couple of years older than me and he'd be the one who'd think up stuff to do, and we'd all do it. Like ripping off a store or smashing car windows or setting fires. He'd supply the drugs and we'd supply the action.

Josie was arrested and put in a county home for girls. That's where we met her while we were interviewing for this book. She said:

When you don't feel too sure of yourself and somebody says, "Hey, you're cool. We like your looks," well then, you appreciate that so much, it makes you feel so good, you just want to be with them. You want people to notice you. I think everybody does probably. If the kid who was class president or somebody who got straight A's wanted to be friends with me, I'd probably have ended up getting straight A's too.

It's important to most people to feel accepted, especially if they aren't getting much support or acceptance at home, or if they're going through a difficult personal experience—like parents splitting up, or moving to a new place, or changing schools, or if a family member has an accident or dies. At times like these, people feel particularly vulnerable, and it really hurts more than ever not to have friends who like you and appreciate you. Josie wrote this poem and gave it to us to put in the book:

LONELINESS

Loneliness is a terrible thing.
It rules, in some way, every human being.
Help, is what some people cry—
Can you just sneer and pass them by?

Feeling Lonely

When you think no one likes you or cares about you or wants to be with you, that *can* be a terrible thing. You may be on the outside of an "in" group and want very much to get inside. You may feel too shy to make friends or perhaps you were rejected by old friends. Maybe you feel like an outcast because your style and opinions are different from everyone else's. These experiences can be very painful and can make you feel very lonely.

Though this may only be small consolation, the fact is that *everyone* has felt rejected and lonely at some time or at many times during his or her life. The following are just a few of the stories we heard about loneliness from teenagers all across the country.

Steven is a fourteen-year-old, originally from New York, but we met him in Des Moines. He said:

I moved to Des Moines in the middle of the year last year and everybody in my new school was going around in their own little groups. It's hard to get into a group of people. I would sort of hang around, but no one would really notice me or pay attention to me. I started making a couple of friends this year, but last year was really tough.

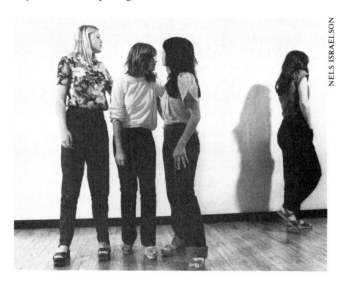

For Danny, a junior from a town outside Detroit, it wasn't anything in particular. He just hasn't found anyone with whom he feels a close connection:

There are a lot of people in my school, of course, and they're nice and all, but I go to homeroom and I sit there and do my work and I walk to my next class and I sit there. I might say Hi to whoever's the person sitting next to me, but I go through the day pretty much by myself. I know most of the people, but no one's really more than an acquaintance.

Sixteen-year-old Polly told us she feels older and more mature than the people she knows at school:

I have some so-called friends, people I hang out with at school, and we can have fun together. But I don't feel close to them. Like when I have a problem I can't go to them because they just don't understand. They talk behind people's backs. You can't trust them. I'm looking forward to college next year. At least I'll meet some new people.

Many people go through periods of loneliness as teenagers. Some told us they don't feel part of any group. Others said they try to make themselves fit in, but it just doesn't work. Stephanie, a ninth-grader from Texas, said that's the way it is for her:

I spent just about my whole seventh-grade year wishing I could be in the popular crowd. I would watch the kids in that crowd and sit near them at lunch and

I'd pray that one of them would call me and ask me to go somewhere with them on the weekends. Well, in the eighth grade I did become friends with them. I went to their parties and dated the guys in the crowd, but I never really felt like I fit in. I found out I wasn't really into drugs and I didn't feel comfortable at make-out parties. So this year I stopped hanging around them. I guess you'd say I'm not exactly in any group now.

Accepting Yourself

Some people we met said they feel "out of it" because they don't think they're like the other teens they know. Brian, a ninth-grader from Cleveland, told us he isn't sure he can measure up to other people's standards:

I'm not a tough guy and I don't like to fight. But in my school it seems like people get respected for their physical strength—I mean boys, that is. Everyone goes around bragging about how many kids they've beat up and how strong they are and how much they work out. I'm not big and I have a lot of fears that keep me from doing the things that those kids do. Like I'm even afraid of roller coasters, and I don't like being in deep water, so I don't really know how to swim. And I always worry that someone will dare me to do something that I'm scared to death of, or that someone will start fighting me and I'll lose. Of course I'll lose. I've never fought before in my life. And then everyone will see how chicken I am and they won't respect me anymore. That's one of my biggest worries—not being respected by the other kids.

A lot of teenagers we met think they *should* be feeling more confident than they do. They're down on themselves for not being tough enough or popular enough or smart enough or attractive enough or talented enough. Nobody told us exactly what "enough" would be; they just know they're not it. They look around and see other people who seem to have it all together, who seem to be attractive and fun to be with and full of self-confidence. And that makes them worry all the more that they're the only one in the world who's afraid to fight, or afraid to stand up and give a speech, or afraid to ask someone out on a date. You may have some of your own private issues that cause your stomach muscles to tighten up and your heart to beat faster.

The truth is, *we all feel that way*. There isn't anyone, no matter how mature, who doesn't feel scared and out of it at times. Some people have learned to forge ahead in spite of their fears. Others know how to cover up their insecurities with well-acted performances to prove how capable or happy or confident they are. Once you start seeing through the performance, you find that, underneath, everyone—at least everyone we've ever met—has the same desire to be liked and respected that you have, and that everyone has the same worry that they may not be able to "measure up." That's one of the secrets most people carry with them throughout their lives. (For more discussion of this see "Feeling Bad, Feeling Better," p. 133.) If you talk with your friends about it, you'll probably find out they feel the same way. That can be a big relief for everyone, and it can help you get over some of the insecurity. Nancy, a seventeen-year-old first-year college student who helped us write this chapter, told us she thinks that's the biggest problem she's facing right now:

The hardest thing is coming to grips with who you are, accepting the fact that you're not perfect. Even if you are really good at something or a really fine person, you also know that there's so much you aren't. *You* always know all the things you don't know. And however much you can fool the rest of the world, you always know how much bullshit a lot of it is.

Accepting Others

How you feel about yourself influences how you relate to other people. That issue came up at one of our meetings in Los Angeles, and Janice, a high school junior, said:

I've been thinking of all the times I've been rejecting of people. Like even in grammar school I'd walk down the hall and go, "Oh, there's so and so, she's weird." Or "Eeuu, stay away from Richard, he's a creep." It was so cruel, but that really happened and I used to do it. People I know did it all the time. I'd sometimes think to myself, That's so mean. I don't want to be like that. But like if *you're* doing the rejecting, then you're not the one being rejected. You know, you don't feel good about yourself being mean, but at the same time, you're so worried about being accepted yourself that you don't stop to think about that for others.

So while some people who are unsure of themselves withdraw and feel lonely, other people, like Janice, go to the opposite extreme. She said she was part of a tight little group that ignored people or talked behind their backs. She said it was their way of making sure *they* were "in," and if their actions made other people left *out*, that just made being *in* even more desirable.

Lots of social clubs, sororities, fraternities, country clubs and other exclusive organizations are based on the idea that if you're in this group you must be great. And that, of course, means if you're not in this group you must not be so great. The same idea comes through in many patriotic or religious organizations: we're the best, we know the right way. Anyone who thinks differently must not be thinking the "right" way. People who insist that they are the best or that their ideas are the *only* right ideas probably worry somewhere deep inside that if they're not the best, then they're nothing.

Sometimes even groups that preach love and togetherness are exclusive organizations in disguise. These groups can be just as closed and rejecting as any other. Jenny said:

> I went to this really liberal, open high school and I was in a special alternative program there. Now that I'm out I realize all the things I don't like about it. What really scares me is that I could never have seen these things while I was in the program. We were such a tight group. We thought of ourselves as so loving and accepting—except we really weren't. We all thought of each other as neat and superior in a way. We'll be friends with you, but we really don't think you're as good as we are because you're not in our program. I really think we could have been led into anything—like the people in Guyana even. Everybody did and thought like everybody else, but we each felt we were choosing for ourselves. If anybody criticized us, we thought, Oh, poor them. They just can't fit in. And some of the teachers in the program got their kicks feeling like they were these great gods. Now that I'm out I think it was irresponsible of them.

You have to stand back a little to be able to balance who you are as an individual with who you are as a member of a group. By standing back, you get a chance to understand what makes you unique. Bill, a seventeen-year-old senior from New England, said:

> In junior high especially, it was like everyone had to be cool and fashionable and taking the right drugs and going to the right parties to be in the popular crowds. I never really fit in and I felt terrible most of the time. Since I've been in high school, though, it's been different. I'm finding some friends who accept me for who I am now. I don't feel I have to dress a certain way or act a certain way to have friends. Now I'm sort of glad that I didn't really fit in in junior high because I know I don't want to be that way anyway. When you're so caught up with fitting in, you lose a lot of chances to find out who you are.

Best Friends

Many of the teenagers we spoke to said they have their most important relationships with one or two close friends. In Wisconsin, thirteen-year-old Sam said:

> A best friend to me is someone you can have fun with and you can also be serious with about personal things, about girls or what you're going to do with your life or whatever. My best friend, Jeff, and I can talk about things. His parents are divorced too, and he understands when I feel bummed out about the fights between my mom and dad. A best friend is someone who's not going to make fun of you just because you do something stupid or put you down if you make a mistake. If you're afraid of something or someone, they'll give you confidence.

It's almost always easier to do something or say something if you have a friend around for moral support. Marlene, a senior from Chicago, told us about her friend Julie:

Julie was on the swimming team with me and she was scared to compete because she thought she wouldn't beat the other person. We were all trying to tell her, "Come on, you can do it," but she always thought she wasn't good enough. And that was the way she felt about everything, not just swimming. Since I was her best friend, I really talked to her. I kept telling her, "You can do it. You're great. Do it for our team." I kept boosting her confidence and, you know, after a while she did do it. We all cheered for her and she was terrific.

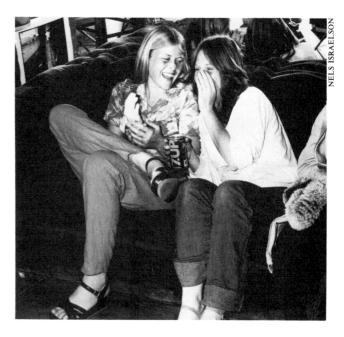

Close friends can give each other confidence and appreciate the best in one another. When you're feeling your lowest, it's especially reassuring to have a friend who'll listen to you and help you through the hard time. In Iowa, sixteen-year-old Sarah told us this story:

> One of my closest friends got so mad at her parents that she said, "Well, I'm going to swallow this whole bottle of pills." I was with her and I just started crying because I hadn't ever heard anybody say anything like that before, and I was scared. I tried to talk her out of it by saying, "No, don't do anything like that. It can't be that bad." I said, "You can talk to me about it." So she did, and it turned out that she didn't really want to do it. She was just so mad. I told her to talk to me about how she was mad and she said her parents just have too tight a hold on her. She feels like she can't hardly move.

Another part of having a close friend is knowing that you can get really angry with each other and still remain friends. It would be pretty hard to have an intense relationship with anyone without having some disagreements. It's healthy to be able to express anger without being scared that it will destroy your relationship. We ran into a lot of teenagers who told us they've had big fights with some of their friends, and when they make up they generally feel closer to each other than before.

Some teenagers told us they don't have any close friends to share feelings with. Several said it was OK because they were able to work out their emotions in other ways. One fifteen-year-old girl we met in Rhode Island is writing a novel. She spends much of her time alone, writing her thoughts and feelings into her book. A senior named Bob who lives in Seattle is preparing himself for Olympic swimming competition, so he works off a lot of his tension through practice. Other people write poetry or meditate or hike or go on long-distance runs, and they are able to learn a lot about themselves and how they are feeling through those experiences alone.

It can get lonely, though, when you feel you really want to talk to someone your own age but don't know anyone well enough. Chris, a seventeen-year-old boy who works at a park in Chicago, told us:

I know a kid who doesn't have anybody at all. His mother's dead and his father's off somewhere and he's living with his great-aunt who doesn't understand him, so he doesn't really have anybody. I met him at the park because he was hanging around all alone, so I asked him to come play on the football team I was coaching. I think he was hoping someone would ask him. After that, whenever he was having a problem he'd come a little early and we'd spend some time sitting around talking about what was on his mind. He just loved to come to that park when I was there. We got to be real good friends.

Chris had this advice for readers of this book:

If you really don't have anybody, it's best to try to go out and do a little bit. Like get into a sport and join a team, or go to a dance class or some after-school club or something. Get interested in something. You don't have to be great at it—just have some fun and be with other people. Then you can find a friend.

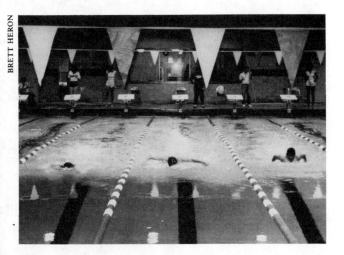

Friendships usually form at school, or at work, or at church or temple. When you see the same people all the time, you have a better chance to get to know them. Kathy, a sixteen-year-old we worked with in Vermont, said:

If you just smile and say something friendly to people, I think it's pretty hard not to meet them. Like at my new job I found at first that people weren't really talking to each other. But then one day one of the girls looked really sad, so I asked if something was the matter and she started crying. We went out to talk for a while and she told me that her dad was in the hospital. Well, after that most of the kids started being real friendly to each other. I don't know why, except maybe once you start thinking about each other as real people with feelings and problems at home and stuff like that, it makes it hard not to be friendly.

There can be a physical closeness as well as an emotional closeness between best friends, as Jennifer, a sophomore from New Jersey, said:

Me and my best friend, Elaine, always go around with our arms around each other or holding hands. And one time some guy yelled out from a car, "Hey, Lesbos." It made us mad for a minute but it really didn't bother us because I mean, if people are going to call you names just because you're holding hands with your best friend, well then, forget them. The only people who are going to judge you are people you don't care about anyway.

Having a close relationship with someone of the same sex doesn't mean you are homosexual, just as having a loving friendship with someone of the opposite sex doesn't mean you're heterosexual. Homosexuality and heterosexuality are different ways people choose to express their sexual feelings toward others. (We discuss sexuality and sexual preferences more thoroughly in Chapters III and IV.)

Best friends often spend hours together each day, sleeping over at each other's home, taking showers together, touching or wrestling or telling jokes or whispering and laughing together. They can do all that without feeling at all sexually aroused.

Sometimes that intimacy does create a kind of sexual tension and friends do start feeling turned on by each other. Some people, like seventeen-year-old Laura from Pennsylvania, told us they have acted on their feelings. She said:

My best friend and I—well—we were like sisters, and you know I wondered about how much I loved her. I'd give her little presents and we called each other by nicknames and we'd both write each other little poems about how much we loved each other, as friends, that is. Her boyfriend was jealous because we were so close. Sometimes we'd fool around and dance with each other, and once we got drunk together and we got a little too drunk and we started slow-dancing together. And I thought, This is weird, you know. But then I thought, Oh, what the heck. So we kept dancing and we kept putting on slow dances and we kept dancing. And then we both fell down and started kissing. I would say we kissed for a long time, maybe a half-hour or so, and then we stopped, and for the next few days we were real formal with each other. When we finally talked about it, she said, "I wish we hadn't done it because you probably think I'm a lesbian now." And I said, "Oh, that's funny. I was afraid you were going to feel that way about me." So we laughed and everything and hugged each other.

Girls often hug and kiss each other without feeling that there's anything "wrong," but Laura said she and her friend felt funny about their experience because it wasn't just friendly kissing, it was definitely sexual.

Lots of people who have very close friendships have had experiences like Laura's. It's not unusual and it doesn't mean anything in particular about a person's sexuality, except that they enjoy being intimate with people they love. Allan, a junior from Massachusetts, said:

My best friend and I used to fool around with sex all the time, and until I was fourteen I never thought anything of it. I just thought it was natural. But then one of the kids in our school got into a scandal by being caught in some gay bar and everyone started talking about fags, and that's when I started thinking there was something wrong with what me and Steve were doing. So we stopped.

In our society boys aren't usually given as much freedom to kiss and hug as girls are, even though boys can of course have the same intense and affectionate feelings as girls toward their friends. In many societies men openly hug and kiss and touch each other. In fact, it's expected that they will be physically affectionate with their friends.

Sexual feelings can be confusing, though. Read the next chapter on changing sexuality, which has information as well as quotes from many teenagers. It will probably help you to sort out your feelings. You might also try talking with a friend or someone you trust. If you feel particularly uncomfortable with some of your feelings or fantasies, read the section "Feeling Bad, Feeling Better" for advice on how to find a counselor or therapist to talk to.

Opposite-Sex Friendships

Some people form their closest friendships with people of the opposite sex. They can confide in each other, go out with each other and have fun together but not get romantic. In Washington, D.C., sixteen-year-old John said:

Sandy's just about my closest friend. I talk to her about everything, especially things I wouldn't talk to the guys about, like if I'm having problems with my girlfriend or something. We tried going out together in the ninth grade, but it lasted exactly a week. We're just not compatible that way, I guess, but it's great to have her as a friend.

A lot of teens said it was a pleasure to have a friendship with someone of the opposite sex, without having to get mixed up in a sexual relationship with them. Mary, a senior from Delaware, described what she especially likes about her relationship with Bill:

I have girlfriends who are fun and stuff, but I just don't feel like I can trust them. There's so much competition between the girls I know, you never know who's going to turn around and spread a rumor about you. Bill is really my best friend. We really love each other, but just not romantically. You know what I mean? It's comfortable. It's really comfortable—no games, no expectations.

In many opposite-sex friendships one person does start fantasizing about how it would be if they were more than friends. Linda, a junior from Colorado, told us that happened to her one night when she was at a party with her friend, Bob. She said:

Well, we'd really liked each other for a long time. We were really close. But I started thinking about him differently that night and I guess I started coming on to him. But he just wasn't up to getting together. He was too bummed out about some things that were going on for him at home. Things got so tense between us at the party that we just ended up going for a walk and we talked about it. We both ended up crying, but it really cleared the air and we got even closer than before. It just wasn't the right time for us to get together. He needed me more as a friend than as a girlfriend. It felt awful at the time, but it really deepened our friendship.

When one person wishes the friendship would become romantic, that can lead to complications unless it's what they both want. There isn't any way to force someone to feel sexual if they don't feel it. Sometimes, though, when people who really care about each other are in a situation that is intimate and cozy, sex does come up. Madelyn, a senior from the Midwest, told us:

Peter and I have been best friends since junior high. And we were always just buddies until one night a couple of months ago we were out at a movie and we came out of the theater feeling different. There was something going on between us and we both felt it. We ended up making love, and it was nice. It was sort of a surprise to both of us, but there was something very comfortable about it, since we knew each other so well. For a while afterwards, though, we both felt pretty shy around each other because we didn't really want it to happen again. I didn't want us to be lovers because our friendship was too special the way it was.

We heard from many teens that they enjoy having a

nonromantic, opposite-sex friendship because it's "neutral." You have the benefit of advice and caring from someone different from you, but you don't have the tension or jealousy or possessiveness that often comes in a boyfriend-girlfriend relationship.

Just because two people like each other in a romantic way, though, doesn't mean they can't really enjoy a friendship together. Several teenagers we met said that their boyfriend or their girlfriend is their best friend too. And most of the married couples we know who are happy in their marriages say it's the friendship and trust between them that makes their marriage so satisfying.

Asking Someone for a Date

Vic, a tall, quiet boy we interviewed at a high school in New York, complained:

> I'm already in the tenth grade and I've never even gone out with a girl, and that bugs me. I'm shy to an extent, but I think I could overcome it if I knew there were some girls who liked me. Then I could probably ask them out or something, but I haven't been able to be friends enough with a girl to give her a reason to like me.

Once people start thinking about dating, meeting people with the intention of asking them out becomes an issue, and shyness can make that a problem. In fact, Vic's complaint is familiar to a lot of the teenagers we interviewed. Many of them feel too shy to ask someone out.

There are lots of reasons for shyness. It can even be an extreme form of politeness—not wanting to intrude on someone else's privacy. Often people are shy because they don't think enough of themselves. Steve, a junior from Pittsburgh, said:

> The way you think about yourself really has a lot to do with how you act. Like you might stop yourself from going up to someone you might want to meet because you think, Oh, I'm not attractive enough or I don't have a good enough personality. You think you won't make a good impression so you're afraid to make an effort. For me, it was always that I was afraid I'd be rejected or—even worse than that—ignored. But what I've learned is that you may have

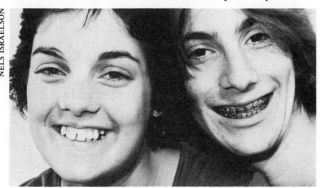

NELS ISRAELSON

something inside you that the other person would like very much. You have to give yourself a chance because if you put yourself down too quick you never get anywhere.

It takes effort to break through shyness, but without that effort it's hard to make contact. You'd always be waiting for someone to come up to you first. Steve said he finally realized that nearly everyone feels awkward and uncertain about approaching someone he or she doesn't know, and that made it easier for him.

A group of tenth-graders we met in Los Angeles were talking about exactly that when we interviewed them. Bill, a fifteen-year-old, had just moved to the school. He said:

> Since I'm new, I feel like it's OK for me to just go up to someone and start a conversation because that's the only way I can get to know anybody at all. When you're starting without any friends, you just have to keep trying until somebody takes an interest in you.

Peter, another boy in the group, said:

> It's not always so easy, though. Like what if you see this girl going to class every day and you want to meet her, so you go up to the class and wait for her to come. Like you plan to be there at the right time so she'll have to pass you on her way and you set the whole thing up. That's really tough for me because I get more of a fear of her turning me down when I stand around and wait. My stomach goes crazy.

Cheryl, one of the girls sitting next to Peter, said:

> I think it's great when someone comes up to me, when they're wanting to meet me. It makes me feel good. But it depends on what kind of energy they give me. If they're nice and act like they just want to get to know me, I like it. But if they just want sex or something, I can tell that too and I usually leave as soon as I can.

In our society it's been boys who've been taught that they're supposed to make the moves; girls have learned that they're supposed to wait to be asked. That's called sex-role expectations; it means expecting boys to act one way and girls to act another. Most teens we spoke to said they're glad things are changing now in this area.

Sex-Role Expectations

You may have learned somewhere along the way as you were growing up: boys play with cars and trucks; girls play with dolls. Or boys get dirty and play rough; girls look pretty and play house. Or boys plan careers; girls plan to get married. Some people have very set ideas about what boys are supposed to do and what girls are supposed to do, and these expectations are passed down from generation to generation.

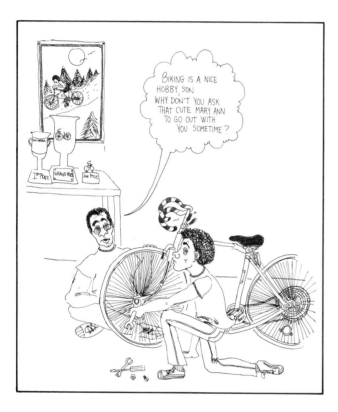

Sex-role expectations limit our behavior. Each of us, male and female, has a whole range of activities and feelings that are normal because we're all human. We have our individual strengths and weaknesses. We each feel like being active sometimes and passive sometimes, and we want to be able to act on our feelings without having to hide them because of what someone tells us is the way boys or girls are "supposed" to act. Many of the teenagers we interviewed said they don't believe people should have to fit those old-fashioned stereotypes anymore.

The traditional male-female roles can especially get to be a burden when it comes to dating. A lot of boys feel the burden of having to be the one to make the first move to

ask a girl out. Max, a fourteen-year-old boy from Philadelphia, said he feels the pressure:

> I think boys have it really hard. Once you get to be a teenager, suddenly everybody expects you to start calling up girls and going out with them. But, hey, I think it takes a lot of courage to call a girl up and ask her out. You know, you always worry that she'll say no, and then you feel like shit. It's not so easy for me to just pick up the phone and act cool. I get nervous.

If you're a girl and you've been taught that you're supposed to wait to be asked, you may sit around and go through the opposite despair. Sixteen-year-old Lee-ann told us:

> Sitting around waiting for the phone to ring is a big part of my life—you know, wondering if some boy's going to call and ask you out for the weekend. Like on Monday night I'll sit there and say to myself, Well, the phone's going to ring by the time I count to twenty-five. Then if it doesn't ring I count to a new number. It makes me so nervous I can't concentrate on anything else and I'm always yelling at everybody else in the family to get off the phone if they're using it.

Like Lee-ann, many said they don't feel as if they have much control over their social life. They think it's up to the boy to make the call, so they have no choice but to sit and wait for the phone to ring. Then they feel rejected if no one calls. Boys at least have to make a move to be rejected; girls can feel rejected by not doing anything at all!

As you can see, we're talking about male-female relationships. That's because most people in our society do have heterosexual dates and heterosexual life-styles. But in homosexual (same sex) dating the same divisions can take place. Some people get stuck in the mover role—always doing the asking, making the first moves, making the plans, and other people get stuck in the waiting-around-to-be-asked role. (You may want to read pp. 112–23 for more discussion of homosexuality.)

It takes some self-confidence to move against traditional values and expectations. Evie said that at her high school in Seattle where people act as if they're interested in changing, she has felt put down by some boys:

> A lot of guys I know don't like it when a girl comes on to them. So that makes me hesitate to make the first move or ask a guy out because I'm afraid that he'll be totally shocked by it and then lose respect for me.

Basically, Evie is saying that she's worried that if she asks a boy out he might say no. That's the same worry Max has. The difference is that Evie has to go against years of tradition to ask a boy out. She's risking rejection as well as being thought "weird," and that certainly takes courage.

Whenever you make a move, especially if it's an original move, there's always the chance that you won't be accepted. It's the same in everything—relationships, job applications, school elections, choosing a college, anything you have to try for. It hurts to be rejected, but as Leroy, one of the teens who helped us edit the book, said:

All they can do is say no. And then you have to say to yourself, Well, nice try, Leroy, you gave it a shot.

Sally, a senior from Boston, explained that to her it's more important to act according to what she thinks is right. And Sally doesn't think that girls should always have to wait to be asked. She said:

I always approach guys when I want to. And I've met very few guys who are afraid of that or who shy away from that. It always blows me away when I run into a guy who says, "I can't go out with you because you asked me, I didn't ask you." I wouldn't really want to go out with someone who was so uncomfortable with himself that he'd feel that way.

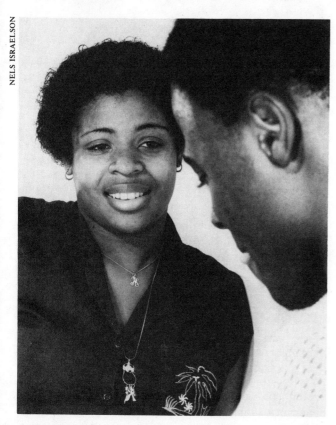

As we found out during our interviews, there are plenty of boys around the country who would appreciate Sally's willingness to move first. In Wisconsin seventeen-year-old Alex said:

I think it's great when a girl calls up a guy to ask him out. A lot of guys are shy, like I was shy for a long time. It was hell for me to ask a girl out. And a lot

of the girls I know are much less shy than I am, so it makes me feel wonderful when one of them asks me out.

The Double Standard

Sex is another area in which traditional attitudes about what's good for girls and what's good for boys can get to be a burden. Kenny, a fourteen-year-old ninth-grader from Pennsylvania, said:

Where I used to live the guys had to go out and get laid. That was the attitude. All right, you're fourteen or fifteen, so go out and get laid. There was real pressure on you, like they'd say, "Whatsa matta, you some kind of sissy?" or "Whatsa matta, you don't like girls?" If you weren't acting like a sex maniac everybody thought there was something wrong with you. But it was the opposite for the girls. They heard, "Stay pure. Save yourself. Don't be cheap."

This is called the double standard because separate and opposite standards are set for boys and for girls. We are judged by different ideas of what's "right" when it comes to sex. Boys are told they're supposed to "get as much as they can." Girls learn that it's up to them to keep their date from "going too far." Whether or not we agree, those ideas create a false sense of what's "normal," and since most of us want to be "normal," it can make us feel we have to conform.

We heard stories about the double standard all over the country, in Des Moines, Los Angeles, Detroit, Boston, New York, Washington, Denver, Seattle, New Orleans, Dallas and everywhere else we visited. Henry, a fifteen-year-old from Texas, told us:

In our school if you don't go around bragging about how far you got and what you did with the girl you were out with, well, then they start calling you fag or queer or something like that. I think it's totally stupid. I think most guys lie about how far they go and what they do just to keep their image up.

Henry said there's a lot of pressure on the boys in his neighborhood to "get laid," and so for many boys, dating becomes a kind of contest: get as much as you can as soon as you can. He says that's considered a test of a boy's manliness.

On the other hand, in Detroit sixteen-year-old Diana said:

You know how it's OK for a guy to go around telling everybody about how horny he is and bragging about how he's going to get some this weekend. Well, if a girl ever said those things everybody would call her a slut.

We're supposed to get the idea that there are "nice" girls who know how to control themselves and "bad" girls who are loose and let boys get their way. Leah, a sixteen-year-old from New York, told us that she's perfectly "nice" by most people's standards. She gets good grades and she's on Student Council and she's going to go to college when she graduates. But, she said:

> I really shocked this boy I went out with because I had intercourse with him so soon. He kept expecting me to stop him, but I didn't. He told me afterwards that he never expected me to be *that way*. I guess he had the image that nice girls don't do that.

Leah said she felt her date would have been a lot happier if she had stopped him, because he didn't really want to have sex with her in the first place. He just thought that she'd think he was strange if he didn't try anything.

The problem with the double standard is exactly that: it doesn't allow people to act according to their own feelings. Many boys said they feel pushed into having sex before they really want to, because they think that's how they're supposed to behave. And many girls cover up and control their sexual feelings because they worry about getting a bad reputation. (See the Sexuality chapters for more discussion on this, especially p. 67).

A lot of teenagers told us that they themselves buy into those attitudes. Girls expect boys to want sex all the time—and think there's something wrong with a boy who doesn't. And boys push for more but expect "nice" girls to stop them. They force each other to keep playing the same games.

All of us feel turned on sometimes and not at others. All of us have a right to choose not to have a sexual relationship until we want it and feel ready for it. And when we do feel ready to have sex, we want to be able to act on our feelings in a way that doesn't hurt or take advantage of anyone, without having to worry that our "reputation" is at stake.

Penny, an eleventh-grader from New York, said she found out how mistaken her attitude about boys was when this happened:

> In one of our classes the guys and the girls had to switch roles for a day. We were supposed to try to imagine what it's like to be the other one and act that way. The guy I did it with said he thought it would be so much better to be a girl because you wouldn't have to worry about knowing what to do or have to be smooth and cool and all that crap. He said the pressure is always on the guy to perform.
>
> I just couldn't believe he was saying those things because I always thought how much easier it would be to be a guy. You wouldn't have to worry about how you looked or how you acted. You could do whatever you felt like doing without worrying about your reputation.
>
> But he said, of course guys worry about their reputation, but it's the opposite kind of reputation. He said they have to put on this big act about how expe-

rienced they are. He told me it's really hard for him to take off his clothes in front of a girl because he gets embarrassed too. He worries about whether the girl will think he's attractive and everything. He worries that he won't do the right thing or say the right thing.

> That really helped me see how guys and girls have a lot of the same hang-ups. If only we would talk more about it with each other, that would take a lot of the pressure off. But everybody assumes the other person has it all together, so everybody's afraid to open their mouth.

Falling in Love

When two people fall in love with each other, they create a kind of joy between them. Each appreciates the other. Each feels content with the other. As their love develops, the level of their trust and commitment to each other deepens. The more they get to know each other, the closer they feel.

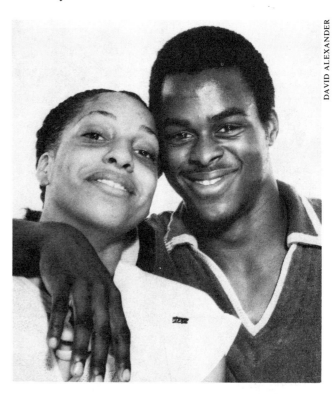

DAVID ALEXANDER

Many people fall in love during their teenage years. Sometimes it turns into a respectful, long-lasting love. More often it is an intense emotional experience that lasts awhile and then changes.

This kind of short-term relationship can be very exciting. Thirteen-year-old Janet told us:

> I went to a party with my boyfriend and at the party I was slow-dancing with another boy and I fell in love with him. I didn't want to hurt my boyfriend's feelings, but I really wanted to be with the other boy.

When he touched me I got shivers all over my body. While we were dancing I felt like we were floating on a cloud.

If you've ever felt the way Janet's describing, you know how intense it can be. Some people find they can't eat or sleep or concentrate on anything other than the person they care about. There's often a lot of fantasy—daydreaming about the other person and making up romantic love scenes in your head. Fourteen-year-old Bruce said:

I'm reading a book or watching TV and all of sudden it's me and Wendy in the story, off alone somewhere kissing and touching and staring into each other's eyes.

Often one person is more involved in the infatuation than the other. Sometimes, in fact, you can become seriously infatuated with someone you don't really know at all. Noelle told us:

In the eighth grade I was really in love with Burt Reynolds. I thought about him every second. I went to see every one of his movies and anytime he was on TV I'd have to stay home to watch. It used to make my parents very mad, because sometimes they'd planned something for the family to do and I would refuse to go because I had to watch TV. I wrote him a couple of letters and once I got a letter back from him. That meant a lot to me, because I just knew that if he met me, he'd fall in love with me too.

It's painful to have strong feelings for someone who doesn't return your affection. Brendan, a sixteen-year-old sophomore from Texas, is experiencing that right now. He said:

I really have a pretty bad crush on my friend's sister. She's a little older than me and I already know she won't got out with me because I asked her and she said no. She was real nice about it, but it was still no. The trouble is, I can't stop thinking that we could really get it on together if she'd just give me a chance. But, you know, you can like somebody all you want. If they don't like you, there's nothing you can do about it.

It's even more painful when you are still in love with someone who's no longer in love with you. Several teenagers we met were going through deep depressions over breaking up with their boyfriend or girlfriend. It can be a very serious time in a person's life. You may feel that nothing else is important, that nothing's worth it anymore. Seventeen-year-old Geri described her feelings this way:

I just feel like my life's over, like there's never going to be anything to smile about again.

Although time has a way of healing the wounds caused by a broken romance, while you are experiencing the grief you may feel like Geri, that you'll never be happy again.

DON'T KILL THE FIRE

Don't kill the fire.
Water is poison, it kills instantly.
It's my child. The flames are the stretched-out hands
Longing for a handshake.
They are twisting impatiently in a graceful dance,
Trying to please you,
Not knowing about their inevitable death.
Oh, baby! What a gullible child!
    it gives you everything
You need: warmth.

It can't ask you questions
It just listens to your overburdened breathing.
    Crackles. It understands you.
Trust it! It's a little sun
    Shining for you in the dark.
You are cruel! Don't feed it with wood
Anticipating its death.
It's just like feeding an animal before its slaughter.
So you can get more fat.

Oh silly! It trusts you.
It takes your generous charity
And gets warmer
    Not like me
    I don't like short favors
Don't kill the fire.
Be tender with it.
Nurse it.
And I promise it'll give you the best of itself.
Be its brother.
Please, please, don't kill the fire.
You are killing all the warmth
    there is
        left on this earth.

—Anonymous

Usually it helps to talk over your feelings with a close friend, or your folks if you feel close to them.

Many of the teenagers we spoke with asked, "How can I be sure I'm in love?" It's an important question that doesn't have a definite answer. Emotions can't be weighed or measured, so everyone has a different definition of what it is to be in love. Seventeen-year-old Becky said:

I've been going with Don since the ninth grade and we've changed a lot together. That's why I know he's right for me. We're really compatible. We hardly fight at all. We really respect each other, so if something's wrong, we can work it out between us. That's not how it always was, so we've come a long way. In fact, I don't think I've seen a better relationship in people my age. But still, sometimes I think, I wonder what it would be like to be with somebody else. I see some guy and I think, Oh, look at him. I wonder what it would be like to be with him? When I think that, it scares me, because I worry about whether that means I don't really love Don.

During the romantic and absorbing first stage of love, you may not have any doubts at all. Everything may seem perfect. Then when questions start coming up—and they *always* do—you may not want to let yourself think about them. You may try to push them aside and get back to the way things were, but without this questioning stage, growth of your relationship is hard to achieve.

Several teens we talked to said they don't want to be disloyal to their boyfriend or girfriend, but they'd like to see what it's like to go out with someone else. That thought can be scary because it might mean breaking up a steady relationship. Seventeen-year-old Nelson, a senior from Los Angeles, said:

I think it would be hard to break up, especially after three years. I wouldn't know where to begin if Debby and I decided to stop going steady. I'd just be out in the cold saying to myself, What do I do now?

Lots of people stay in relationships because they're afraid to break up. It's comforting to know that you'll always have a date for the weekend and that someone cares about you and is choosing to spend time with you. But fear—fear of being alone, fear of going out with new people, fear of hurting the other person's feelings, fear of being rejected—is not a healthy basis for a relationship. If your love is going to grow, you have to get past fear.

Sometimes people even allow the comfort of a steady relationship to lead them into marriage before they have cleared up their questions. They confuse feeling glad to be with each other with wanting to marry each other. Elizabeth, a second-year college student from Colorado, is very concerned about that distinction. She told us:

I've been thinking about it so much lately, and I'm beginning to realize that I'm just not ready to make a commitment. There's no way I could settle down right now. There's just no way. My boyfriend is much more ready to settle down. He's older than me, and he's done more already, so he feels more prepared, I think.

But it's really hard for me when I'm around these friends of mine who really think they love each other enough to get married. It's a lot of pressure on me because it makes me feel like I want to be in love like that too and settle down. It seems so romantic. They seem so sure that their lover is the person they want to be with for always and always. I just don't know that yet. I don't think I feel that way. Sometimes I wish I did, but I just don't. I've got too many other things I want to do first.

Love can seem so wonderful, so romantic, but making a long-term commitment to someone is a serious matter.

Doubts are natural because so much is at stake. Take the time you need to examine your questions and explore your fears. If you can be open with each other about what you're doing, that will help a lot.

Some people may say, "Forget it. Love can conquer all." But the question isn't whether love can conquer all. The question is, Are you ready for marriage?

Marriage

With the divorce rate so high, some of the teens we spoke with said they don't trust marriage. They said they can't see any reason to get married. Carol-Anne, a senior from Ohio, said:

I never think about marrying anybody. In my entire life I have seen one good marriage. That's disgusting.

Sixteen-year-old Aaron said:

The only reason I can see getting married is to raise a family, and right now I don't think I want to have kids anyway.

You may feel the way Carol-Anne and Aaron do. Perhaps your own parents are divorced or separated, or maybe you know lots of other couples who are.

Some people agree with the singing group Pink Floyd, who say that our lives force us to build walls around ourselves. Instead of making commitments, we barricade ourselves behind our own private wall built of disappointing experiences.

Marriage is really a leap of faith across that wall. Friendship is another leap of faith, and so is parenthood, certainly. When two or more people make a commitment to each other, it's based on faith that they will respect each other and not take advantage of each other, that they will protect each other. There aren't any guarantees.

Marriage is a partnership, and like any partnership it works only as well as the two partners allow it to work. Before you decide to get married, look at the partnership you have and ask yourself if it is one you will be able to live with.

It's usually difficult to know at age eighteen or nineteen what you will want for yourself at age twenty-five or thirty. People change a lot during those years. That's why many teenagers we talked to are choosing to wait before making a long-term commitment. Larry, a seventeen-year-old senior from Ohio, put his feelings this way:

I'm looking forward to going away to college next year even though me and my girlfriend think we want to get married someday. I'm ready to meet some new people and have some new experiences. Not to take away from what I have, just to find out some more. I can't imagine getting married before I find out as much as I can about myself.

SEXUALITY

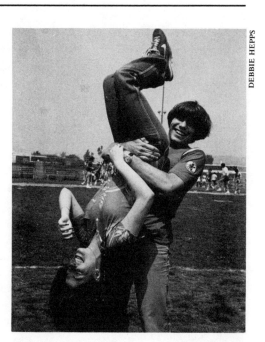

People often think that being sexual means making love with someone. They think you aren't "sexual" until you actually start having sex. Watch any naked baby and you'll see this isn't true. Babies explore their bodies, love to be held and stroked, and often fondle their genitals when they can find them. From the beginning, we are all sexual.

Being sexual can mean having sexy thoughts or feelings, loving to be touched, enjoying the way other people's bodies look, touching your body in places that feel particularly good, making up romantic or sexy stories in your head that you might or might not ever act out, kissing and touching someone you feel attracted to. All these things can be part of your sexuality. In fact, if and when you do make love with someone, you will continue to be sexual in these other ways, too. Sexuality is much fuller and more varied than just lovemaking.

The body changes of puberty often bring stronger sexual feelings. You may find yourself thinking more about sex, getting sexually aroused more easily, even at times feeling preoccupied with sex. Several teenagers described walking down the street or sitting on the bus feeling as if their whole body was on fire with sexual energy, and excitement.

Sometimes people don't feel sexual at all. They get busy, or excited about sports or school or music or a job or something else in their lives, and don't even have many sexual feelings. It is sometimes said that teenagers are all wild about sex. You know from yourself and your friends that this isn't necessarily true. You may not even be thinking much about sex at this point. This doesn't mean that you aren't or won't be sexual, but that right now you are putting your energy into other things.

*Because different teenagers are at so many different places about sex, we are writing this section with no as-*sumptions *about you and what you have or haven't done.* You may be having lots of sexual feelings these days or not many. You may or may not masturbate: that is, spend private time with yourself touching your penis or clitoris and making yourself feel good. You may have kissed or not, French-kissed or not, taken your clothes off with someone or not. You may not have made love with someone, or you may have just started.

You may have been taught that sex before marriage is wrong, or that it is OK. You may be amazed that some fourteen-year-olds who talk in this section have made love already, or amazed that some eighteen-year-olds aren't interested. You may be attracted to people of the opposite sex or people of your same sex, or both. You may have friends who pressure you to go all the way, or friends who say people who "do it" are dirty. You may be excited about reading a chapter on sex, or a little shocked, and even worried that it will make you feel that you "ought" to be doing or feeling something you're not.

Our main aim in this section is for you to feel good about your sexuality and what you do with it. This includes everything to do with you as an individual person: your feelings and daydreams, your physical sexual responses, your sexual exploration with yourself. These are aspects of sexuality, whether or not you are being sexual with someone else.

We also hope the discussion here will help you know how you want to bring sexuality into your relationships: to feel good about being sexual with someone else when you are both ready for that, to say no when that's right for you, to hurt as few people as possible (including yourself!).

In this section teenagers talk about the things they do and feel about sex. We hope what they say will help you understand your own feelings better—whatever they are.

MOVING AT YOUR OWN SPEED

> At any point in this sexuality section we may be talking about something that you don't believe is right, or that you haven't done or felt. Maybe you will someday, maybe you won't. Our main message is this: Move at your own speed. Do only what you are sure you want to do, or at least as sure as you can be. As a seventeen-year-old boy said, "If you're in doubt, wait!"

Don't be surprised if you're not always sure what you want. Sexual feelings can be intense and confusing. It is often difficult to be perfectly "sure" and "decided" about what you want to do. Maybe you will decide only *after* trying something that you wish you hadn't. If this happens, you can stop. Perhaps having decided not to do something, you'll wish you had. Sometimes you will conclude that postponing any decision at all is the best way to handle your mixed feelings.

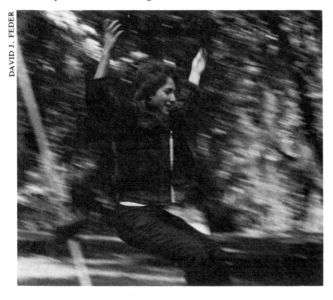

DAVID J. FEDER

People make mistakes. In fact, a lot of what we learn comes from making mistakes. Some mistakes in sex are serious, and we hope this book will help you avoid those. Others are just part of learning.

Where sex is concerned, teenagers get pressure from all sides. Some people say, "Don't do XYZ—it's wrong!" Other people say, "Do XYZ—it's great!" XYZ in this case might be masturbation, French-kissing, oral sex, sleeping with someone of the same sex or the opposite sex. Your parents, friends, school, government, church or temple will all have something to say about sex, and their views are often important. But when the moment comes, you are the one who has to decide. Or, if you are involved with someone else, you and that person decide together.

Reading a book like this and talking honestly with your friends may help you be clearer about what you are ready for and what your values are. Whatever you do, we encourage you to be decent to yourself and the people you are sexual with. This means:

—Not letting yourself be rushed into anything.
—Not rushing someone else into anything.
—Not feeling you have to prove how great you are by how much sexual experience you have.
—Not blaming yourself endlessly for mistakes.
—Taking responsibility. This means using birth control if you need it, and telling a partner if you have a sexually transmitted disease (and getting treatment immediately).
—Feeling free to enjoy what you do once you have decided to do it.

Moving at your own speed is important, because sex can feel terrific if you are ready and not so great if you are not. This is true of everything from masturbation to kissing to making love. A seventeen-year-old girl from the West Coast had this to say:

> I have at least fifty, maybe even sixty, more years of being sexual, and I'm sure I don't have to worry about doing everything right now.

III EXPLORING SEX WITH YOURSELF

LEARNING ABOUT SEX

Much of what we learn about sex isn't what is told to us directly. We learn by watching what goes on around us. Some things we just absorb, depending on who's in our family. Karen, a fifteen-year-old from California, said:

I remember taking showers with my brothers all the time, so I always knew how boys looked naked. Then when I got in about the sixth grade and I started knowing about sex, and we had those sex education movies, I'd think to myself, Oh yeah, that's like my brothers.

Lots of children go beyond Karen and do "research" on their own. Polly is from New York:

There was this one girl in our class—her name was Nancy—that me and my girlfriends used to play doctor with and she was always the patient. We would make her take her pants off and we'd pretend to stick her with things, like giving her a needle, you know, and we'd go up to this room we have in our attic where we knew we could be private. Even now I can remember it being sort of thrilling to me that she would take off her pants.

Like Polly, you may have games you used to play that let you do some early exploring of bodies and sexual feelings. Jeff remembers:

I was always experimenting with sex, ever since I was really little. Like even at nursery school, it made no difference to me whether it was with a boy or a girl, we'd roll around together and feel each other and get naked together. It was no big thing, just fun. And of course it felt good. My mother wasn't too crazy about it, though. She kept asking me why didn't I go out and play or ride my bike or something. She wasn't mean or anything, she just let me know that she didn't think it was so cool to be doing what I was doing.

Maybe Jeff's mother was uncomfortable with his sex play because *her* parents had reacted that way when she was young. Indirectly she was teaching him something about sex. Maybe a question entered his head: "Is what I'm doing OK?"

Coleen's mother was more strict:

My mother came into my room and found me masturbating one day when I was ten, and she couldn't handle it at all. "Don't do that!" she said. "It's wrong! You'll hurt yourself!" I was terrified. For years whenever I masturbated I felt this shame, you know?

Coleen's mother had probably been taught that masturbation was wrong, and was passing on the message (for more on this, see p. 80).

Parents also teach us about sex by how they are with each other and how they feel about their own sexuality. For example, some parents are comfortable being openly affectionate in front of their children. For others, sex is a more private thing, and their kids rarely see them even kiss and hug. This might make you more shy and private about sex. If your parents talk freely and in a relaxed way about sex, this will make a difference.

We also learn by how our parents handle nudity. If your parents are strict about nakedness, they may teach you to feel your body is something to hide. If they are more relaxed, you may be, too. But some people whose parents are very open about nudity feel as they get older that they want more privacy for themselves.

People also learn about sex (as we mentioned in the "Changing Bodies" chapter) through books, movies, magazines, jokes, advertising, locker rooms, friends. These sources sometimes give you inaccurate information, however, and may carry attitudes about sex that make it seem dirty. Watch out for "commercial sex." It's often associated with exploitation in one way or another.

The "facts" of sex may come from courses in school,

sex manuals, discussion groups, talks with parents or counselors. Often you learn the most when you first start having a boyfriend or girlfriend. But how you *feel* about your body, as opposed to what you *know,* comes mostly in the indirect ways we've described—especially from the attitudes you pick up, and from how the people who are important in your life respond to their own sexuality and to yours.

FEELING BAD ABOUT SEX

Our bodies are sexually responsive. Our skin is sensitive to touch. Our minds get turned on to sexy pictures, thoughts and fantasies. Sex connects us to other people: being with someone we like or love a lot and feel attracted to can be a great delight. But along with the pleasure and joy that sex of all kinds can bring, people often feel bad or guilty about what they are doing.

Feeling *private* about sex is different from feeling guilty or bad. Nearly everyone feels private—or shy sometimes—about sex no matter how old they are. No amount of sex education will change a certain natural mystery there is about sex. A father of a fifteen-year-old girl said:

No matter how open and informative I've been with my daughter about sex, she still keeps her sexual feelings very secret. So do I, in fact. With all the information you can have, sex is still pretty awe-inspiring. Sexuality is such a powerful influence in my life that I always feel a certain privateness about my sexual feelings. This seems right to me.

But sometimes we are made to feel guilty as well as private. Lots of teenagers talk about feeling ''dirty'' or ''sleazy'' about some part of their sexuality. As a fifteen-year-old boy said about masturbating, ''I always wonder, Am I the only pervert, or is everyone doing this?'' And Cedric, a seventeen-year-old from Providence, said, ''When I had my first wet dream, I was really excited about it, but I felt guilty at being so excited.'' Several girls spoke of feeling some shame when they started their periods. Boys and girls mentioned feeling ashamed sometimes about having a sexual body and sexual impulses.

These guilty feelings may come because some influential person or group in your life believes that a certain sexual act is bad, and has taught you to think so. Society has disapproved of sex outside of marriage, of homosexuality, and of certain sexual practices like masturbation and oral sex which are just for pleasure and having nothing to do with creating children. Rules have been made about these things, and we are told not to break the rules.

Our Western culture has been negative about sex for centuries. Maybe this started back when there was no dependable birth control and having sex usually meant pregnancy. Also, sexual feelings are powerful enough to make people do things that they later wish they hadn't. Some of the rules about sex may come from fear of this power. Sex also brings pleasure, and some people believe that physical, sensual, sexual pleasure is just plain wrong or sinful. And finally, some religious traditions have called the body ''bad'' and the spirit or mind ''good,'' which has made many people feel guilty about being sexual at all.

These negative voices don't stop us from being sexual—they just mean we often feel bad about what we do. We who are writing this book believe that a lot of society's moralistic attitudes and rules about sex can make people feel *unnecessarily guilty* about feelings and activities that are part of being human. This can have some unfortunate effects. For example, some of us who felt guilty about masturbating as children—let's say, a parent caught us and told us it was a bad thing to do—may find we have trouble enjoying ourselves later on with a partner. Young men who feel guilty about sex may have problems with coming too quickly (see p. 111), and girls may have trouble enjoying lovemaking. It's hard to let yourself go and feel all the pleasure if some part of you is thinking, I shouldn't be doing this.

A couple may have trouble talking openly to each other about sex because they feel somehow they ''shouldn't'' be having sex at all. And many teenagers say that often they ''forget'' to use birth control because they feel a little guilty about having intercourse. They don't want to use birth control because that means ''getting ready'' for sex, admitting to themselves what they are doing. Feeling guilty, then, makes them risk pregnancy.

It will take all of us time to get over unnecessary guilt about our sexuality. We hope this book will help.

Everyone has values about sex—that is, everyone thinks some things are right and some wrong. Those of us who wrote this book do too. But our values are somewhat different from many of the traditional ones. To us, being sexual and having sexual feelings is part of who we are, and part of what we bring into loving someone else. Sex can bring energy and closeness and fun. It draws people to each other. Our concern is with how we *use* sex. To us it's bad if you do something that hurts yourself or another person. Here are some examples:

Maybe you are doing something that's not right for you, or that you're not ready for. Leah, who's sixteen, said:

Anything you're not sure you're ready to do, you feel dirty. Say you're twelve or thirteen and a boy touches your breasts and you weren't sure you wanted him to, you'll feel dirty. It's the same with screwing someone later on, if you're not sure.

Maybe you are pressuring someone into doing something they aren't ready to do. Boys often pressure girls because they are under pressure themselves from their friends and the macho culture to ''get'' as much as they can from a girl. At its worst, this pressure is rape (see p. 124). Girls also sometimes pressure boys to go further than they want to in sex. They may do it indirectly by implying that a boy isn't manly if he doesn't want to do more than kiss.

Maybe you are hurting someone by what you are doing. For example, pretending to be ''serious'' when you're not, or fooling around with someone else's boyfriend or girlfriend without thinking whether someone will be hurt. Where love and romantic relationships are concerned, there may always be some hurting, even if you usually try to be good to people in your life. But there are limits beyond which you know you are hurting someone unnecessarily.

Maybe you're not using birth control. Maybe you have gonorrhea or herpes or some other sexually transmitted disease (STD—see p. 216) and haven't told your partner or gotten treatment.

As far as we are concerned, it makes sense to feel bad about doing things like these because they are harmful and inconsiderate.

SEX ON YOUR MIND: SEXUAL FANTASIES

Everyone has fantasies or daydreams or dreams in our sleep. We all spend time wondering, hoping, wishing, fearing and imagining. Fantasies are like stories that come into our mind in which we are often one of the main figures. When you begin to have stronger sexual feelings and attractions, a lot of your dreams or fantasies may become sexual too. If you find yourself dreaming about your teacher, or imagining a passionate romance with your favorite singer, or wishing you could run away with your best friend's brother, don't be surprised.

Fantasies are a safe way to explore your feelings. Fantasies are thoughts—they are under your control. You don't have to act them out unless you want to. Thoughts can't hurt other people; only actions can. Jerome, who's fifteen, put it this way:

My fantasies are all about things I'd never really do in real life—in fact, that's almost the definition of a fantasy for me: something I'd never really do. Then I feel free to do it in my mind without feeling guilty. Usually the things in my imagination would be real embarrassing to me, really humiliating if I was ever in one of those situations. Like lying naked in the lunch yard and having everyone standing over me, pointing at me, laughing at me. Or, they are dreams about hurting someone else, like pulling someone's clothes off. I know I would never do those things, but just fantasizing about them makes them exciting. It's like having something and not having it at the same time.

Jerome knows that thinking about something doesn't necessarily mean he wants to do it. He's just enjoying some of the less explored territory of his mind.

Here are three other fantasies people told us. Like Je-

rome's, they are about imaginary situations that are very erotic (sexually exciting) to the person having them:

I dream about diving into a swimming pool full of red jello. I swim around and swim around and it's thick and cool, and I bury my face in it. It feels so far out.

I dream about being covered in whipped cream and some stranger comes and licks it all off.

Whenever I'm on the subway I have this fantasy that all the women are naked. They have their shoes on and their purses and packages and everything, but no clothes on.

Thirteen-year-old Kathleen's fantasies are more about a real-life situation. They make the limits of her life more tolerable:

I think about my boyfriend all the time. Like especially when I'm watching TV or reading something romantic and they're kissing, then I think, Oh God, I wish he were here. We barely ever get a chance to kiss, because we're not allowed to in school, and that's about the only place we see each other. My mom thinks I'm too young to have a boyfriend, so she doesn't let him come over. I mean we've tried to see each other, but it never works out. So mostly I just spend my time dreaming about him and what it would be like to be alone with him somewhere—just the two of us. Sometimes I practice kissing with my pillow, dreaming that we're making out.

When Kathleen finally gets to be with her boyfriend, maybe things will be as terrific as she has imagined. This was true for Dan, who's sixteen:

Sometimes you fantasize about somebody you really like and then you find out that they really like you too. That happened to me with this girl I used to go out with. I used to daydream about how wonderful it would be to be with her and then we really did get together and it *was* wonderful.

For Oliver, however, the fantasies were better than the reality:

When I was in junior high school I found that my fantasies were a lot more pleasurable than the reality. In my imagination I could make things work perfectly and be with just who I wanted to be with but the reality of it at the time wasn't anywhere near as great. In fact I was really awkward with girls and had trouble getting it on with them—but in my fantasy world I was really smooth.

While your sexual feelings are blossoming, you may get a fierce crush on someone completely impossible. It may be a teacher or camp counselor, the youth director at the Y, someone several grades ahead of you in school, or a performer. Darcy told us:

When I was ten I used to have such a crush on Sean Cassidy. I used to daydream about him all the time—

in school, while I was walking home, before I went to sleep. I really thought I would meet him and he would fall in love with me—if only we could meet. I would sit around and plan how to meet him.

Crushes like this are fine if you don't suffer too much over not being able to have the person you yearn for. They give you a chance to explore your sexual feelings.

A fantasy may be about someone of your own sex (a "homosexual" fantasy). This may mean that you are trying out feelings and possibilities that you will never choose to act on. It could also mean that you would like to have a sexual relationship with someone of your own sex—anything from kissing and hugging to making love (see p. 112 for information on homosexual relationships). Many people have a homosexual relationship at some point. For some it is a brief experience; for others it is a way of life.

Having same-sex fantasies, however, doesn't predict one way or the other whether you will have a homosexual relationship in the future. Eric, seventeen, told us:

> I have a dream sometimes that I'm lying on the beach and these two big muscley guys come over to me and tell me what a great body I have. They stick around talking for a while and then we take our suits off and go swimming. I wake up excited and feeling sexy.

Sometimes we dream or fantasize that sex is being forced on us. These fantasies can be repulsive or scary even though they are sexually exciting. *Do I really want that?* the person asks in a panic. The answer is usually no, but people do worry that fantasizing something means you really want it. Gloria speaks for the fears of many girls:

> I have these fantasies about being raped, like when I'm walking home from school I imagine that I'm pulled into a car and this man with dark hair and blue eyes pulls off my skirt and underpants and forces me to have sex with him. Right there in the car. It scares me to think about that because it makes me wonder if I really want to be raped.

Rape is an ugly reality in our lives these days. Real rape is very, very different from fantasy rape. It is a violent, not a sexual, act (see p. 124). Yet many women who have been raped actually wonder if *they* are responsible, because they have occasionally had fantasies of sex being forced on them. *This is not true at all.* Rape fantasies often reflect real anxieties about being a female in today's world.

Rape fantasies can also be a way of letting you imagine yourself having sex. Our society often makes teenagers feel guilty about having sexual desires. Sometimes the easiest way to picture having sex with someone is to imagine that it is forced on you. This may become clearer when you read these fantasies:

> John (seventeen): A lot of guys I know have this same fantasy about being with a couple of really huge women who are whipping them and forcing them to get undressed and have sex with them. In my fantasy it's always in a sleazy motel room and there are two women who hold me down and take turns with me.

> Susan (nineteen): I have this very exciting daydream about a woman and a man coming to my house and making me have sex with both of them before I can leave.

> Gary (fifteen): I fantasize about older women. I like the idea of being seduced by an older woman, someone who knows what she wants, so you don't have to be put in that decision-making position. I get really turned on thinking about an aggressive woman who'll just lead me through the steps.

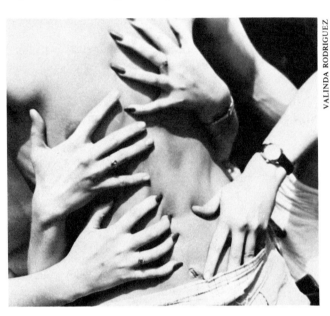

VALINDA RODRIGUEZ

These fantasies all have the same theme. Thinking about being forced into sex or being seduced lets you enjoy the turned-on feeling without having to imagine yourself being the one to start it. People also have fantasies of being hurt—whipped, tied up, beaten—and of hurting others. Again, these are ways of exploring sexual feelings, not a statement of what a person wants in real life.

Fantasies are mostly fun. If you have fantasies about things that frighten you, remember that fantasies are often a way your mind has of dealing with your real-life fears. However, occasionally a person will find herself or himself spending nearly all day and night in fantasies. They may come to seem more real than reality. Or your fantasies might be so strong and so vivid that you fear you might actually act them out. This is especially scary if they are fantasies of violence, of hurting someone or of letting yourself be hurt. In cases like these, it is a good idea to talk about your fantasies and fears with someone you trust—a parent or other relative, or a teacher or counselor. See Chapter VI for ways of deciding whom you would most want to talk to.

MASTURBATION

Masturbation usually means touching, rubbing or squeezing your penis or clitoris, to give yourself sexual pleasure. Sexual thoughts and fantasies may fill your mind at the same time. If you keep it up long enough, you will often have an orgasm—rhythmic waves of muscle contractions in your genitals which feel very good. Masturbation is something you do with yourself, a way of giving pleasure to yourself, of loving and being tender to yourself. It also helps you to get to know your body's sexual responses.

Many teenagers told us that masturbating lets them enjoy their sexuality when they aren't in a relationship with someone or if they don't want their relationship to be sexual. But masturbating is also part of your relationship to yourself even if you are with someone else.

Not everyone masturbates, of course. Lots of people have never done it or don't want to. You may read this section to see what other people do, and decide it's not for you at this point in your life. As Cecily, sixteen, said:

I wouldn't masturbate, but if someone else does, that's their decision.

Most babies and little children masturbate. They touch themselves all over, exploring this part and that, finding the places that feel especially good. Greg, who's seventeen, said, "I've always masturbated, at least for as long as I can remember." Beth, who's sixteen, remembered:

When I was little I used to rub against things, like the corner of my mattress or this one stuffed animal I had which had a perfect nose for rubbing against my crotch. So I would go around rubbing this animal against me all the time. I don't think I really had an orgasm, it was more like after a while I would just get tired and stop.

Many children stop this kind of body play when they get to be a few years old, often because a grown-up pulls their hands away or tells them that touching themselves "there" is bad. Other children continue to have a good time masturbating privately. Sam, who's eleven, said:

I like sleeping with my hand down there; I guess it just helps me feel relaxed. Sometimes I don't even know I'm doing it, but I'll wake up and that's where my hand will be.

A lot of people rediscover masturbation when they get to be teenagers and find their stronger sexual feelings need an outlet. A fourteen-year-old boy from Washington state told us:

Around the time when I was just starting junior high school I was changing a lot and feeling really sexual and learning all about sex. All this tension started building up, and for me masturbating was a way of releasing it. It still is.

Emily also discovered masturbation in junior high:

You know, I never even knew that girls could masturbate. I mean I probably did it when I was a baby, but I don't remember. One day I overheard a conversation some kids were having at school, and one guy asked a girl if girls could masturbate and she said "Of course." And she was telling him how great it felt and everything, so that night when I was in bed I started feeling around down there and I started getting these sexy sensations and I got really aroused. Right on that bone was the part I was pressing, I guess sort of rubbing. It felt amazing and I kept rubbing until these spasms of incredible feeling started happening. I couldn't rub after that because it was too tender, so I just lay there feeling good. I can't imagine how I went all those years without trying this before!

Privacy. Most people we talked to agreed that they like to masturbate in private, when they are alone with their own thoughts and feelings. Some mentioned masturbating with a friend. But even then, they wanted privacy from others. As Josh said:

It's a pretty vulnerable position to be in—caught with your hand on your cock, lost in your fantasies, working away at it. I don't think I'd want my mother or sister walking in on that!

Getting privacy can be hard, especially for kids, and especially in big families or if you share a bedroom with someone else. (Masturbating or not, time alone with yourself is important.) Darell had an upsetting thing happen:

One time I walked into my little brother's room to talk to him and he was whipping it and I scared the shit out of him. You know, he started yelling at me to get the hell out. He really was embarrassed—I mean really embarrassed. Probably he felt like he was doing something he shouldn't have been doing. I couldn't help laughing, but then I told him it was cool. I told him, "Hey, man, I do it too, you know." But he acted like he was getting busted for robbery or something.

Most of us get upset if our privacy is interrupted in the middle of a sexual experience. Even if we don't think what we are doing is "wrong" in any way, we may feel exposed, embarrassed, even ashamed: there is a natural privateness about sex.

How People Masturbate. Touching yourself is one of the most natural ways to explore your sexuality, to find out what excites you, what places are the most sensitive. There are lots of ways to masturbate because it's a very personal thing.

Girls usually rub around or near their clitoris, since that is the most sexually sensitive part of their body and can be stimulated with the slightest touch or pressure (see p. 25). But many also enjoy touching their breasts and other erotic (sexy) places at the same time. Some girls enjoy putting their finger in their vagina. Some girls like to wet their fingers with saliva before rubbing around their clitoris. Some masturbate using a spray of water from the shower or faucet; some rub against the sheets or pillow or some other soft object. Others use a small massaging machine called a vibrator on their clitoris and in their vagina. Some don't use their hands or an object at all but squeeze the muscles in and around their vagina and anus. For some, fantasies are enough. Ellie had this experience:

> One time when I was sixteen I was on this bus and I was sitting right over the wheel where it was vibrating a whole lot. I was fantasizing about this guy that I had just seen in the street and I was getting more and more into the fantasy. I was wearing a skirt, so my thighs were touching and rubbing together, and with the vibrations and everything I was so aroused that I had an orgasm, right there on the bus. In the middle of everything.

Boys usually masturbate by rubbing or stroking or pressing their penis and testicles. Some boys don't touch their penis with their hand at all but use sheets or a pillow or something else to rub around their genital area. Others tighten and release the muscles around their anus and pubic area. Still others bring themselves to orgasm by fantasy alone. Lots of boys combine fantasy and penis massage, as this fourteen-year-old describes:

> When I'm beating off I can get so much into a fantasy that it's almost like I'm really in it. There's this one very sexy girl that I always picture. I always watch her at school with her boyfriend. But when I'm masturbating she's with me, you know what I mean, and it's a real shock when I come out of it, after I come and I open my eyes and see my own room in my own apartment. What a letdown! But it sure is great while I'm into it.

How Much Do People Masturbate?   Some people don't masturbate at all, others not much. But for some it feels so good that they do it a lot. Bob, fifteen, was talking about this in a discussion group in Pennsylvania:

> Sometimes when I masturbate a whole lot I begin to feel like I must be a sex-starved maniac or something. You know you always hear that if you masturbate too much you'll end up crazy. I don't really believe that, but a lot of the time I feel like I should stop myself from whipping it too much.

Bob doesn't have to worry. Masturbating doesn't hurt you, and you can't really do it "too much" unless you make yourself sore, or unless you find yourself doing it so much that it interferes with other things you want to be doing.

Masturbation: Is It Wrong/Bad/Sinful/Dangerous/or Perverted?   People are more accepting of masturbation these days. But many adults grew up believing that mas-

turbation was wrong and actually harmful to the body. Max ran into this theory head-on:

> My grandparents gave me this book about bad little kids who masturbate. One of the bad little kids went blind, and another one had his thumbs cut off. Can you believe that? There was no doubt about the message in that book: *Don't Masturbate*. It was lucky for me that my parents were cool and didn't do that number on me.

If your parents or grandparents have punished you for masturbating or told you it would hurt you, it's probably because that's what they were told. Some doctors a generation or two ago thought it was harmful. Of course we know now that it isn't. Adults have also disapproved of children masturbating because it is sexual—it turns you on, it feels good, it lets you explore your sexuality. The thought that their children are doing something so sexual makes some parents uneasy.

Even today, however, the idea that masturbation is bad creeps in—and not just from adults. Ed told us this:

> When I was about thirteen I masturbated a couple of times but then I heard from the other guys that it would sap your strength and that it leads to becoming a pervert. So I sort of gave it up.

Ed's friends have misled him. It's too bad that he feels he has to fight his natural sexual urges.

Boys seem to talk about masturbation more than girls do, but it's often in a joking way that doesn't exactly make you feel great about what you are doing. Boys' slang words for masturbating have a joking and sometimes violent tone to them: jerking off, beating off, whipping it, pounding the pud, slamming the ham. These terms don't express the tenderness that you can feel when masturbating, when you're enjoying being alone with yourself and getting into your fantasies. That side of masturbation is probably less acceptable to talk about. The joking shows that even though boys are talking about it, they aren't completely accepting it as a good thing to do. Gene, a sixteen-year-old from New England, described this:

> Even if you know it's normal and all that, you still lock the door! You don't go around advertising that you're doing it. There are all those jokes like, "What are you doing after school today?" "Oh, I'm going home to beat off." You know, Ha-ha-ha. That kind of thing. Everybody does it, but they sort of pretend they don't.

Caddie, fifteen, describes her changing feelings about masturbation:

> When I was really little, my best girlfriend and I would sleep over at each other's house and we'd masturbate together in the same room. We even had our own name for it. We certainly didn't think there was anything wrong with what we were doing: it was just

something we did that felt good. But in about fourth grade I found out more about sex and I realized that masturbating was *sexual*. Then, as far as I was concerned, it was definitely not OK to do anymore—especially not with somebody else in the same room. After that I used to feel guilty when I was doing it, like it was kind of humiliating, and I tried to stop myself. Then last year when I heard from a lot of my girlfriends that they do it too, I felt better about it.

Caddie learned an important thing here (besides getting to enjoy masturbating again): talking with friends can help, because so often you find you're not alone in the things you were worrying about.

Masturbation and Lovemaking. Some people believe that masturbating will keep you from being able to enjoy sex with someone else. In fact, if and when you decide to make love with someone else, you may find that having masturbated helps you enjoy lovemaking more. It teaches you what makes you feel good, and you can communicate that to the person you are making love with.

Some people believe that once you are in a sexual relationship with someone else, you shouldn't masturbate anymore, and that masturbation isn't "as good as" sex with another person. But that's not the way it is: masturbation isn't better or worse, it's different, as fifteen-year-old Angela described:

You know, you can have a boyfriend and everything, even lots of boyfriends, but when you're home in bed at night and you feel sexy right at that minute, what's wrong with doing it yourself? Sometimes people think you only masturbate because you don't have anybody to go out with and so you have to get off by yourself. But I don't see it that way at all. One thing doesn't have anything to do with the other.

SEXUAL RESPONSE

Our bodies are alive to sexual feelings. We respond physically to a sexy thought, a scene in a movie, a kiss, the prospect of being with a person we're attracted to. A boy's penis may get hard or the lips of a girl's vagina get wet. These are the first signs of response to sexual excitement. Often it stops at that. If the excitement dies down, your penis will get soft or your vagina will stop making extra lubrication. But if the excitement keeps up, your whole body will go through a series of responses that are almost identical for males and females.

We will describe this process, sometimes called the sexual response cycle, so you can recognize what is happening in your body when you are sexually aroused. This is what the cycle is like: a buildup of excitement, a climax of excitement (called "orgasm" or "coming"), then a time when your body returns to a normal relaxed state. People don't always go through the whole cycle. For each person, each time, it may be a little different: you may get excited

and not have an orgasm, for instance, and your body will return to normal more slowly. *There is no particular pattern your body and feelings "should" follow.*

The first phase of sexual response is when you are getting excited. A boy's penis gets hard and a girl's vagina gets wet because extra blood from nearby blood vessels flows into areas of special spongy tissue inside the vaginal walls or in the penis. This tissue swells up, making the penis longer, wider and erect (as we described in detail on p. p. 13). The swelling makes the walls of the vagina "sweat"—that is, a liquid comes out from them and flows down to the entrance. A girl's clitoris also swells a bit and gets erect. In fact, her whole pelvic area has a full, aroused feeling. This swelling is called "vasocongestion," and the same process takes place in both boys' and girls' bodies.*

During this phase your breathing and heartbeat speed up and your blood pressure rises a little. A girl's vagina gets slightly larger and longer inside, and her breasts may swell slightly. People can stay in this excitement phase for a long time, moving in and out of it as the stimulation varies.

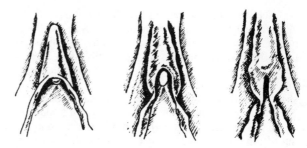

CLITORIS DURING SEXUAL EXCITEMENT

If the stimulation keeps up—if your penis or clitoris keeps getting stroked or your fantasies keep going—you will move into another phase in which you reach a high level of body tension and sexual arousal. Your muscles tighten, especially around your pelvic area and buttocks. A boy's testicles pull in closer to his body, and a girl's clitoris pulls in under the hood of skin attached to her inner lips. In this position, her clitoris can be stimulated by friction from the hood, if a finger or a penis is moving in and out of her vagina and rubbing against her inner lips.

If you stop suddenly once you get this excited, your pelvic area may feel congested (swollen, full) for a while until your body gets back to its regular unstimulated state. This is what boys sometimes refer to as "blue balls." It isn't going to physically harm you, but it can be unpleasant. If it happens to a girl, her pelvic area may ache.

*It is fascinating to realize that this same swelling process happens inside both boys' and girls' bodies. It reminds you that our sexual organs start out identical inside the mother's body and don't become male or female until a few weeks after the fertilized egg attaches to the uterus and starts to grow.

Orgasm ("coming," "getting off," "climaxing") is the second phase. At the peak of sexual excitement and muscle tension there is a sudden series of muscle contractions all along the penis or all through the vagina and clitoris. It lasts about ten seconds but sometimes feels longer. An orgasm releases the body tension that has built up, and usually feels really good. An orgasm can be an intense release of energy, during which you might make wild movements and sounds that express the pleasure you are feeling. Sometimes it can be a peaceful flow of warmth over your whole body. At other times it is a ripple of thrilling sensation moving through you from head to toe.

Since a boy nearly always ejaculates during orgasm (that is, semen spurts out of his penis) and a girl doesn't ejaculate, a few of the sensations are different. For a boy, there is a moment just before orgasm when the liquid (semen) that's about to come out gathers together and there's no turning back: orgasm feels inevitable. It's a great feeling, according to most boys. Then a wave of muscle contractions along his penis pushes the semen out fast in a few spurts that feel terrific all through his body in the same way a girl's orgasm does. Richie described it this way:

> As I feel the orgasm coming I forget about everything else and get lost in this feeling that starts in the tip of my penis and spreads all over my body. It's like my body begins swimming all by itself, like there's something in me reaching out, welcoming the pleasure. As it becomes really intense my body begins shaking with excitement. The sensations take me over, and just at the peak of it I can feel this pulsing at the base of my penis and I feel the sperm shooting out of me like I'm sending it off, far away. It's amazing.

Dorie, who's sixteen, described an orgasm too. You can see that the sensations are much the same:

> How does it feel to have an orgasm? Well, for me it's like this buildup of excitement—you know, everything starts feeling better and better and with me, my fantasies get really vivid. Then as I get closer and closer to coming, it's like all my muscles tighten up, especially around my butt, and I feel tingly all over. All my concentration is on my clit because that's the place that is responding to every movement. I kind of cheer myself on in my head, Come on, come on, you're getting closer. Then I get to the point where I know it's going to happen and my whole body relaxes, and with that I feel this flood of sensation—I don't know how to describe it—it's like these waves of pleasure that just take me over. When you're having an orgasm, you're just focused on that. Total involvement in that; nothing else exists. It's the most wonderful feeling of just being alive in your body without your head getting in the way telling you things. For me it's very peaceful.

After orgasm your muscles relax, the swelling in your penis or vagina goes down, your breathing and pulse return to normal. This phase may take half an hour, maybe more. For many people it is a relaxed, quiet, tender time, either alone or with someone else. After orgasm, most boys have a period of time during which they don't get an erection again. It can be as short as five minutes or less, or as long as several hours.

Having an orgasm can be one of the best experiences you have in your life. It can be exciting and show you a powerful part of your own nature. When you share the experience with someone else, it can make you really value each other and be proud that you can give somebody else so much pleasure and grateful to the other person for the joy he or she has given you.

If You Don't Have Orgasms and Want To

People can have orgasms when they masturbate, or through fantasies, in dreams, in sex play or lovemaking with another person. But doing any of these things doesn't always bring an orgasm. Any one of them can feel good, even if you don't come. Some people don't have orgasms often or at all; others have orgasms when they masturbate but not with someone else; some seem to have orgasms easily and frequently. There's been a lot written and said about orgasms recently, and many teenagers (especially girls) complained of feeling they "ought" to have them. "Having an orgasm" can become a *goal* that pressures people and makes them feel bad if they don't achieve it.

Susan, who's fifteen, said something we heard from a lot of teenage girls:

> I hear all the time about orgasms and how neat they are. But I don't think I've ever had one.

Julie, seventeen, didn't know what an orgasm was:

> I knew that there was this thing called a climax, because you read about it in books. It would say, "And they came to a climax." But I never knew that it was *someone's* climax. I didn't think women had orgasms at all. Then one time making love my boyfriend said, "Did you come?" and I said, "I don't know," because I didn't know what he was talking about.

Some boys have never had an orgasm, but a lot more of the girls we talked to hadn't had orgasms yet. Many of them worried about it. "Will I ever come?" "Is my body built wrong?" "Am I too screwed up about sex?" "Why do guys come so easily and I don't?"

It is not surprising that some girls and women have orgasms less easily than boys and men do. First, there's anatomy. A boy can't miss his penis. He touches it several times a day to urinate. Most boys discover masturbation, and it is pretty easy for them to figure out how to do it. But a girl's clitoris, and certainly her vagina, are more hidden. Also, she may be taught as a child not to touch her genitals.

Then there is sex education, or lack of it. Most girls are never taught that they have a clitoris and what it is and does. Since orgasm usually depends at least in part on a girl's clitoris getting stimulated, not knowing about your clitoris can make orgasms pretty hard to have. Girls may be taught that their vaginas are the passageway for babies being born, but *not* that vaginas are sexually responsive as well.

Thirdly, girls in general are brought up to be less accepting and proud of their sexuality than boys are. This is part of the double standard we've talked about. A teenage boy finds that his sexual adventures are usually tolerated or even encouraged. (Of course, this is often hard for the boys who aren't interested!) A girl, however, is told she must be the one to say ''No!'' and to hold off a boy's sex drive. She rarely hears about her own sex drive. So it can be hard for her to let her sexual responses flow freely, and to let go enough to have an orgasm.

If you are comfortable with masturbating, it can teach you about orgasms. Girls are often taught that some man will come along sooner or later to teach them about sex and to give them pleasure. Many girls assume they aren't supposed to find that pleasure for themselves. This makes some girls shy about masturbating, so they miss a chance to learn about orgasm. It can also make them expect too much of their partner.*

Sooner or later, if you want to have orgasms, you most likely will. Since girls' bodies are all built pretty much the same way, there isn't any reason to think that you won't. For many girls and women it takes time, even some months or years of getting used to being sexual.

Orgasm is a part of our sexuality that everyone deserves to enjoy if he or she wants to, but for both girls *and* boys, feeling that you *have* to have orgasms to be a ''liberated'' person can add to the confusions and pressures that many of us feel about sex. Try not to let yourself feel pressured to come.

---

*What about orgasms in sex with a partner? We will talk about this in the section on lovemaking, p. 82.

IV EXPLORING SEX WITH SOMEONE ELSE

Loving someone and wanting to be closer, having a friendship that suddenly opens up to sexual feelings, feeling sexually excited by someone, getting just plain curious about sex—all these are reasons why people start exploring sex with each other. For you, "exploring sex" might mean kissing and hugging someone you're attracted to. It might mean staring at each other a lot, or touching each other's bodies, or taking your clothes off with each other. Later, it might mean giving each other orgasms, or even making love. *This chapter makes no assumptions about what you have and haven't done!*

Bringing sex into a relationship between two people nearly always changes how they feel about each other and themselves. This can be true even of a first kiss. Sometimes you may find your body aching to touch someone but wonder whether to do it or not. Deciding about sex isn't always easy, and this chapter will show how a lot of different teenagers try to handle the decisions.

Sex can bring pleasure and fun and passion and closeness. There's the rush of good feeling when you share a good sexual experience with someone you care about, and you discover more and more about each other. Or when you finally get to try out the things you've been hearing and dreaming about.

But sex can bring pain, too: for example, if someone's feelings are hurt; if someone you trusted goes around telling people what you did together; if it's not as great as you'd expected it to be; if you worry that you can't "perform" right; if you get a girl pregnant or get pregnant; if you get VD; if the person you are crazy about doesn't care as much for you. Painful feelings about sex are among the most difficult that the teenagers we met have to cope with.

We hope this chapter will help increase the pleasure and make the painful times less frequent.

IN LOVE

We laugh
  not because it is funny,
  but because it is funny
  to feel so happy.

We rant and rave,
  not because it is dreadful,
  but because it is dreadful
  to hurt so badly.

And when we love, at love,
  our bodies communicating
  in their own clandestine,
  coded way . . .
  We sigh—
  not because we are frightened
  but because it is frightening
  to become each other
  for one moment,
  and still,
  in the instant's shrieking sharpness,
  to remain obliquely outside.

Forever together . . .
  and yet,
  together
  alone.
  and then,

We kiss,
  not because it is loving,
  but because it is loving
  that makes us want to.

—Michael Scott

WHEN DOES IT START?

Exploring sex with someone else starts early for some of us and a lot later for others. When you start will depend on how strong your sexual feelings are, what your standards are for when you want to start, who your friends happen to be, whether you are close to someone who also wants to explore sex, what kinds of chances you get.

Some people we interviewed started experimenting with sex when they were in grade school. Usually it was not so much a matter of ''being in love'' with someone as of playing around with a friend and finding out about sex. Maria told us:

In the fourth grade me and this boy in the next grade used to meet in the garage in our apartment building where there were these storage rooms, and we'd spend hours down there making out and fooling around.

Sixteen-year-old Joe said:

My dad's *Playboy* magazine got me familiar with looking, and this girl in my fifth-grade class got me familiar with everything else. We used to sit around and talk about sex and stuff and then we'd be playing around with each other, like making out and exploring each other.

Often this kind of sexual exploring is with a friend of your own sex. Lisa remembered:

I had my first sexual experience when I was seven years old. It was with my best friend. We were constantly together—we went to school together, we played together, everything. Then one day we started fooling around and touching each other all over. For about a year, we'd sleep over at each other's houses and do this.

For Connie, playing around sexually with boys at an early age was more of an adventure than a sexual experience:

When I was eleven, me and my best girlfriend were with some boys who were fourteen—we looked about thirteen ourselves. That night we were making out and the guy I was with was feeling my breasts. I wasn't getting off on the feeling of it myself as much as I was thinking, Wow, look what I'm doing; wow, I'm making out; wow, he's feeling me up; wow, I can't wait to tell Jill about this! For me at that point most of the excitement was in the fact that I was doing what I was doing.

Other people don't try out these experiences so early. Wendy remembers:

In my sixth-grade class on Monday morning there used to be all this whispering and giggling about these few kids and *who* had done *what* over the weekend.

Who had kissed who, what happened when the lights went down at so-and-so's house. I was out of it. Sometimes I wished I weren't, but mostly I was just busy with everything else.

Between the ages of twelve and eighteen, more people start getting interested in sex. Some people go steady, some have a few girlfriends or boyfriends, others go to an occasional party. Marge and Paul talk about this:

Marge: I changed so much in this past year. In the seventh grade I used to think it was gross to see a boy and a girl making out at a party. It was just about the same as going all the way in my mind. But this year we all make out at our parties, and everybody I know has boyfriends. I have two.

Paul: At thirteen I was into everything wild. I was in a gang and we were bad, we got in a lot of trouble. Our gang was so tight, nobody else counted, not even our families. So girls were far from my mind then. Now at fifteen, I'm a lot different. I'm not hanging out with a gang of dudes anymore, I have a girl and she's real important to me. We're into each other real deep. And a lot of the other dudes feel the same way too; they all have girls now.

Many people don't get into sex of any kind with someone else until they are older—in high school or out working, or at college, or later. Johnny said:

I'm pretty quiet and I changed schools a lot because my family was always moving, so I never really got into any crowd or got to know anyone real well. So I didn't have any girlfriend until this year. I'm seventeen and I met this girl who's a little older than me. I met her where I work at the market, so we just about see each other every day. She really has helped me get over some of my shyness. She takes the lead a lot because she's had other boyfriends. We really like each other a lot.

Flo, who's a senior in high school, remembered:

I was in the eleventh grade the first time I really made out with someone. Before that it was just some kissing games at parties when I was much younger. I was so much slower than a lot of my friends.

Not Yet. Many of the teenagers we interviewed said that sex with someone else just isn't important to them at this point. Most of us have times during our lives when we aren't much interested in sex. Sports, dance, photography, mathematics, cars, writing, work that is very hard or very absorbing—all of these can fill our lives so that there is little room for anything else. Donna, who is fifteen, said:

Right now my whole life is skating. I ice-skate about seven hours a day, and that's all I think about and I want to do.

Teenagers who have definite goals for themselves often

put off having sexual relationships. Tina, a sixteen-year-old from Detroit, said:

> I have other things going for me right now. I'm just not into sex. I was into it when I was younger, but now I'm more involved in my schoolwork and my photography. I have a lot of plans for myself and this is no time for me to be messing around with boys.

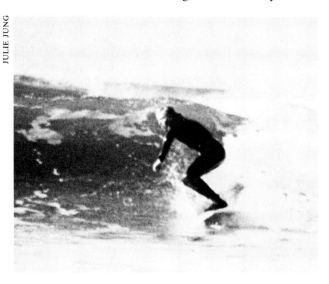

JULIE JUNG

Or you may have no special reason at all. George, fourteen, feels neutral about sex:

> Every time I see my grandfather he wants to know if I have a girlfriend. It's like he wants to ask me, "How's your sex life?" but he doesn't come right out and say that. Well, I don't have a girlfriend now and I don't think I'm going to have a girlfriend for a while yet. I'm just not into that. Not now anyway.

George's grandfather may sound familiar to you. There's a lot of pressure to be socially active, if not sexually active, by a certain age.* If everyone around you is talking or thinking about sex all the time, or if your friends are all getting sexually involved and you don't want to, you might worry about being different from them. But you owe it to yourself to respect how *you* are feeling, to listen to what your body and emotions are telling you. One of the nicest things about your sexuality is that it will be there for the rest of your life, to be enjoyed when you are ready.

Will It Ever Happen? What if you want to be more active socially and sexually but you're not getting the chance? This can be an especially painful question if it gets mixed up with worrying that you aren't popular. Some people wait for a relationship to come along, and feel OK about waiting. Some jump into sex more casually. Some people wait, and feel frustrated. They may wonder

*The pressure is to be *hetero*sexually active, too, which often makes teenagers with homosexual (same sex) attractions feel out of it. See "Exploring Sex with Someone of Your Own Sex," p. 112.

whether they'll ever find someone they like who likes them back, and who wants to be sexual with them.

If you worry that you'll never have a close relationship or get to explore sex with someone else, all we can say is—judging from the talks we've had with teenagers—you have lots of company. In fact, some of the people you know who *talk* about sex a lot may be feeling the same as you underneath. Loneliness is one of the hard things about being human. Masturbating and enjoying your sexual fantasies can let you feel your sexuality without having to depend on someone else. But it's usually not just sex we want, and not only a relationship with ourselves, important as that is. We want someone who will be especially close and caring with us, whether that includes sex or not. Building enduring relationships is something that most people hope for, work at and learn about all through their lives, and waiting may be an important part of this. Like everyone else, teens mostly don't want to settle for relationships they don't feel good about.

WHEN AND HOW FAR: MAKING DECISIONS ABOUT SEX

Whether it's a first kiss, a French kiss, touching his penis, stroking her breasts, or making love, deciding what you want to do sexually with a certain person isn't always easy. At its best, the choice comes out of your relationship. It is something you both choose, as a way of expressing how you feel about each other and bringing you closer. But deciding about sex is not always so clear, or so mutual. It's often done in a split-second—at a party, in a car, on the beach, with parents about to come home or the movie about to end. You're excited, the other person is excited, and your bodies are reaching for each other—whether for a long kiss or for something more. Thoughts may rush through your head: What will she/he think of me? What will my friends think? Will I be glad or sorry? If I don't do it now, will I get another chance? Sometimes you consciously make a decision, sometimes you just go ahead, or stop, because your gut tells you to.

"Being sure" is something the teenagers working on this book talked about a lot. Leah, a high school junior in Boston, said:

> Say you're thirteen or fourteen, with a guy feeling your breasts or something. If you're not sure, you feel dirty.

Manuel, sixteen, said, "I sometimes wonder whether I'll be glad the next day." On the whole, people feel better about themselves if they are doing what they know they want and are ready for. But sexual feelings are often so strong and confusing that it is hard to be sure.

How "sure" do you want to be when you try something new? What can you learn about or think about in advance so that you can trust your split-second decisions to work out right? Reading books like this and talking with your friends may help you do some thinking ahead of time so you know more what you want and what your limits are. But we all learn by experimenting, and part of experimenting is making mistakes. Some mistakes in sex are serious—especially if they involve pregnancy, disease or your good feelings about yourself. Fortunately, most mistakes just teach us what not to do next time. As Beverly, a fourteen-year-old from Detroit, said:

Once you make a mistake and it really hurts you, you know you're not going to do it again. You gotta learn from your mistakes. You gotta learn how what you do affects other people around you.

Considering the Relationship. You don't have to be in a relationship with a capital R in order to want to make out or, for some people, even to go further. But whether or not this person is the love of your life, you'll probably ask yourself some questions before you want to share your body and feelings. Here are a few of the questions teenagers told us they ask themselves:

—How tight are we? Do I love this person? Do I like this person? Do I trust this person?
—How much can we talk about what's going on? Do I know what she/he is thinking? What will she/he think of me?
—If I don't do it (whatever "it" is), will I lose her/him?
—Is he/she using my body or does he/she care about me?
—Will she/he go tell everyone tomorrow that we made out tonight?

Knowing each other well and caring about each other usually makes any kind of sex better. But not everyone has—or wants—one single boyfriend or girlfriend. Many teenagers who talked with us have no one special person; some have several friends, many have no one at all, and some are trying out sex more casually with people they don't know very well. Angie had never made out with anyone, and decided it was time:

Me and my cousin—I was sixteen and she was seventeen—were at the amusement park and we saw these two gorgeous guys. We were following them for a while and then I guess they knew, so they turned around and we asked them if they wanted to go on the roller coaster with us, and they said OK. Then we went in one of those spook-house rides where it was dark inside. The guy I was with put his arm around me and I was so pleased and I could tell that he wanted to kiss me, but he was kind of afraid of what I would think. So I kissed him, and then that led him to French-kiss me and then he put his hand under my blouse and felt my breasts. It was really nice; I really enjoyed it. It was like so much fun and it was so safe,

because I mean, how much can you do on a haunted-house ride at the amusement park?!

Because the boy in the amusement park was a stranger, Angie had to think about "safety." On a haunted-house ride with her cousin there, Angie felt the situation was "safe" enough to let go and enjoy her feelings. You might not have made the same choice. Judging what is safe enough for you—physically and emotionally—is an important thing in exploring, and especially in enjoying, sex.

With *casual sex* and any kind of pickup scene at beaches, bars and so on, the teenagers we talked with told us the one thing to remember is that *you can't count on the other person to care about you.* So you have to take care of yourself. This means trying to keep out of situations where you'll feel used or hurt. It means preventing pregnancy and venereal disease if you have sexual intercourse. As one girl said:

When you're playing around with a lot of guys you don't know well, you gotta watch out for yourself first of all, because you're the only one who's going to watch out for you.

THE DIFFERENT INFLUENCES, OR "VOICES"

How does a person decide about sex? Picture yourself in a situation where you are trying to decide what to do sexually. Put yourself inside your head, and imagine the "conversation" going on in there. There are probably many "voices" in this conversation, each with an opinion about what you *should* do. These are the pressures and influences on you as you decide how far to go. Teenagers talked to us about a number of "voices" they respond to.

Voice One: Parents. If your parents or other adults who play a parental role in your life have talked to you about sex, their voice may be saying, "You're too young to be in the back seat of a car with a girl!" or "Enjoy yourself, but just don't go too far!" or "Boys won't respect a girl who's easy" or "Do what you think is best, but just be sure" or "If I ever catch you making out with that kid again I'll . . ." If you feel your parents are overprotective their message may not be helpful. If they seem to fear your sexuality, or if they don't want you to be sexual *at all* until some distant time, you may feel you have to tune out their voice entirely. Or it may be strong enough only to make you feel guilty. But if your parents seem to trust your judgment and basically just want you to take care of yourself, their voice of carefulness can help you make decisions you will be glad about. Whatever your parents' voices say inside your head, they will probably be powerful, because parents are so important in our lives.

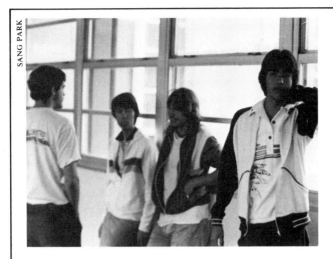

SANG PARK

Voice Two: Friends. Your friends' voices are probably very important to you at this point. What they say may differ, depending on whether you are a boy or a girl.

Inside a boy's head, the friends' voices may be saying, "Go ahead! Get her to go as far as she will!" or "What are you, some kind of wimp, that she hasn't even let you inside her bra yet?" or "They always say no, but they don't mean it!" or "Show us you're a man!" Josh complained:

> If I don't get a girl to make out with me on the second date, I'm just not making it, man. The guys will wonder if something's wrong with me.

Josh may not *feel* like making out right then, and what's ironic is that his friends may not either. But they think they ought to and he feels the pressure. Daniel, a ninth-grader from Washington, talked about the image many boys feel they have to live up to:

> I know a lot of guys who feel like it's a sickness to be a virgin, and they can't wait to get over it. It starts real young, like in junior high, especially for guys who have older brothers who had reputations as being sex symbols. They feel like they have to keep up the family image. And then there are whole neighborhoods where everyone is supposed to be a macho man. That's a lot of pressure, you know. You end up feeling like there's something wrong with you if you don't go in for that.

Hearing these "voices" that say "Get what you can" doesn't mean that you have to obey. Greg, sixteen, explained:

> The big goal for me is just to be with the girl I like, not to do anything in particular or get anyplace, just to be with her.

In a girl's head, the friends' voices may encourage her to go ahead *or* warn her to stop, depending on what's expected in her particular crowd. Up until a certain age—usually in junior or senior year of high school—the girls who spoke to us said that they and their friends were pretty harsh judges of girls who were more active sexually than they were. Kerri said:

> Up until junior year there were only two girls we knew weren't virgins. We were always going up and asking them these questions. Then afterwards we'd talk about them like they were dogs or something.

And Julie said, "With the kids I'm with I feel pressure not to get into sex." So when a girl is about to make out with a boy, her friends' voices inside her head might be saying, "Watch out! You'll get a bad reputation. We'll gossip about you if you go any further. We'll call you a slut." This shows that friends follow the double standard, too: very often a boy's reputation is made by how sexual he is, and a girl's reputation is ruined if she is too sexual. This is unfair to those boys who don't especially want to get into sex, and unfair to girls who have thought about it and know they do want to.

Sometimes the friends' warning voice is a welcome and helpful one. Susan, a young teenager from Des Moines, said:

> I've never been in an experience where I might have to compromise my morals, because most of the people I hang out with feel the same way I do. I know I want to be a virgin when I get married, and that's all there is to it.

Betty, who's thirteen, describes how the idea of "reputation" helps her make judgments about herself and other people:

> I don't want to go to one party and make out with one person and then go to another party and make out with someone else. You get a terrible reputation that way. I know some girls who do that, and all the boys are after them because they're known as loose. Even boys can get that reputation—that they'll make out with any girl. I wouldn't want to waste my devotion over some guy like that.

Worrying about your reputation can keep you from being true to your feelings, but it can also be a helpful guide in the uncharted territory of sex and relationships.

The pressures on girls may change at some point during high school. Kerri, who spoke earlier, went on:

> Now, in the senior year we're all talking about sexual experiences, and the people who haven't experienced sex are left out.

Suddenly all your friends may seem to be experimenting with sex, and their voices in your head may say, "You're so behind the times, kid—go ahead and try it!" or "You'll be out of it if you don't have any sexual adventures to talk about!" or "Being a real woman means at *least* doing X, Y or Z." This sounds more like the voice that so many boys have been hearing all along. It makes a lot of girls go further in sex than their body and feelings tell them to—just because everyone else is doing it. (Of course, everybody else might not be doing as much as they *say* they are.) This is the voice of what gets called the "sexual revolution" or "sexual liberation." It says, "Sex is great, everyone is doing it!" It can be just as oppressive as the voice that says, "Girls shouldn't be sexual."

Voice Three: The Media. From TV, magazines or movies, you'll have a lot of sexy images in your head that may influence your decision. The glamor-

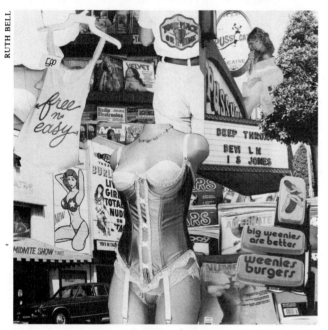

Society influences our feelings about sex.

ous love life of movie stars and popular singers makes us feel we're pitiful if we don't have at least one gorgeous admirer hanging all over us. In advertisements, the media voice says: "Buy this deodorant and you'll have lovers falling at your feet." Or, "If your love life isn't dazzling, then your body must be unattractive." The ads seek to make us feel inadequate about our bodies and our sexuality so we'll buy their products. By making us feel that a successful love life and a perfectly desirable body are the most important things in the world, the media voice makes us rush into relationships we might otherwise think twice about. It's probably the least trustworthy voice in your inner conversation.

Voice Four: Religious Attitudes and Beliefs. For some people, including many teenagers, religious attitudes about sex are very important. Many Catho-

lics, Protestants, Jews and Muslims believe that sex outside marriage is sinful. Their voice may say, "Wait, wait, wait. These feelings you are having belong only in marriage," or "Oral sex and homosexual relationships are sinful." You will have to decide for yourself how important these messages are for you.

Unfortunately, many people find that when the religious voice says a great big "NO!" it isn't very helpful, and just makes them feel guilty. Here's how it gets expressed in Doug's school in a fairly conservative community:

> I think my school treated sex like it was a drug. You know, *Don't do it!*—you might get brain damage. Like it was some illegal sinful thing that shouldn't be tried.

If the voice that reaches you from religion tells you that *all* sexual feelings and activities outside marriage are wrong, you may feel like rejecting it completely. This is a loss, because you may miss a lot of guidance. For instance, when religion tells us to "treat other human beings with love and respect" or to "love your neighbor as yourself," it helps us see when we are hurting someone else. Religion also helps us see and value the importance of *love* between two people.

Voice Five: Your Own Needs. Your own feelings and needs are important. If you find yourself listening only to the *other* voices in making decisions about sex, then try to listen harder to yourself. Of course, needs are often contradictory, and yours may confuse you. But it's important to figure out as best you can what *you* want to do—whether or not you decide it's the best thing in the end. Your needs may say, "I am horny and I need some sex"; "I am lonely and I need some affection"; "I love this person and want to express it sexually"; "I'm feeling uncertain and pressured and I need to wait"; "I'm feeling worried about birth control"; or "I don't know what he/she is thinking and I must know that before I go ahead." Going ahead with sex can meet some of these needs; waiting can meet others. If affection or reassurance or acceptance is what you need, then sex may not be the answer. And if what you want will hurt someone else, you'll have to reconsider.

Chip, a sixteen-year-old from Santa Barbara, finds this voice a valuable guide:

> I'm very religious and so is my girlfriend. Both of us agree that we'd rather wait until we're married to do some things, because we just feel that you make more of a deep commitment to each other if you wait.

For both boys and girls, the double standard can keep you from knowing and acting on your needs. If you are a boy who feels shy about sex but your

RUTH BELL

friends are pushing you to prove yourself, you may not feel free to move as slowly as you'd like to. If you are a girl with strong sexual feelings, you might worry about acting on them. Lucy, sixteen, wanted to move her hips against her boyfriend in a way that excited her—she called it "grinding"; others call it "humping" or "blue-jean pumping":

I remember the first time I tried grinding. I was really horny and I wanted to really bad, but I didn't want to because I was embarrassed. I didn't know if he knew what I was doing, and I didn't really know what I was doing. It kind of seemed like screwing to me. I thought, What is he going to think? Will he think I'm sleazy? What will I feel about it afterwards?

Sometimes it's next to impossible to know in a split second what Lucy wants to know: how you'll feel about what you're doing after you've done it. You'll make mistakes, as everyone does. Try to balance what your own feelings are telling you with what will be good for you and the other person in the long run.

Voice Six: Your Own Standards. Most teenagers told us they are working on developing their own standards and values about sexual activity, figuring out what they themselves think is right and wrong. The voice of your standards may say, "Remember what you decided about pressuring someone into sex?" or "You always said you wanted to know someone well before doing X, Y or Z." For instance, a fourteen-year-old girl from Michigan reported:

When I was with my boyfriend and we were making out, I was feeling so good and so close to him, but also, another person inside me was saying "Just don't get undressed, don't make

love," so I think that means I have some control. I'm even kind of disappointed that we went as far as we did, because I wonder if he's going to try to get me to go on and on and on. I said to myself I definitely would not go all the way until at least eleventh grade.

Jerome, seventeen, who is gay, developed his standards the hard way:

After getting into an ugly triangle last year, struggling with this other guy over a guy we both liked, I promised myself never to mess around with someone who's got another romance going. It's giving me some lonely Saturday nights, but a lot less heartache.

Your ideas about what's right may change, of course. Paula remembers:

In sixth grade my friends and I made a pact that we would never ever French-kiss anyone because it was such a gross thing to do. Needless to say, we all broke the pact sooner or later.

Standards never stay exactly the same. They grow as you do.

As you get more experience in knowing yourself in relationships, the voice of your own standards will probably get wiser and stronger, and you'll come to trust it more. Trusting yourself is in fact a big part of making decisions. For instance, until you have some experience, you may not think you can go only as far as you want but no further. You might think, If I go as far as touching her breasts, maybe I'll get out of control! or Once I French-kiss him there will be no turning back. As you get some experience, including making mistakes, you'll learn how far you can go to without getting carried away. You'll learn what your limits are, what you can handle, what seems right for you.

Balancing the Voices. Hearing even a few of these voices at any one time can be a real challenge to your ability to decide for yourself what you want to do. Rhonda, seventeen, put it this way:

We're at the age where we're having real sexual feelings and we want to act on them, but my conflict is that I can't just be natural about it—whatever that means—because the feelings I have get so mixed up with outside pressures and standards. It gets pretty complicated, so that sometimes I don't know what I'm *really* feeling and wanting, and what I'm feeling and wanting just because I think I'm "supposed" to be feeling that.

If it's any consolation, knowing what's right for you usually gets easier with age and experience. You become more able to weigh the opinions of your parents, friends,

media and religion against your own feelings and values, so that you come up with decisions that you're pleased about in the long run.

Blurring the Voices: Drugs and Alcohol. Getting drunk or high is one sure way to drown out the inner conversation about how far you're going to go. It can get you in trouble, as Nell, a junior from Iowa, described:

The decision comes at the start when you get high. Once you are past a certain point, you can't make decisions anymore. A lot of junior high girls I know only have sex on weekends when they are drunk or stoned.

Linda, a sophomore from San Francisco, put it this way:

At our school most sexual relationships start at parties. Being loaded makes a lot of difference, you get a little crazy. When I'm really drunk or really stoned, that's when I'm more likely to get involved with someone at a party. That's when you have to watch out, because you can't trust anybody when they're loaded. You can't trust yourself, either.

Some people use drugs the way Leni, nineteen, used to:

When I was sixteen I learned about sex all the wrong ways. I never knew what I was doing and I never got any pleasure out of it. And I was always so afraid everyone would see I didn't know what I was doing, so I had to get drunk and stoned to get me through.

Several teenagers working on this book said that in their school the pressure to get into drugs or alcohol is as strong as the pressure to get into sex. Together, they can be a devastating combination. Jeff, seventeen, said:

Last summer my girlfriend and I got crazy on beer and dope at this beach party. I had a package of rubbers in my pocket, but when we rolled off into the dunes to fuck, they stayed in my pocket. It was wild at the time, but not in September, when she told me she was pregnant.

Susan, a senior, said:

It's happened to me. Guys will try to get you to drink or to have a toke or whatever, and if you're not used to it, you feel more relaxed and what they're saying to you doesn't seem as crazy. You don't say to yourself, Oh, I would never do that, like you would if you were sober or playing with a full deck. And they start talking to you and you think, This guy digs me—he really wants to be with me. And you're just not as careful as you should be.

Melanie, eighteen, had a similar experience:

I go to bars with my friends sometimes and get drunk, and a couple of times I went home with this older guy who started putting the moves on me and I was too dizzy to stop him. I didn't even enjoy the sex or anything. I felt dirty and mad afterwards, but it was like the booze led me on.

Some people say that sex feels better to them when they're high, but others don't like the way they act sexually when they've been drinking or doing drugs. The chemicals can affect the way people relate to others in a negative manner. Joanne, sixteen, told us:

When you're drinking, all your cares go away and you're just in it for you. I guess you don't care much about the guy except to get him to do what you want.

In addition to blurring your ability to decide what you really want, being drunk or high sometimes makes sex not too great anyway. It often dulls a person's sexual responses and makes boys unable to get or keep erections. Sometimes it gets in the way of being able to communicate while you're together with someone physically. If you've made out with someone or had sex only under the influence of drugs or alcohol you ought to try it sometime when you're not high. You may like it better—especially if you're with someone you *want* to be with.

Being Pressured to Go Further. It's nice when both people in a relationship want to move at the same speed, but this isn't always the case. Usually the strongest pressure comes from the person who wants to go further. A lot of teenagers told us that if their partner really wants to do something, it is hard to say no, no matter what the other voices inside them may be saying.

Elsa, a fourteen-year-old from Denver, said:

The first time I was with this boy we were at a party together, and we started making out. And then, all of a sudden, there were his hands on my chest. I felt really funny about it, because it wasn't my idea, it was his idea and he sort of rushed into it. Since it was the first time we were ever together I felt like it was too fast, but I let him do it, because I didn't exactly know how to tell him not to.

Three teenagers in a discussion group found that they had similar experiences:

Penny (sixteen): If I'm out with somebody for the first time and we double with two people who are boyfriend and girlfriend, of course they're making out, and I feel like, God, I don't want to make out with this guy. I don't even know him. But then he wants to because the other couple is doing it and so I end up either doing it and not wanting to or feeling like I'm some kind of prude or something. That's the pits.

Matt (fifteen): You know, I've been at parties where everybody's sort of coupling up and there wasn't really anybody I wanted to be with, but it would work out that I'd be with some girl and I'd feel like we were supposed to be making out or something. Because everybody else was doing it. After a while I'd be thinking to myself, Hey, get me out of this. But she's coming on strong and you feel like you'd be a heel to drop her. So I go along, even though I'm not really feeling anything.

Jeffrey, sixteen, agreed with Matt:

You're at a party and you're making out and she wants more. You know what I mean. And you're thinking, Wow, what is this going to get me into? I don't want to have a relationship with this chick. But if you don't go for it she thinks you're really weird, and the story gets out that you're queer or something.

The point is that instead of *guessing* what the other person wants to do, it pays to check it out directly.

Sometimes the hardest time to decide what's best for *you* is when someone is luring, coaxing, seducing, pleading with, or even manipulating you into going further than you feel like going. A sophomore from Iowa wrote, "This confuses the hell out of my inner voice.'' People use lines like: ''You would if you loved me,'' or ''I'll get blue balls (see p. 81) if you don't make me come,'' ''I'll ditch you if you don't,'' ''Why can't you loosen up and enjoy life?''* Girls use lines too, but boys use them far more often. You have to feel pretty sure of yourself to be able to resist arguments and threats like these and do just what you want to do. Mary Ann, sixteen, had an effective answer:

> The guy I was out with the other night was coming on pretty strong and like he was getting real excited, but I wasn't really into it. He kept trying to get me to rub his penis; he even told me he had blue balls and wouldn't I do something to help him out. I was so pissed. I couldn't believe he actually used that line on me. So I said, ''I'm sorry about your problem. Why don't you masturbate?'' I think he was embarrassed by that because he just sort of dropped the subject after I said that.

Most of us have gone further than we want to at one time or another just to please the person we're with, or to keep our ''cool'' reputation, or not to make a scene. However, since the whole enjoyment in sex is feeling good, if you're not feeling good about it then there's really no point in doing it. If you do get pressured into something, as one girl said, ''Afterwards how you feel will tell you what you really wanted.'' The next time maybe you'll do it differently.

Sometimes a person will feel not just pressured or pleaded with, but *forced* into going further than she/he wants to. This frightening experience happens mainly to girls, and can involve an acquaintance, a stranger, a boss, even (in cases of incest) a relative. If you feel you are being forced to do *anything* in sex against your will, try to get away from that person as quickly as possible. (See the section on ''Sex Against Your Will'' for more information.)

SAYING NO

There are a lot of reasons for saying no in certain sexual situations: you don't want to be sexual with the person you're with; you don't want to do a particular thing; you aren't feeling turned on; if it's intercourse, maybe you have no birth control. You'd be going against what you want for yourself if you didn't say no under those circumstances.

Even though you are loving the person you're with, enjoying what you're doing, and feeling very turned on, you may *still* want to say Stop—if you feel yourself getting carried away and you have certain limits beyond which you don't want to go.

*Sol Gordon has put hundreds of these lines and some handy answers in a paperback called *You Would If You Loved Me* (New York: Bantam Books, 1978).

Often when two people are just getting to know each other in a sexual situation, they may experiment until one of them says, ''Stop, that's far enough!'' If nobody says anything, they may both assume there's no problem.

Many teenagers who talked with us find it hard to say ''No'' or ''Stop'' to someone else. For instance, how do you say it gracefully and still have the person believe you? As Judy pointed out:

> When I tell a guy that he can feel my breasts but not my vagina because that's my limit right now, often he'll act like I was talking about the weather or something. He just keeps on going, as if I didn't mean what I said.

Rob answered her:

> It's like a game. My friends told me that when a girl says no she doesn't really mean it. So if a girl tells me quietly to stop, and doesn't yell out loud about it or hit me over the head with it, I'm not supposed to listen. It's a game to find out if she really means it.

Here is the double standard again: girls are expected to say no whether they mean it or not. So girls like Judy end up having to say it *loud* in order to be believed, and it becomes a scene. Brad, too, has to say it loud to be believed:

> If I tell a girl I want to stop, or I don't want to get into sex right now, some girls are cool, but some can't believe a boy isn't a sex maniac.

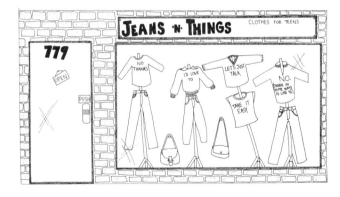

Another question: How do you say ''Stop'' without hurting the other person's feelings? Brad went on:

> My girlfriend and I went through this whole thing last weekend because we were getting pretty carried away and I wanted to slow down and she thought that meant I didn't dig her. Thought she was ugly or something. When all I said was ''Let's cool it and go out for a walk.''

Ideally, the person you say ''Stop'' to won't feel hurt or rejected. Ideally, you'll be able to explain that your not wanting to go on doesn't mean that you're putting the other person down. But there is a lot of meaning attached to sex, even if it's only a kiss. People's feelings get hurt easily. If that happens, it's good to be able to talk about the hurt feelings, but this is easier if you know each other well than if you don't.

> Saying no is often just plain awkward. But it's less awkward than going ahead with something that will make one of you feel bad.

Another big question is: When do you say it? If you say ''Stop'' too far in advance, you feel like a wet blanket. If you say it too late, you're called a tease. Boys talked about how frustrated they get when a girl waits until the last minute to say no. Bill put it this way:

> I wish if a girl wasn't going to touch my cock she'd tell me ahead of time so I wouldn't get so incredibly turned on just imagining it about to happen. Here she is all passionate one minute and then it's ''I've got to go home,'' just like that, and I'm left panting.

What Bill doesn't know is that the girl may be waiting until the last minute because of the wild debate going on inside her head: ''Yes!'' ''No!'' ''Will I be sorry?'' ''What will he think of me?'' ''Just be sure'' and so on. He can't hear the inner argument, and only feels its results. Michelle, sixteen, said:

> I don't know how many times I've been called a cock teaser, because when it gets right down to inter- course, man, it's ''negative . . . no way . . . I won't do it.'' I might get as far as taking my pants down, and then I'll chicken out. Because when it gets right down to it, that's where you start getting scared. These rushing emotions go through your head, like ''Oh, my God!'' and maybe you're feeling guilty and maybe you're hearing your mother's voice in your head saying ''Don't do it! Keep your reputation!'' So many times I've gotten right down to it and just left.

Given all the pressures on her, Michelle can't be blamed for ditching out. After all, girls are ''supposed'' to be the ones who set the limits. But her boyfriend can't be blamed for feeling angry and frustrated either. Because they hadn't talked about where they would stop, they were in a sense leading each other on. Ron, seventeen, said a challenging thing about this:

> They say guys push sex on girls. But when my girl- friend is making out with me real hot and heavy and I'm getting turned on out of my mind, and then she says ''That's it'' I could go through the ceiling. I'd be *crazy* not to try to keep her going. Is that pushing? Or is she teasing me beyond my endurance?

Pushing any kind of sex on someone, of course, *is* wrong, but you can understand how Ron feels.

What can help people avoid these frustrating last-minute scenes? Trying to *talk in advance* about how far you want

to go with each other makes a big difference. Talking about sex isn't so easy in this culture, however. It can be awkward if you don't know each other well, if you are shy, if you are feeling guilty about your sexual desires. But it's worth the effort. (See p. 107.) *Getting rid of double-standard thinking* would help, too. If boys and girls didn't feel that they had roles they were ''supposed'' to play, it would be easier to talk honestly about what they did and didn't want to be doing. There wouldn't be so much guessing about what the other person is going to do. Pete, a sixteen-year-old from Los Angeles, said:

> You know, I think so much bad communication goes on between guys and girls just because everyone ex- pects the guy to move first. He's supposed to call up for a date, and he's supposed to initiate all the sex, and he's supposed to know what to do. That's such a drag. Like I'm not into coming on too strong, that's just not my style. I don't believe in pressuring people into things, and I don't want to pressure my girl- friend. But she doesn't think the girl's supposed to be aggressive, especially not in sex, so she's always waiting for me to make all the moves. And since I don't want to pressure her, I usually hold back. I would feel a whole lot better if she'd let me know what *she* wants some of the time.

WHAT DO PEOPLE DO?

The things that people enjoy doing together sexually are limited only by human imagination and ingenuity. What *you* do will depend on what you are ready for, who the other person is, what he or she is ready for. (See the sec- tion on ''When and How Far.'') But whether it is kissing or making out or going all the way, it is amazing how much people worry about whether they are *doing it right*. Most of us feel pressure to perform well in school, sports,

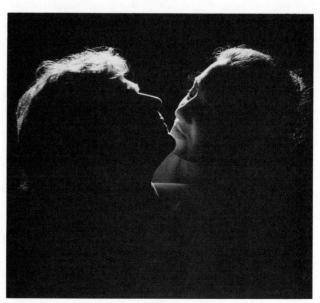

GREG NEWMAN

work—and we carry that into what we are doing sexually! Holly, sixteen, said:

> When I'm making out with my boyfriend, I feel like a part of me is watching from the outside and saying, "How's your technique tonight? Are you turning him on? Are you doing it right?" When that voice shuts up, I have a much better time.

Pablo, seventeen, advised:

> I think you should stress in the book that sex should be an enjoyable thing and partners shouldn't worry about performing. I have trouble forgetting about what I "should" be doing and just enjoying it.

So the theme of this section is: *Sex is not a performance!* You have no audience, no judges. There is no "right" way. Once you're both pretty sure that you want to be doing whatever you're doing, the point is to explore what makes you and the other person feel excited, close, satisfied. People aren't born knowing how to be in a sexual relationship, so you have to learn a lot with each partner.

DETOUR

arms to legs
grasping
making cups
with our bodies
we roll
like one ball
following
the stains
of sweat

each crease
explored
with tongue
with touch
and mapped,
coded, diagramed,

we missed
the correct exit
followed
the wrong trail
and now
stumble
into uncharted
territory

this new land
lay fallow
and we
exhausted
can't find
the road back.

—Amy C. Rosen

Feeling that you ought to know how to do it just keeps you from enjoying it. Telling each other about what feels good is the best way to learn what's "right" for the two of you. Even with kissing, what turns one person on may not be great for someone else—or what feels good in one mood may not in another. It is a matter of learning to flow freely with your feelings and your partner's.

Kissing. There's kissing: like kissing a relative hello, kissing your parents good-night or kissing a rabbit's foot to bring you luck. And there's *kissing:*

> Annie (fourteen): The first time I kissed my boyfriend we didn't have to say anything to each other, we just felt this thrill run through us. Just being so close to him, holding him, it was like we were part of each other.

> Ben (thirteen): When we were in the sixth grade we'd play spin the bottle or post office and you'd always hope that you got the girl you liked. Then you'd take her into the closet and kiss her and that was about the most exciting thing you could imagine. It was amazing.

Because lips are so sensitive, pressing your lips against the lips of someone you like can be a thrill. However, as with everything else in sex, sometimes our expectations are too high. Peter, fifteen, warned:

> Somebody should tell you that fireworks aren't going to go off on your first kiss. At least they didn't for me.

A lot of people enjoy opening their mouths while they kiss, and using their tongues to touch the other person's mouth and tongue. This is called French-kissing, or Frenching, or, in some places, tongue-kissing. It is a more intimate way of kissing. Laura, sixteen, talks about it:

> I used to think there was some special trick to French-kissing, like you had to know what to do with your tongue, and since I didn't know what to do, I never wanted to French-kiss. Even after I was going out with someone for a long time, I always avoided that. Then one boyfriend I had just told me to open my mouth while I was kissing him, you know, not really wide but just with my lips parted, and he sort of slid his tongue into my mouth and started touching my tongue with his tongue. I liked it. I mean, it was really sensual.

Ethan's introduction to French-kissing was a surprise:

> At camp last summer I met this girl who was a little older than me and we started liking each other. The first time we kissed she stuck her tongue all the way in my mouth and I threw up all over her.

Like any other sexual activity, kissing feels good when you want to do it. You may know the person well, or you may hardly know the person at all, but as long as you are choosing to do it, kissing can be really nice. When you don't want to do it, or when you are with someone you don't want to be with, kissing may not be so pleasant.

Andrea (fourteen): I rinsed my mouth out the first time somebody French-kissed me. I was kissing this guy good-night after our date and he just stuck his tongue in my mouth. Just like that. It took me totally by surprise and I didn't like it one bit. I never went out with that guy again!

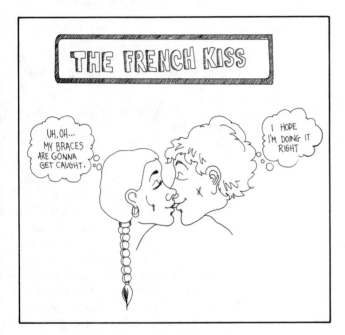

Kissing is pretty intimate, and sometimes you just may not feel like doing it. That's OK. It's not your obligation to kiss anyone, no matter what the circumstances. You don't owe anyone a kiss.

Making Out

Making out is more than a kiss. Jennifer, fourteen, from the Midwest, told us about the first time she and her boyfriend made out:

When I was with my boyfriend and we were all alone for the first time, we were making out. We were out in a park where it was real private behind a bunch of trees and I was feeling so close to him. We were French-kissing real long kisses, so sometimes I had to pull away to catch my breath. He was rubbing my back and I was rubbing his. We must have stayed there for an hour, just hugging and kissing and rolling around, but then I had to get home, so we had to stop. When I got to my house, my lips were all red and swollen from so much kissing, so I went in and washed my face with cold water. I don't think my mother noticed because she didn't say anything.

Making out with somebody is pretty intimate, and Glo-

ria, seventeen, and her boyfriend always feel some shyness:

When we first started going out, we would flirt and make eyes at each other, but he didn't touch me and I didn't want to start anything. This would go on until it was almost time to go home. I was so excited I wanted to jump him at this point. Finally we would start laughing and tickling each other and then start making out. We always have this embarrassing moment before we fall into each other's arms. He always got home late and got in trouble.

Bob and Sue talked about some of the pleasures and minor hazards of making out:

Sue (fourteen): When Bob and I are making out, I get so into it I just lose myself in kissing and hugging and licking and sucking his face and neck and the soft inside part of his arms. And he does the same to me.

Bob (fourteen): Yeah, it feels terrific. But last Saturday night she gave me a hickey on my neck—you know, a big red mark that stays there for days letting the whole world know what you've been doing.

Sue: Isn't a hickey a small price for feeling so good?

Bob: But you didn't get the hickey—I did!

Barry, seventeen, is gay:

I remember making out with a guy for the first time. We used to play basketball in the lot down the street and then come back to my place for a soda. This one time we were clowning around with towels drying off each other's sweat, and we started leaning up against each other. It was real exciting and real tender. We hugged and kissed for a while, then we went for a walk to get used to what had happened.

Barry and his friend went out for a walk, but when you're making out, it's not always so easy to know when or how to stop. Mary Ann, fifteen, told us:

I was rubbing his back and then his stomach and he took my hand and put it down between his legs. I felt this hard thing there under his pants. My God, it must be his penis, I thought. This must be what it feels like! I could tell he wanted me to touch it, but I didn't want to yet. Just then my parents got home, so we had to stop anyway.

Petting/Fooling Around

When you're feeling really excited, one thing seems to lead to another. If you go beyond hugging and kissing to "feeling up" (touching the girl's breasts) or to rubbing the other person's penis or clitoris, you are moving past what most people call "making out" into what some people call "petting" and others call "fooling around." You may or may not want to go that far. *You certainly don't have to, no matter how much you like the other person.* (See p. 92

for a discussion of being pressured and some thoughts on saying "Stop.")

Toni, fifteen, was ready to go further. She told us about the first time her boyfriend touched her breasts:

> He put his hands on my back and pulled out my shirt and put his hands underneath. Then he moved them around to my front and they were on my chest. It felt like this wonderful tickling. He put his hands inside my bra, and at first I felt a little embarrassed because my boobs are so small, but it really felt good, so I didn't really mind. All this time we were kissing and hugging each other.

Jerry, a sixteen-year-old from Washington, described how it was for him:

> I was feeling my way slowly, trying to catch on, wondering what was going to happen next. My girlfriend was more experienced than I was so there were times when I felt like she might be wanting me to do something more than I was doing. But it wasn't like she was sitting there waiting for me to make all the moves. That was a relief. She took my hands and sort of led them around to her chest. I really got into feeling her breasts. I unbuttoned her blouse and put my hands on her bra. Then I unhooked her bra and put my hands on her bare skin. It felt incredible.

Reading about Toni and Jerry, you might be saying, "Things don't go that smoothly for *me* most of the time." Getting into what some people call "heavier" sex increases the chances for misunderstanding what someone wants, or wondering if you are performing well, or for feeling bad about what you did. Remember that sex is not a performance, and that good sex usually takes knowing each other pretty well.

Touching Each Other's Genitals. For some couples, petting includes touching each other's genitals. Brian described a time with his girlfriend:

> She put her hands down my pants and I just about couldn't control myself. But I held back for a while because it was feeling so good I wanted it to last. She started masturbating my cock and I couldn't hold back anymore. After I came, we held each other really tight for a while, just lying next to each other. Then she took my hand and put it down her pants, and after a while she came too. It was great.

This is sometimes called "mutual masturbation." If you and your partner want to give each other orgasms like this and wonder how, you can read the section on sexual response and orgasm—but remember that *a book can't tell you exactly what will feel best*. You can find that out from each other.

Making each other come may be part of petting for you, or it may not. It depends on what you are both ready for. You can see that other teenagers who spoke in this section expressed a lot of tenderness for each other without giving

each other orgasms, so it's not something you *have* to do in order to be close.

Most people find that having an orgasm with someone else through petting is much more intimate than kissing or hugging or other kinds of making out. It can make you feel vulnerable to that person in a certain way, as if you have shared something very private. It can make you feel more emotionally involved. You may or may not want this. It is also, when you're ready, a wonderful way of giving each other pleasure *without worrying about pregnancy.**

Oral Sex

A group of New England teenagers who helped us on this chapter were talking about what it should include. Elaine said:

> I think you should have some stuff about oral sex, because a lot of people think, Oh, that's gross, or It's not good for you, or whatever. Some people feel that oral sex is bad or dirty.

Enrico added: "Yeah, say that like everything else oral sex takes some getting used to, but once you are used to it, it is very rewarding." But Marilyn jumped in, "Tell them they might *not* like it too. Tell them to brush their teeth afterwards, man!" As you can see, there are different opinions on oral sex.

Oral sex means using your mouth and tongue to stimulate someone sexually, usually by kissing and sucking their genitals. It is a kind of lovemaking that many people find very pleasurable and exciting (and it doesn't risk pregnancy). Many others don't feel comfortable with it at all and never have oral sex; or even if they have oral sex, they don't enjoy it. The important thing to remember is that what you do should feel right for *you*. If you don't want to have oral sex, you shouldn't. It isn't your "duty" to do it. You needn't let yourself be pushed into it, and you shouldn't push anyone else into it.

In some ways, oral sex is the most intimate kind of lovemaking. You are exposing your genitals to someone else's mouth, eyes, ears and nose, opening a part of you that you may feel shy about. Maybe, like many of us, you grew up hearing that penises and vaginas are secret, a little dirty, and not to be touched. You might say in your head, "I think genitals are fine," but when it comes to getting that close, you may feel embarrassed or hesitant, or downright repulsed. You may not be able to imagine ever feeling comfortable enough with someone, or with your body, to want to do it. There are so many ways that we can give ourselves and each other sexual pleasure that there isn't any reason to feel you have to do something that seems

---

*The only thing to be careful about is making sure none of the fluid from the boy's penis gets near the entrance to the girl's vagina. Sperm can swim, and pregnancy has been known to happen when a boy just ejaculated near or on the vaginal lips.

disgusting to you or that you really don't want to do. You may always feel that way, or maybe someday your feelings will change. There are years and years ahead to try things if you want to.

Licking or sucking a man's penis is technically called fellatio (fel-*lay*-she-oh). Slang terms for fellatio are: giving head, blow job, going down on, creaming. Johnny, who's sixteen, told us:

> I think there are lots of ways of making love. Me and my girl aren't into chancing a pregnancy, we don't want to have to deal with that. So we find other ways to get each other off, and for me, when she goes down on me it's great. I've had intercourse before and I think this way is just as good, maybe even better.

If the boy has an orgasm during oral sex, his semen (the fluid that spurts out of his penis) will end up in the girl's mouth unless one of the partners moves away at the last minute. Most girls we talked with who had tried oral sex said they didn't like the taste or the feeling; they were relieved to find out from each other that the boy doesn't have to come in their mouth and that, if he does, they don't have to swallow the fluid. Many girls also spoke of feeling suffocated during oral sex and not liking it much. They gave each other some support for saying no.

The girls in the New England discussion group thought that, on the whole, boys want oral sex done to them more than girls want to do it. "Hey, baby, will you give me a blow job???" one of them imitated. "Finish me off, honey, will you?" repeated someone else. From the resentment in their voices, we could sense that they sometimes feel pushed to have oral sex when they don't feel like it much. If, instead of saying no, they go ahead and do it under pressure, it's not very pleasant at all. Sometimes, because it feels so good, a boy will put pressure on a girl to try to persuade her to do it. Remember when we said, "You don't owe anyone a kiss"? Well, you don't owe anyone oral sex either. And, as Henry said (he's eighteen): "If she's not into it, I don't really dig it much, anyway. It's not as good if she's just doing it to please me."

Licking or sucking a girl's clitoris and vagina is technically called *cunnilingus* (cuh-nih-*ling*-gus). Slang terms used to describe cunnilingus are: eating, eating out, going down on. Since a woman's clitoris is the most sexually sensitive part of her body, this can bring her intense pleasure. Many women say it is the most enjoyable part of lovemaking for them. Donna, a seventeen-year-old, told us:

> I was with this guy who said, "Let me do something to you that I think you'll really like." And that was when he went down on me and started licking me. I was really kind of embarrassed at first, because I didn't really know what he was doing. But it felt really, really good, and I relaxed and just got into it.

You may have heard of the slang term "69." This refers to a couple turning their bodies so that each can do oral sex with the other at the same time. Some people like this, and others prefer to take turns. There is no "right" way in sex between people who are choosing freely to do what they are doing.

It can be hard to imagine that someone else could enjoy having his or her face so near your genitals. Girls seem to wonder about this more than boys do. Girls who have seen all the advertisements for vaginal deodorants may worry that their natural body smell is offensive. "Does he really think it smells good down there?" one girl asked. But boys wonder about how their genitals smell, too. It's a natural worry when you first start oral sex. Gloria put into words what a lot of people think:

> I was always brought up, as a little kid—you don't put things in your mouth, not your fingers, not pencils, not anything except food and your toothbrush. So to all of a sudden be asked by a guy to put his penis in my mouth makes me feel gross. That's why I won't let a guy go down on me. I always feel like it's smelly and dirty down there.

You may not want to have oral sex at all, and that's fine. But if you do, you don't have to worry about "dirtiness." All you need to do is wash yourself with soap and water. As Nancy said, "If you're going to try oral sex for the first time, you should be clean." If you are with someone you care about and decide you want to try oral sex, you'll probably find you like the natural smells and liquids. Also, part of the pleasure of oral sex comes from being able to relax and stop worrying about how you look or smell.

Some people disapprove completely of oral sex. They think of it as "perverted" and "immoral." Some people with strong, traditional religious beliefs believe that any kind of sexual practice other than sexual intercourse between husband and wife is forbidden by the Bible. If members of your family or community believe this, you may choose not to have oral sex now, or maybe ever. Or you may decide that you don't agree with their view. This is the kind of hard decision that all of us end up making as we find our way (sometimes stumbling) toward how we can best express our own sexuality.

Some people disapprove of oral sex because they think, mistakenly, that only homosexual couples do it. These people's homophobia—that is, the irrational fear of homosexuals—makes them believe that these acts are therefore "perverted." In fact, some states still have laws on the books (rarely enforced) that outlaw oral sex; the few times these laws have been used, it has been to harass homosexuals. Of course, many gay and lesbian couples enjoy oral sex, but they don't have a corner on the market—many heterosexual couples do as well.

As far as we're concerned (we've said it before, but with oral sex it bears repeating), the only time any sex is perverted or immoral is if it is being forced on someone, or someone is doing it under pressure. *If you find yourself having oral sex because you think you owe it to your partner, we think that's wrong.* It's a misuse of your sexuality, and a misuse of an act which, in other circumstances or another relationship, could be a source of pleasure and passion and closeness.

Sexual Intercourse

A sexual relationship involves the pleasure of being near someone who excites you, someone you may care a great deal about. It can mean feeling aroused in every inch of your body. The two of you might spend hours feeling and touching and kissing and looking at each other. You might bring each other to orgasm. You can hold each other and be quiet with each other and be naked with each other. Sometimes as part of that sexual relationship a boy and a girl will want to have intercourse.

We do not assume that you want to have sex at this point. Many teenagers we met told us they want to wait until they are older. Whenever you do choose to have intercourse, we hope you will consider it carefully and do only what you feel is best for you and those you care about. If you *are* having sex now, we hope the information here will be helpful to you. If you are not, we hope this section will answer questions you may be curious about.

NOTE TO READERS WITH GAY AND LESBIAN EXPERIENCE: Although some gay men who have anal sex refer to it as "intercourse," in this chapter we are using the word "intercourse" to mean *heterosexual* intercourse (between males and females). We will use "lovemaking" to refer to things that gay *and* straight couples do. Even for heterosexual couples, however, intercourse is often not the main thing they do or even their favorite part of making love. Lovemaking is much more than intercourse. Some of the topics in this section on intercourse will be relevant to many couples, whether gay or straight: for instance, issues about deciding, communicating and the first time. We have included quotes from teenagers with gay and lesbian experience where we have them. For more, see the section "Exploring Sex with Someone of Your Own Sex," p. 112.

Deciding about Intercourse

In one sense the only difference between intercourse and all the other things people do in sex is that in intercourse a boy's penis goes into a girl's vagina. But that simple difference is a major one for most teenagers. The decision about intercourse is bigger, tougher, and often more confusing than any of the others. If you are considering having intercourse with someone, we suggest reading "When and How Far" (p. 86) for the basic issues in deciding how far you want to go with someone. Here we will present the extra issues that teenagers told us about in the special decision about intercourse.

Having sexual intercourse means the risk of *pregnancy*. As Brian, a seventeen-year-old from Massachusetts, said:

> My girlfriend and I do just about everything but actually screw. Neither one of us wants to get into that, since we're not ready to deal with the possibility of her getting pregnant. I don't know what we'd do if that happened.

If there's even a *chance* of your having sex with someone, it's time to look into *birth control* (see p. 159). Intercourse also means an increased risk of *sexually transmitted disease* (see p. 216).

Emotionally, having sexual intercourse often means making yourself more vulnerable, more open to intense feelings of joy and hurt. Andy, seventeen, remarked:

> When my girlfriend and I started making love, our relationship changed somehow. We were closer, but not completely. In fact, when we had fights we felt further away than ever, and things she did hurt me more easily. We got thinking about the future too. It was like crossing a bridge to another shore.

Some people don't feel ready for that extra vulnerability. Molly, fourteen, explained:

> Breaking up after you have intercourse is much harder, I think. Especially for the girl. How could you face the guy afterwards, knowing that you'd done that with him? I don't want to have intercourse until I really fall in love with a guy and know we won't break up.

Molly will probably find that you can never "know" for sure that you won't break up. But there *is* a kind of sureness and closeness that most people want to have before having sex with someone.

Traditionally in our culture, people have saved intercourse for a long-term, committed relationship—usually marriage. Many teenagers today believe that waiting like this is right for them. Many of the teenagers we spoke with, however, are open to having sex without being married. Some are more casual about it than others, but most of them have certain *conditions* that are important to them before they will do it. For most, it has to be with someone who is willing to share responsibility for birth control and preventing VD. For some, it has to be with someone they plan to marry. For others it must be someone they love or whom they know well and trust. Marilee, a ninth-grader from Detroit, said:

> Making love means something to me. It means really loving the person you're doing it with and it means not feeling bad that you did it even if the two of you

break up. I'm just not ready for that yet. I'm only fifteen and I think that's way too young to be getting so involved with somebody. I just can't see myself handling that kind of a relationship.

Dexter, a sixteen-year-old from the same city, added:

Before I'd do it with some girl I'd want to know her really well. I'd want to respect her and I'd want her to respect me. If you're going to be that close with someone, then you really want to feel something between you, you want to care for each other.

Greg, a gay seventeen-year-old who read over this chapter while we were working on it, said:

Bars are one of the only places that gay guys can meet, because usually we can't be open in school or at work. At this one bar I go to sometimes there's a pickup scene that I hate. After one evening of conversation and some dancing, I feel pressured to go home with some guy and go to bed with him. But I don't. Because what I'm looking for is a good relationship. Then I'll get into making love. That's the order I want it to go in.

Boys get a lot of pressure to "score" with their girl-friends, but many don't want to. Denny, a tenth-grader from Denver, said:

I don't believe in that "fuck'em and leave'em" thing. People put too much emphasis on guys always trying to get some. For me, if I find someone I feel real close to and we want to do it, then we will. Otherwise I can wait. I sure as hell won't do it just because somebody's pushing me.

These four are all speaking about *standards* or conditions they have for when they feel ready to have sex.

One standard that people have differing opinions about is *virginity*. A "virgin" is defined as someone, male or female, who hasn't had sexual intercourse. Virginity, especially for girls, is widely thought to symbolize purity, virtue and honor.

In many cultures and ethnic groups it is considered a disaster for the family if a girl loses her virginity before she marries. One Chicana from Los Angeles said:

My father was just about ready to beat up my boy-friend because he thought he was taking advantage of me. He thought we were going to "go all the way." He saw us making out in the backyard and he won't let us see each other anymore. So now we have to sneak behind his back to be together.

And a boy from the Midwest said:

My parents were pretty serious with me about sex. They really tried to get me to see that my girlfriend's reputation would be at stake if we had intercourse; that if anyone found out, she would be considered "damaged property." Can you believe that—Damaged Property?

In the past a woman's virginity has been seen as a sign that she is a man's property—her father's and then her husband's. That is a difficult idea to accept these days when we are working so hard for equality between women and men. (By "equality" we don't mean that men and women are the same, but we do mean that no one belongs to anyone else, and that women's and men's and boys' and girls' actions should be judged by the same standards.) We who are writing this book believe that women are *not* the property of their husbands, just as men are not the property of their wives. We are people, not property. Protecting a girl's virginity to keep her as pure "undamaged" goods for the person she will eventually "belong" to just doesn't make sense.

Many parents stress virginity not so much for family honor as for fear of pregnancy or concern about their child feeling used or hurt. These are certainly legitimate worries. Parents are usually more protective of their daughters than their sons, however, because girls can get pregnant, but also because of the double standard in all matters of sex: in many families boys are not expected to stay virgins, whereas girls are.

In making your decision about whether to keep your virginity or not, you will undoubtedly be influenced by your family's ideas and have to wrestle with whether you agree with their beliefs.

The idea of virginity makes a lot of people feel guilty about having sex. It sometimes makes sex a contest between boys and girls, with boys pushing for intercourse and girls "defending" their virginity. It sometimes makes people get married before they are ready to, just so they can have sex. You may think, as many people do, that we should stop thinking virginity is so special, and make our decisions about sex for other reasons.

The idea of virginity is still important to many people, however. It is probably a big help to both girls *and* boys who don't want to rush into sexual intercourse and need some guidance, or a reason for waiting. Also, having sex with someone can be a big step, and the idea of virginity can remind you to respect this. In this case, virginity isn't so much a matter of "protecting the property from damage" as guarding your sense of yourself and what you want for yourself.

Pressures. There is probably more pressure to *have* sex these days than not to. Several teenagers who spoke with us had regrets about giving in to pressure. Wanda, who's now in college, gave in to her boyfriend:

I was thirteen and I only did it to keep my boyfriend. He kept hinting that he was going to break up with me if I wouldn't do it. But afterwards I kept thinking, What am I going to tell my kids? I felt like I was too young and I was really sorry that I did it, especially with a jerk like Ricky, who obviously didn't care about me very much anyway.

Charles, a tenth-grader from Washington, gave in to expectations everyone seemed to have of him as a boy:

> If a guy says no, he better have a good excuse, like an overdose or a heart attack or something, because the pressure is really on you. Like when you're making out with a girl and she wants it and you don't—maybe you think there's a chance she might get pregnant, or you just don't want to get that involved with her, or maybe you've never done it before and you're frightened. You have to really hope that the girl's mature enough to understand that. And the one I was with wasn't. So I went ahead and fucked her, but I felt like a piece of crap the whole time. And I was really afraid for the next four weeks that she was going to call me up and tell me she was pregnant.

Trish, sixteen, felt the pressure of "sexual liberation"—the idea that to be cool you have to have sex. She spoke bitterly:

> I felt dirty, I really felt dirty. I felt that I had deceived my mother in a way, too, because she had always told me, "Wait till you're sure, wait till you're sure." And I wasn't sure. *I just did it because everyone else was doing it.* And it didn't feel good, and I didn't like it, and I thought it sucked all around.

Because of the pressures and the possibilities of getting hurt, a group of high school students in Boston wanted us to be careful that this book didn't pressure teens to have sexual intercourse. Here are some of the things they said:

> In your book you should say some things about not having sex early. Say that it's OK to have sexual feelings, to get horny or excited, and *not* to go out and do it. . . . If you don't have sex with somebody, you don't have to worry about getting pregnant. . . . You don't have to worry about what you're supposed to do, or if you're pleasing your partner. . . . If you have a partner and you build into it instead of rushing into it, the act itself feels a lot nicer. If you rush into it, you feel like a piece of shit afterwards. . . . You wouldn't have to worry, Did I do this right, did I do that right, was I being used, should it have happened. . . . If you're worried about it at all, then it wasn't right. . . . The slower the better.

They were talking mainly about *taking care of themselves*—trying not to do something they'll feel bad about, wanting to be as sure as they can. And, as one of them added:

> I don't see why everybody's so hung up on intercourse. There are so many wonderful ways of turning each other on without putting a penis anywhere near a vagina.

Waiting. Angela, a twenty-year-old from Oregon, told us this:

> In the eleventh grade I became aware that everybody I knew was having sex, and I hadn't yet. All my friends, even the holdouts, were starting to talk about doing it with this guy or that, and I thought, Oh my God, I'm so backward. And people would say to me, "You're not worldly; you're not a woman; you can't understand what we're talking about because you're still a virgin." In my head I could say, That is such crap, how can they say that about me. But underneath it was hurting me and I was thinking, What's wrong with me? I spent a lot of time the next few years thinking about what it would mean to me to have intercourse with a guy. I just knew that I couldn't make love with someone I didn't love. So I waited. Then this year, my second year at college, I started going out with someone I really care about. We have fun together, we like the same things, and we respect each other's opinion about things. We've started talking about making love and it feels OK to me. I feel ready. Even though we aren't thinking about getting married or anything, I feel good about us making love.

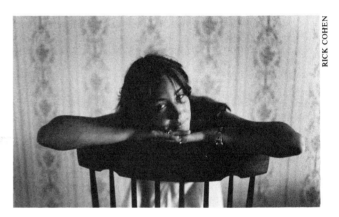

Deciding not to have sex *can* mean the end of a relationship, though usually that means the relationship wouldn't have lasted much longer anyway. Candy, seventeen, from New York, reported:

> I was going out with this guy and we were having fun together, but he really wanted to have sex and I really didn't want to. I just felt like I wasn't ready—like I wasn't in love with him the way I wanted to be before I'd do that. I gave it a lot of thought. I talked to my mom about it, and she really helped me to feel good about my decision. So all of a sudden this guy stopped calling me—this guy who had been all along telling me how much he loved me and everything. I didn't really feel bad about his not calling me anymore, because I knew that if sex was all he wanted, then I didn't really want to go out with him.

Just because you've had sex before doesn't mean you have to do it again until you want to. Tony, seventeen, from Kansas City, said:

> I feel this way about it. I'm just not into making love anymore. I did it a few times when that was the thing to do, you know, but I didn't really like it. I don't need that, man. But all my friends are telling me,

Hey, what's wrong with you? You weird or something? They say, Oh, that's why you're breaking out in pimples, you don't get enough sex. But that has nothing to do with it. I haven't done it now in a couple of years, and I'm not planning to do it again until I want to.

Emily, seventeen, added:

I always felt like after I had broken up with the guy I had sex with the first time that it was just sort of expected that every time I went out with somebody I was going to have intercourse. And especially if it was an older guy. Every time I was with an older guy they've always said, ''Well, if you've already had sex anyway, why wouldn't you want to do it now?'' Like once you're not a virgin anymore, what's the difference? Once you've had it you're automatically supposed to do it all the time from then on. I felt like that for a long time until I realized that it's up to me. I mean it's up to me not to do it if I don't want to. You have the right to say, Hey, I don't feel like having sex with you.

Having Sexual Intercourse. *Like so many things in sex, intercourse can be great if you want to be doing it and trust the person you're doing it with—and awful if you don't.* Having intercourse can be an amazingly intimate experience, a way for two people to express their deepest feelings of love for each other, and to risk being extremely vulnerable. More simply, it can also be an act of affection, pleasure and friendliness. Sometimes intercourse is passionate, sometimes awkward, sometimes funny, or playful, or tender, or sorrowful, or frustrating, or even dull. Sometimes you're in the mood for it and sometimes you're not. It's also something people tend to enjoy more with experience, and with a partner they know and trust.

We have so many expectations, so many fantasies about what IT will be like. It seems like everything we've heard or seen or learned about sex is all pointing in one direction: toward sexual intercourse—which, in slang, people call fucking, humping, screwing, home base, going all the way, making it. The importance of intercourse has been so exaggerated in books and magazines and movies that people forget it is only one part of lovemaking. Teenagers also get so little information about it that they often don't know what to expect. Even teens who have had intercourse say there's a lot that they don't know. The teenagers who advised us about this chapter said, ''Be straight about it. Tell what it is, who does what, the different ways people might feel, the problems and what to do about them.'' And a couple of them added, ''Be sure to say it's not always what it's cracked up to be.''

What happens in intercourse. Michelle, a thirteen-year-old from Los Angeles, said:

I've been trying and trying to envision it, but I still can't exactly figure out how two people actually get together. I know the girl spreads her legs, but I don't know what happens after that.

Another thirteen-year-old, named Matt, added:

In my sixth-grade class it seems like we talked about everything. I mean like we talked about rubbers, birth control, VD, everything. The teacher told us a lot of stuff. But then a little later on I saw some people actually doing it, you know, making love, and I thought it was pretty weird-looking.

In sexual intercourse the man's erect penis goes into the woman's vagina and moves in and out in a way that ideally stimulates both of them. The couple can be lying down, sitting, standing up, or on their sides. Any position that is comfortable for both of them and in which the vagina and penis can fit together is a good position for intercourse. If they are lying down, either the man or the woman can be on top, depending on which is most stimulating for both of them. Each couple will find the positions they like. It is especially important to find a position in which the woman's clitoris gets good stimulation (see below).

Usually a lot of kissing and stroking and licking and hugging goes on in the lovemaking before intercourse. This is good, because for a woman, especially, it's best to be very aroused when intercourse starts. Sometimes one or both will have an orgasm in this time. All of this is sometimes called ''foreplay,'' but we're avoiding the term because calling it foreplay makes it sound as though everything a couple does in sex is just leading up to the ''goal'' of intercourse. These other forms of caressing and lovemaking are great, with or without intercourse, and often bring just as much satisfaction and closeness as intercourse can.

When both are ready for intercourse, one of the partners usually reaches down to guide the penis into the vagina with his or her hand. ''Ready'' for a man is when he is excited enough to have an erection. A woman is really ready a while *after* the lips of her vagina get wet, when her whole pelvic area is feeling full or swollen, and aroused the section ''Sexual Response,'' on p. 81, will help your understanding of this). When the penis is inside, the couple move their hips and lower body so that their pelvic areas rub against each other, and so that the penis pushes into the vagina and then pulls partly out again (sometimes called thrusting). This moving together can lead to orgasm for one or both of them, unless they decide to stop.

You might come almost immediately, shortly after the penis enters the vagina, or you might go on for five, ten, fifteen minutes or longer. Generally it takes a man a shorter time to reach orgasm than it does a woman, since his penis gets *direct* stimulation from the movements they are making. The woman's clitoris, however, gets only *indirect* stimulation from the thrusting of the penis in her vagina: the penis moves the swollen inner lips around the vaginal opening; these inner lips are connected to the hood of skin over the clitoris; the hood moves, rubbing the clitoris. The outer third of the vagina *is* sexually sensitive, but the clitoris is the most important in orgasm. When she heard about this difference in men's and women's body design, one girl exclaimed, ''That's not fair!'' Actually it's not fair only when people define lovemaking as involving *only* putting a penis into a vagina, and assume that what satisfies a man will satisfy a woman.

To have an orgasm during intercourse, a woman may want the man to rub around her clitoris more directly with his hand, or she can rub it herself at her own speed. She may find a position in which her clitoral area gets lots of pressure and rubbing from his body. Many women also find that they do not have an orgasm during actual intercourse, and prefer to reach orgasm by oral sex or other kinds of touching. There's no one way to reach orgasm. What works is what's right for you.

Sometimes one or both partners won't reach orgasm, which is fine if they don't feel the need to. There is a whole lot to enjoy in intercourse whether or not you come. If you don't come and want to, see p. 82 for some suggestions.

Often one person will reach orgasm before the other. Even though a lot of novels talk about the thrill of reaching orgasm together (called ''simultaneous orgasm''), it doesn't have to happen that way to feel good.

During intercourse a couple can experience great closeness, sharing each other's rhythm and excitement. They can adjust to each other's pace. Each one can move in a way that is stimulating to herself or himself as well as to the other. This double joy of giving and getting pleasure is one of the special things about intercourse. But, as many teenagers mentioned to us, don't expect it to be wonderful every time.

Pregnancy. When a boy has an orgasm and ejaculates, his semen, which usually contains millions of sperm, spurts out into the girl's vagina. If the couple isn't using birth control, these sperm will swim up into her uterus and fallopian tubes where they can fertilize an egg. If a sperm enters an egg, the girl is pregnant. So if you're having intercourse and don't want a pregnancy, *protect yourself and your partner by using birth control.* Worrying about pregnancy is one sure way to ruin sex—you can't relax and enjoy it and feel all the sensations if somewhere in your mind a voice is agitating: ''Is she going to get pregnant?'' or ''Am I going to get pregnant?'' Since getting and using birth control is sometimes hard, see the section on birth control (p. 159) for some information and support.

The first time. Tony, a seventeen-year-old from Hartford, spoke for many people:

> Since I haven't had intercourse yet, I worry about what will happen and whether I'll be able to perform.

There are a lot of stories that the first time you have sex you come in five seconds because you're so excited, and you let your woman down.

There are lots of fantasies and expectations and, as Tony said, worries about what the first time will be like. From what the teenagers we interviewed said to us, sometimes it's great, sometimes it's terrible, and usually it's somewhere in between. Steve, who's sixteen, described his first time:

> My first time definitely lived up to my fantasies, not so much the physical fantasies because it was so much faster than I thought it would be, but the emotional fantasies. It was the night before my sixteenth birthday and we were both virgins. We were both scared, but I knew it was right because we really cared about each other. We had talked about it for a long time and we both really wanted to do it. My girlfriend came over to my house. My parents weren't home, so we didn't have to worry about anybody walking in on us. We were making out and we were both getting so turned on because we knew what was going to happen. I didn't really get all the way inside because she was so tight, but it felt amazing anyway. I was so excited that I came right away, so it only lasted a few seconds. The best part was being together afterwards and not being uptight about it. We went out to dinner after, and just being with her was really special for me. It was totally emotional, much more emotional than I had expected.

And Nancy, sixteen, remembered:

> When I had intercourse for the first time it was because I really wanted to do it. We talked about it and sort of planned when we would do it. We tried to make it romantic—you know, with candles and everything. I went out and got myself a diaphragm and I practiced putting it in. The actual intercourse wasn't as great as I thought it would be, but the part leading up to it and the part being together afterwards was really nice.

Sexual experiences are so personal and different depending on the particular circumstances that these two descriptions may not be at all like yours was or will be. Steve and Nancy did, however, mention some things that many people talked about. They both were sure they wanted to do it. They both managed to get enough privacy. (This is very important. See p. 106 for more on privacy.)

A third thing that Nancy mentioned was *birth control*. This is essential. (We wonder what Steve and his girlfriend were doing about it.) Often the first time is the hardest time to use birth control, because you're so excited and maybe nervous and possibly shy. But sperms and eggs don't care about first times: a girl's body is as ready to get pregnant then as at any other time. It is a shame when someone's introduction to having intercourse brings the heartache of pregnancy—but it happens. And although neither Steve nor Nancy mentioned it, you need to be careful about sexually transmitted diseases, too (see p. 216).

Steve mentions some problems that often come up the first several times you make love: a tight entrance to the girl's vagina, or the boy coming more quickly than he wants. See p. 111 for more on these very common problems.

Sexy novels make a big deal about the pain and anguish a woman feels at the climactic moment of the "tearing" of her hymen in first intercourse. It's usually not so dramatic—Nancy doesn't mention pain at all—but it *can* be painful, and it makes sense to take it slowly.

Many people say that the physical part, the actual intercourse, isn't so terrific the first time. Intercourse doesn't automatically feel wonderful to both people involved. We have to *learn* about intercourse, just as we have to learn how to swim or ride a bicycle or play tennis. So although it can be exciting to be naked together and it can be a great turn-on to anticipate that this time you're really going to go all the way, when it comes down to really doing it, you may find that you're disappointed.

Francie, seventeen, told her teen discussion group:

> When we went to have actual intercourse, it wasn't exciting anymore. My legs were starting to shake, and he couldn't get in at first. I was just lying there going through this pain. Finally I just said, "Let's go. Do whatever you have to do, just go all the way in because I'm getting tired of this. Maybe it will go better once it's all the way in or something." It just wasn't great. Then afterwards we were lying there and that felt better than the intercourse—hugging and kissing each other. I didn't like intercourse at all.

Ron, sixteen, said:

> The fantasies that I had about it were way off. I imagined real vivid things like heavy body sensations and getting lost in passion and feeling like we'd love each other forever after experiencing this together. And what really struck me was how different the reality was. Somehow I had the idea that things would just happen, like you'd just do everything real smoothly without much effort. But that wasn't the way it happened at all. In the first place it really seemed to hurt my girlfriend, she was really tight and I had a lot of trouble getting in. And once I did get in, it wasn't like we were carried away with passion. I came and it was over and that was that. I have to say it wasn't at all what I expected.

Sheri, who's seventeen and from New England, said:

> The first time I had intercourse I was lying there thinking, You mean this is IT? Am I supposed to be thrilled by this? It wasn't that it hurt me or anything, because it didn't. It just didn't feel like anything to me. I figured there must be something wrong with me, so I didn't say a word to him.

It is understandable that Sheri would feel that something is "wrong" with her. Since for so many of us intercourse has been built up in our minds to be the most fantastic part of a sexual relationship, if it doesn't feel as great as you expect it should, you might be confused and think you are unusual. You might worry that you're the only one who doesn't enjoy intercourse. Girls, especially, may see that the boy is enjoying it and wonder why it isn't feeling the same to them.

One discussion group made us promise to make it very clear that people sometimes don't enjoy intercourse. As they said:

> Kids always think, I'm *supposed* to be feeling this way or that way, and they feel bad if they don't. So you have to tell people that there's no one way to feel in intercourse.

It will be too bad for Sheri and her boyfriend if she doesn't tell him how she felt, because if he doesn't know, it will be hard for them to do it differently the next time. Lots of people of both sexes get into pretending to enjoy intercourse, when in fact they don't. A nineteen-year-old who's now in college said:

> Everyone's going around wondering why they aren't having the greatest sexual experiences in the world and nobody's saying anything about it.

For more on talking about sex, see p. 105.

Of course, many teenagers do have nice experiences their first time. Lois, a sixteen-year-old from Portland, Oregon remembered:

> It was nice because we were at my house in my own bedroom and we knew each other really well. We'd been naked a lot together anyway, so that was no hassle, but before this time I had felt definitely that there was no doing it until you were married, or at least engaged, so we never did. But then, when my ideas started changing, I realized I didn't know when I wanted to get married, or even if I ever wanted to, and that seemed like too long a time to wait.
>
> Since we were both virgins, I felt really comfortable, like no one was expecting me to know anything. We just figured it out for ourselves and I have to say it was really a great experience. I felt like we were in it together, like both of us really cared about helping each other to have it be good.

Cindy, seventeen, described making love with another girl for the first time:

> The first time Paula and I made love I felt real awkward and hoped she wouldn't notice. I kept thinking there must be something special that girls do. At one point we both cracked up because I finally said, "Hey, Paula, I hate to say this but I don't exactly know what to do." She just kind of took my hand and put it on her, and I was feeling so excited and loving

that pretty soon I just let my hands move all over her body and it was fine.

And Ethan, a high school senior from Michigan, said:

> The first time I did it was with someone I didn't know real well so I was surprised that she wanted to do it. She was more experienced than I was, she'd done it before, so I was thinking, Hey, this is my lucky night. I was so hot to try it, but at the same time I was thinking, Hey, what am I supposed to do now? I was like wondering how this thing was actually going to come off. She sort of helped me guide it in, and it was this amazing feeling. I just closed my eyes and started moving. She was moving with me and it felt so good. The next day at school I wanted to tell everybody, but I was cool.

LEARNING ABOUT SEX / TALKING ABOUT IT / ENJOYING IT MORE

Just about everything that two people do together in sex takes some learning. We often forget this. We think we should "naturally" know how to do whatever it is—kiss, make out, help someone have an orgasm. Often we feel embarrassed if we don't. But although sexual *feelings* may come naturally, what we *do* with them doesn't.

Just because you are feeling excited from your head to your toes, or because you love somebody, doesn't mean you will know what to do, or that sex will be great. Sex is basically a way of communicating between two people, and there are some things that help: time, for instance, and trust, and privacy, and information, and a chance to talk about what's going on.

This section is about some of the things that teenagers told us help them to enjoy sex more and to know themselves and their partners better.

Learning about Sex with Someone Else

A lot of what we learn about sex is through experimenting. For most of us the first time we do anything we're not exactly sure what we're doing. Charlie, who's fourteen, said:

> I had my big chance with this girl I liked a whole lot, because we were at a party on the couch together and we started kissing. But I didn't know what to do. I mean, it was so romantic, but I didn't know how to be romantic. I felt really out of it.

Abigail, seventeen, explained:

> Part of the growing-up thing is that you don't know what to do. I mean you're just learning everything. You know, like I used to think that just touching a guy's penis made him feel great. And people would say, you know, you have to be really careful because a penis is so sensitive, so then I'd be really careful, like just touching it so lightly he could hardly feel it.

No one ever told me anything different until just recently one guy said, "Don't worry, it's not going to break."

In sex, a lot can be learned over time, like what feels good to you and your partner, how lightly or hard to kiss or rub or squeeze or press. Generally it's different for every different person. There aren't any rules except to be honest with yourself and your partner about what you like and what you don't like. People can teach each other what to do.

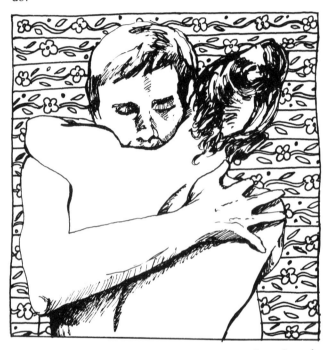

Sometimes what feels great to one person doesn't to the other. Sometimes what turns you on turns your partner off, or it even hurts. Mack, a fifteen-year-old boy from Ohio, said:

> Me and my girlfriend were making out and for the first time she let me put my hands under her bra. I felt like I just wanted to squeeze her, but I was worried that that might hurt her. It felt so good to me, I didn't know whether to let myself get carried away or not. She told me to stop when I pinched her nipple. She said it didn't feel good, but it felt great to me.

Breasts and penises and clitorises are very sensitive, and can bring a great deal of pleasure during sex. However, if you squeeze or rub too hard, you can cause your partner pain. A girl's clitoris and nipples, and the tip of a boy's penis are especially sensitive to being rubbed too hard, although, of course, "too hard" only means what feels too hard to that person. In general, when two people are first learning about each other, it's best to go slowly and gently until you both feel comfortable and trusting of what's going on.

How do you tell someone if what he or she is doing is

hurting you or not feeling so great? Often you can do it without words, as Paula did:

> My boyfriend was trying to masturbate me, but he was doing it too hard and it hurt me. So I sort of put my hand on top of his and showed him how to do it. Now he's getting to be an expert.

Sam told us:

> The other night Donna kept rubbing me after I came. It had felt so terrific, but all of a sudden after I came it hurt like crazy. I shouted "Ouch! Stop!" But then I thought, Uh-oh, kid, you maybe made her feel bad. She was just trying to do something nice. When we talked about it, she said it was cool—how was she supposed to know unless I told her?

Sometimes you may hesitate to ask your partner to stop or change what he or she is doing. You might think it will hurt his or her feelings. This will be true only if your partner thinks he or she *should* know how to do everything in sex. Too many of us grow up feeling that sex is a performance, and if you say, "Please don't do that," you might come across as criticizing the performance. But we all owe it to each other to help sex *not* be a performance. And we owe it to *ourselves* not to put up with something that hurts!

Sex Roles. Boys often feel they *should know* what do do. Jim, fifteen, confessed:

> When I get with my girlfriend, I think, You're the guy. You're supposed to know the moves. And here I am all tangled up in her bra trying to get it off. I don't know any more than she does.

Boys carry a lot of performance worries into sex, because they are taught that a boy should somehow know everything and teach his partner. Frank, sixteen, wants this to change:

> At our level in high school there are so many games that you end up playing. Especially the guy, because we're "supposed" to know everything about sex. Man, if a girl ever seduced me—that would be beautiful. It's so much easier for me when the girl lets me know what she wants. It's hard for a guy to know how to turn on a girl, so it's great when she lets you know. It's just cutting out the bullshit, it's admitting that we both want to do it and we both want to enjoy it.

Girls can enjoy sex just as much as boys do. Girls get horny and girls get turned on just as boys do. But there's a kind of unwritten rule that a lot of girls learned as they were growing up: it says, "Follow the boy's lead, especially in sex." That's the rule that gets us into trouble. That's the rule that makes boys feel they have to know what they are doing. That's the rule that keeps girls from initiating sex and calling up boys for dates and showing boys how to move and where to touch. That's the rule that

makes it hard for a girl to tell a guy how to make sex better for her.

Things are changing. As girls get more accepting of being sexual, and as they feel less judged by others for being sexual, they can start to initiate more and speak up about what they do and don't want. And boys can feel more relaxed about learning *with* their partners.

Talking about Sex

When you are learning something new in sex or learning about a new partner, talking helps. Even if you have been with the same person for a long time, it is natural to want to know if the other person liked what you did, or whether you felt the same kind of sensations. You can tell how things feel to *you,* but a lot of the time it's hard to tell how your partner is feeling. That's why being able to talk with each other about sex is so important. Talking is also indispensable when you are deciding with someone how far you want to go.

Linda, sixteen, told us of an experience that shows how unpleasant and alienating it can be if too much is left unsaid:

> I was over at my boyfriend Mike's house and we were lying on his bed kissing and everything, and he took my hand and put it down his pants so I could feel his penis. But I didn't know what I was supposed to do, I had never done that before. So I was just touching it lightly, sort of tickling it. Then he started moving my hand up and down, so I figured that's what he wanted me to do. But I was afraid of hurting him. He was totally quiet through the whole thing. He didn't say a word, so I didn't know if I was doing it right, but he got really excited and closed his eyes and had an orgasm. The weirdest thing was that afterwards he just got up and didn't say anything about it. I wanted him to say something. Like I wanted to know did I do it right. It was new to me, I wanted to talk about it, but of course I didn't say anything because he didn't say anything. So right after we acted as if the whole thing never happened.

Many couples don't have much practice in talking about sex. Robert, a senior from Iowa, is frustrated by the lack of talking:

> It takes so long for things to happen just because each person's waiting for the other one to say something. It's so stupid. You keep wondering, Well, should I do this or should I do that. Or, Will she like this or doesn't she want me to do that. All that time wasted when if we could just talk to each other you could clear it up in a minute. But it's so hard to talk. I have this image that sex is supposed to be silent, just lovers looking into each other's eyes and knowing exactly what to do. Well, that image really fucks me up a lot because I hardly ever feel like I know exactly what to do.

A lot of people say they feel awkward talking about sex with their partner—especially if they don't know the person really well, and often even if they do. Talking about sex feels embarrassing. Maybe, as Robert said, it seems that sex should come naturally. Or, it seems that sex should be romantic—and talking ruins the romance of it. Or, if you aren't sure you want to be doing what you are doing—if you are feeling unsure at all or guilty at all—then talking about it might seem to bring it all out in the open too much. Or maybe you think you don't ''deserve'' to have it be better. Or it seems ''selfish'' to ask.

Louise, a seventeen-year-old girl from Idaho, gave another reason why speaking up about sex is difficult:

> Can you imagine making out with a guy and being able to say, ''Oh, I don't like that, Oh, I wish you would do this.'' I think that's ridiculous. I'm not comfortable enough with my own body to be able to tell some other person about it.

In lots of ways she's right. Before you can teach someone else what feels good to you, it helps to learn about your body yourself. Even then, you may think that what really turns you on is weird or different from what turns on everyone else, so you don't say anything. Or you may think you ought to be enjoying some sexual activity you've heard other people talk about, but really it doesn't do anything for you. You may not feel comfortable taking your time getting excited because you fear your partner's impatience and you worry about ruining the ''mood.'' All these things and more keep people from being honest with each other about sex.

Sometimes it is tempting to *pretend* to be into it, because you think sex is ''supposed'' to feel automatically wonderful. Joanne, eighteen, speaks of the special kind of loneliness this can bring:

> Sometimes when I'm fooling around with someone and he's really into it and I'm not—I mean, if it's not feeling good to me and I kind of wish I weren't doing it—then I feel alone and out of it. But I never know what to say.

Girls tend to pretend more than boys do, because they have been taught to be afraid of hurting boys' feelings. Boys, too, talked about making out or even making love when they weren't in the mood. But •*pretending isn't a good idea*. It might feel awkward at first to say what's really going on, but if you *don't* there's no way things can change.

''If we can't talk about sex, maybe we shouldn't be together,'' you might say. Sometimes this is true. If you don't feel close or trusting enough to share your inner feelings with someone, it may mean you would rather not be with that person at all. Maybe it means you need to become better friends before you go any further into sex. But don't be too hard on yourself. You can feel friendly and

comfortable with a person and *still* feel awkward talking about sex. We certainly aren't brought up being encouraged to do it, and it takes practice.

Talking with your friends or in a boy-girl discussion group can help. Just getting so you can say ''penis'' or ''vagina'' or ''clitoris'' or ''orgasm'' out loud to someone else without blushing is a big step for many people. Finding out in such a group that your feelings aren't unusual or weird can also reassure you.

It can also be good to talk with your partner about sex sometime when you're not in the middle of it—before or after, or on the next day when you're walking together or doing some work together. Then if there's something you want to change or aren't comfortable with, it doesn't come across like an on-the-spot criticism. And it doesn't feel like an interruption.

Appreciations are important, too. Talking about the *good* things improves a sexual relationship just as much as talking out the problems. And finally, it helps to *know* that talking about sex is an important thing to do. It doesn't solve everything: some problems or disagreements persist painfully no matter how much talking you do. But it can help.

Privacy

Privacy makes a big difference in any kind of sex, but it's often one of the hardest things for teenagers to get. Meg, seventeen, complained:

> It's so hard for teenagers to fool around in privacy, so you never can relax. At least I can't—I'm always worried about making too much noise and someone hearing us. Like once we were in a car with this other couple and you can imagine what that was like. Everybody trying to pretend that the other people weren't there. I was so uptight I could hardly close my eyes, and anytime my boyfriend made a sound I was going ''Shh, shhh.''

Richard, sixteen, said:

> A lot of times people our age have sex pretty rushed—like, their parents are going to be home in an hour. It kind of messes things up.

Teenagers have such a hard time getting privacy that often they end up making out or even having sex in a car (if they can get one) or in a public place at night, or with a relative in the next room. This is unfair. Not having privacy rushes you sexually; it might even rush you into going further without having time to think whether you want to. It keeps you from the kind of gradual learning about each other's bodies that is so important. It can make you careless, too. One teenager wrote to us:

> THIS IS IMPORTANT! If you're having sexual intercourse, lack of privacy contributes to not using birth

control. If this fantastic, unexpected opportunity arises, who wants to pass it up???

Lack of privacy also robs you of the time and space to talk about your relationship or even just to enjoy being close. Francie, who is in a lesbian relationship, said:

Because girls aren't supposed to be in love with each other, Dorie and I have to be *incredibly* secretive about sex. Once people started to know or suspect about us, we couldn't just sleep over at each other's houses the way girls always do. We hardly ever get private time together to hug and kiss and play around.

Heather pointed out the emotional consequences for her:

My boyfriend was over tonight and we were downstairs kissing and fooling around. Then my father came home and my boyfriend was rushing everything. He jumped up and got his clothes all neat. He talked to me but didn't touch me for hours until he kissed me good-night. I felt very lonely, and missed lying in his arms basking in his affections.

Making Lovemaking Better

NOTE: This section is mainly for people who have decided to make love and want to learn about enjoying it more. Many of the readers of this book probably don't plan to have sex soon, and won't need this information right now. We include it for those teenagers who do need it. There is no point in rushing into intercourse. Deciding to have sex with someone is a big decision, often with many consequences. If you're thinking about it, see "When and How Far" (p. 86).

Time, caring and trust are most important to improving lovemaking. This is true for homosexual as well as heterosexual couples. Sex often gets better as a relationship goes on, where two people care about each other's well-being and get familiar with each other's bodies and needs. With more casual partners the initial thrill might be great, but there's no time to work out problems and learn about each other's rhythms and preferences.

Few of us are taught anything about lovemaking as we grow up. Eliot, who is twenty-two now, looks back on how little he knew when he started:

When I was first starting off to have sex it was real straightforward: get a hard-on, stick it in, come, and that's that. It was a real selfish thing in the beginning. At that point, fucking was my main concern. It's like proving something to yourself and to the world: I'm a man, I have sex, I come. But actually, even though I was physically getting off, I wasn't really enjoying sex the way I had fantasized it would be. I had a nagging suspicion that I wasn't really making love, you know. I didn't know anything about how to give someone else pleasure, and what was worse, I didn't even know that there was anything to know!

Eliot and his lover started from scratch, and learned gradually how to make sex enjoyable for both of them. Sally, too, learned with her boyfriend how to make it better:

The first few times we did it, I didn't feel very much. He used to come real fast, before I would even start to feel turned on. Before we started having intercourse, we used to have really great sex together, so we talked a lot about what we could do to make intercourse better. We decided to not just rush into fucking, but to spend time with each other first—you know, kissing and making out and everything, like we used to. Now I get turned on before we do it, and my boyfriend tries to make himself last once he's inside. He holds himself back until he feels like I'm really into it too. I think it's really important to him to make it good for me too.

Sally and her boyfriend have discovered one of the most valuable things to learn in sex: as she said, not to "rush into fucking." Many couples who used to make out for hours on end stop making out much at all as soon as they "graduate" to intercourse. Intercourse becomes what one girl referred to as "Wham, bam, thank you, ma'am." But for most people lovemaking seems to be better when you don't rush so much.

Lovemaking also gets richer emotionally if you make good use of the hour or so afterwards when a couple tends to feel more tender and close than perhaps at any other time. Sometimes you may want to drop off to sleep right away, or you may need to rush away, but staying awake and talking or listening to music or just being together after making love can be really special. As Connie, seventeen, said:

I think the best part of everything is right afterwards, when you're just lying there together. That's my favorite part.

Couples also learn from experience not to make love when one person doesn't feel like it. Moods change and sexual appetites go up and down. People sometimes go for days or weeks at a time not being much interested in sex. Both girls and boys talked about times when they are not really into sex for themselves but go along with it to please their partner. That's fine when it doesn't happen all the time, and when you and your partner care about each other. But there are few things worse in sex than making love when you're having to force yourself.

Some other helpful factors are discussed elsewhere in the book. It helps when a couple doesn't feel pressured about having orgasms (see p. 82). And, of course, it can increase sexual pleasure dramatically to *have and be using dependable birth control* (see p. 159).

One of the things that help lovemaking get better over time, especially with the same partner, is getting used to each other's bodies and to being naked together. At first, being naked with someone else, even someone you like a lot, can feel strange. Maxine, who had just had sex for the first time a few months before, asked the girls in a mixed discussion group, "How about how you felt when you were just standing there naked in front of this guy? I felt so *stupid!*" Every girl in the room laughed. One added:

I think the most embarrassing thing about having intercourse is that you have to get undressed. At my age, you feel kind of modest—you don't even let your family see you. And I think I look better in clothes than underneath.

Jeff agreed:

When my girlfriend looked at me the first time with the lights on, I thought, Oh, no, she's going to change her mind about me.

Another girl in the group felt differently. She said:

The first time I was getting ready to take my clothes off in front of my boyfriend I was a little nervous, but I was thinking, now he can see what I really look like. I guess you could say I'm proud of my body.

Other teenagers said they felt awkward at first with the noises of sex, the stickiness of the come, the smells, the odd positions, the thrusting and the heaving and the sighing.

The embarrassed feelings usually disappear with time and knowing each other. As Katie said:

At first, when me and my boyfriend got together, we just got into sex without really looking at each other. It was quick and sort of embarrassing, and neither of us got much out of it. But now it's so neat. We spend time checking each other out, really looking at each other, exploring each other all over.

For Bob, talking and laughing during sex was what made him more comfortable:

The second time I had sex it was great. We talked and laughed through the whole thing and it kind of eased the tension. When it's just grunts and noises and silence, you feel kind of dumb—so silent you can hear yourself moving against the bed, and it's weird.

The nice thing about getting more comfortable with yourself and your partner is that you're able to relax and enjoy it more. Talking and laughing and grunting and screaming and telling jokes and sharing secrets can be a wonderful part of lovemaking. It's a risk at first, but after a while opening up can be a big relief. For everyone.

COPING WITH PROBLEMS IN SEX

Nearly everyone has a problem with sex at some point, though when *you* have one it may not be much consolation that millions of other people have had it too. Most of the problems that teenagers have in sex go away pretty easily with time and experience, especially if you don't get too upset about them.

It is important to remember that YOU DON'T HAVE TO PUT UP WITH PAIN OR FRUSTRATION IN LOVE-MAKING. Lots of people keep their sexual problems to themselves for months or even years, and do nothing about them because they feel embarrassed or undeserving. But it is important *and possible* to work on most sexual problems. So if something hurts or bothers or frustrates you in sex, bring it up. It may seem embarrassing at first, or seem to be a "complaint" or an "accusation," but it is worth the initial awkwardness. Iris, seventeen, found this out:

I told my boyfriend the other night that I wasn't really getting off on our sex together. I was pretty tactful and gentle, but he just about freaked out. I could tell he was more embarrassed than anything else. He sort of got angry with me and said, "You mean you've been faking it all this time?" And so I said yes and we argued for a while, but then we got to talking about it. He really wanted it to feel good for me. He felt bad that I'd been keeping that a secret from him and he felt kind of dumb that he hadn't figured it out—but I was a real good actress about it. Now we feel like this weight is off our shoulders because we have it out in the open and we're going to try to do something about it.

A sexual problem is usually a concern for *both* people, and calls for patience and understanding and humor on both sides. Some people find themselves with a partner who is good to them in other ways but insensitive to their problem in sex. Sometimes you can be too worried about the problem to be of much help. If despite time and information your partner seems unwilling to work with you on a problem, then you may not be able to work it out in this relationship.

What if your partner is having a sexual problem? It can be upsetting if someone you care about isn't enjoying sex with you as much as s/he could. You may wonder what you could do differently or whether it is your fault. It's important not to take it too personally. You *may* be contributing to the problem in some way, but often it has little to do with you. Many problems with sex come from poor sex education or society's attitudes toward sex or a person's own anxieties. As a caring partner, you can help, but it's not all up to you.

It can be especially tough if your partner is too embarrassed to talk with you about it, or pushes you away because of it. Donna, seventeen, gave an example:

When my boyfriend and I started having sex, he would come right after he got in me. It was a real problem because he was so embarrassed about it. He acted like he failed or something. He never really talked about it, but I could see how humiliated he felt because he wouldn't look at me afterwards. It happened a couple of times and then he just stopped calling me. It wasn't nearly as bad for me as he imagined, so I didn't understand why he didn't want to go out anymore. Finally I saw him in school and asked him why he had stopped calling me. He was shocked that I didn't understand. He said he felt so embarrassed and uncomfortable about it that he never wanted to see me again. I told him that I didn't mind that he came fast. I knew we could figure a way to make it work for me too. He was really relieved.

Donna was brave enough to ask her boyfriend what was going on, and he was willing to try again. Unfortunately, some relationships end completely when one partner or the other backs away because of a sex problem. Our hope is that as more people learn how *common* these problems are, and worry less about performing, and stop stressing intercourse so much, this kind of embarrassment and humiliation will disappear.

Problems for Girls

Pain with Entry of the Penis. Pain when the penis enters the vagina usually has one of these causes:

—the girl hasn't had intercourse before, or not often, and her vaginal opening is still not stretched open enough;
—the girl is not yet sexually aroused enough to lubricate, so the vaginal entrance is not as wet as it could be;
—she has a vaginal infection;
—she is so anxious about sex that the muscles at the entrance to her vagina are tightening.

Some girls are comfortable even the first time they have intercourse. Some feel real pain at first, and some even bleed as their hymen gets stretched. The soreness and tightness usually go away, but you can help yourself and your partner have an easier time by stretching the vaginal opening for several weeks before starting intercourse. This is done by putting a finger into the vagina and gently pushing from side to side. And you can proceed slowly with intercourse. One girl told us:

I just couldn't do it at first because it hurt me so much. So we worked at it, you know. We'd try and then stop for a while, then try again, then stop for a while. After a few tries it didn't hurt anymore.

It is important that your partner be sensitive to the fact that you are hurting. A sensitive partner will not try to force his penis inside.

There are a small number of girls whose hymen (see pp. 26–27) is so closed that no amount of gentle stretching seems to work. If that is the case for you, a doctor can increase the size of the opening with a simple operation.

If the lips of a girl's vagina are too dry for the penis to go in easily, it probably means she is not ready, not sexually aroused enough for the natural lubrication of her vaginal walls (see p. 27). If there is still not enough lubrication, you can buy some K-Y jelly at a drugstore (not Vaseline, which can be irritating) and put some on the boys penis, or use a lubricated condom (the condom will protect you against pregnancy, too).

If your vaginal opening is stretched and there is enough lubrication and you still feel pain, see a doctor or nurse at a clinic. You could have a simple vaginal infection (like monilia or trichomoniasis) or a sexually transmitted disease like herpes (see p. 224). Or perhaps you are allergic to the birth control cream or suppository you are using, or to the condom the boy is using. Or perhaps you have been douching too much.

Sometimes a girl's vagina gets so tight that it's just about impossible to get a penis or even a finger inside. The muscles in the opening of the vagina tighten up and keep it closed. It's your body's way of saying, "I'm not ready or willing to have intercourse right now." (Sometimes this happens when a doctor is about to put her or his fingers in to examine you, but this is rare.)

A tightening up like this can happen for many reasons. Maybe you don't really want to have sex with this particular boy or maybe you just don't feel like having sex at all at this point in your life. You may have some bad memories about intercourse that are keeping you from opening yourself up to the experience. Perhaps you don't feel comfortable at the moment—maybe you're afraid somebody's going to walk in on you or that someone will punish you for what you're doing, or maybe you're worried about getting pregnant or catching a sexually transmitted disease. Whatever the reasons are, they are important to take seriously. If your body says to you, "I don't want to do that," listen to your body and try to discover why it's giving you such a strong message.

A small number of women suffer from this vaginal tightening even when they seem totally comfortable and ready and excited. If this happens to you, it would be good to get some professional help, either from a sensitive and experienced gynecologist or a counselor. Check *Our Bodies, Ourselves* and the chapter in this book called "Emotional Health Care" for some suggestions.

Not Reaching Orgasm. A number of girls we spoke with didn't know exactly what an orgasm was. Many had never had one, others not with a partner. Many girls and women never have orgasm in actual intercourse, however, and prefer to come through other forms of lovemaking.

If you don't reach orgasm with a partner, you might consider what your feelings and emotions are. You may not come *if:* you don't really want to be having sex at all; you are feeling uncertain or tense; there's no privacy; you are worried about pregnancy or an STD; you haven't had intercourse before; you are uncomfortable about being naked; your partner is new. Try to figure out what exactly is making you anxious.

It may help also to read the sections on orgasm and masturbation (pp. 82 and 79). It could be that you aren't getting the kind of stimulation you need.

Girls sometimes worry about not reaching orgasm. Carolyn, eighteen, said:

> I think there's something wrong with me because our sex life is good—neat and comfortable and open, and he does everything so that I can have an orgasm, but I never have one. I don't know what it is.

Girls are not brought up to be very proud or assertive of their sexuality. *There is nothing wrong with you* if it takes some time—even years—for you to learn about sex and to feel at ease letting go.

Timing can play a big role. For orgasm, a girl usually needs to have stimulation until her whole pelvic area feels full and aroused, not just when the lips of her vagina are wet. If the boy puts his penis in too early, he may come and lose his erection before you have come yourself. Fiona told us:

> You get your images of what sex is like from the movies where it's always so romantic and it always takes so long and seems so passionate. That's not the way it's been for me. If it takes my boyfriend two minutes to come, that's long. I don't think I've ever had intercourse that lasted five minutes, and it takes me longer than that to get turned on.

Fiona's experience is very common: most teenage boys come quite quickly. Yet the longer the thrusting movements last, the more likely a girl is to reach orgasm. Many boys say that lasting longer makes orgasm feel better for *them* as well. (See p. 111 for some ways boys can learn to hold off their climax.)

Sometimes squeezing and releasing the muscles of her vaginal entrance around the penis will bring a girl to orgasm. And if the penis goes in very deep it can touch nerve endings far inside the vagina which for some girls is very pleasurable. On the other hand, for some girls this deep penetration hurts. You and your partner can try different things. And if you don't reach orgasm during intercourse, there are lots of other ways of making love.

You may feel hesitant to do anything about not having orgasms. You may feel shy about moving your body in ways that will stimulate your clitoris, or about touching yourself to help yourself come. You may feel it's selfish to ask a guy to please you, or too pushy to show him where and how to touch you. After all, girls are brought up to be passive in sex. But it might be nicer for both of you if you *do* take some responsibility yourself for reaching orgasm. This can be a relief for the boy. Jerry, eighteen, is from New Jersey:

> You know, if it doesn't feel good to her—I mean, if

she's not really getting off on what's happening and she just lays there—then that's no good. But if she wants it too, if she's turned on and wanting it for herself, hey, well then we have a thing going.

Still, it can be hard for a girl to become more assertive in sex. Dorothy, a sixteen-year-old from San Francisco, said:

> My boyfriend always says to me, "OK, tonight you're going to be the aggressive one." He plans it and wants me to take over, but for some reason I can't do it. I like being the one it's done to. I like following his move. That's what I'm used to, and the other way doesn't feel right to me.

Helping yourself have orgasms in lovemaking may be something that you are not comfortable with right now. You have to move at your own speed, in this as in everything else.

Taking the pressure off. Orgasms can feel wonderful, but trying too hard to have one (or, for your partner, trying too hard to help you have one) can get in the way of enjoying sex. This is true whether or not you are having actual intercourse, and whether your partner is of the same or the opposite sex.

It's important for each partner to learn what stimulates the other, and to pay attention to her or his pleasure as well as to her or his own. But sometimes giving your partner an orgasm can become something you feel you have to do well or else you're no good. Both Evelyn and her boyfriend felt the pressure of this. Evelyn, seventeen, said:

> Every five minutes if I made a sound he'd say, "Are you going to come?" Then he'd say, "What if I do this, does it feel better?" I knew he was really concerned about making it good for me, but I got feeling that I'd *better* come or he'd feel like a failure. When I didn't come, he was disappointed in himself.

In a situation like this, try to do whatever will take the pressure off both of you. After all, lovemaking is just that—love-making—and even though orgasms feel good, they aren't the most important thing. If the girl wants to stop, she can say she is tired, or say that she's not going to come right now. He might feel relieved to hear it. She may feel tempted to fake orgasm just to get it over with and to give him a "success," but in the long run faking it isn't a good idea.

Amy, who is seventeen, talked about the place of orgasm in her relationship with her boyfriend:

> I don't like it when we are always all caught up in trying to get each other to come. Sometimes I just like to be with my boyfriend without being sexual that way. We just lie with each other and talk to each other. We spend a lot of time talking about things that are important to us and about ideas we have. Mostly we end up making out even then, but it's a different kind of feeling. It's not just that purely physical feeling, it's more loving.

Problems for Boys

Not Getting or Keeping an Erection. Not being able to get an erection at a critical moment is one of the things that the boys we spoke with worry about most. Tony, seventeen, gave an example:

I was out with this girl and it became pretty clear to me that she wanted it and I wouldn't have minded obliging her, but I couldn't get it up. I thought about every sexy thing I could think of and nothing did it for me. So in the back of my mind I was panicking, thinking, "What if she goes around telling everybody that I can't get it up?" That same thing happened to me a couple of times before, and I sure as hell didn't want to be stuck with that kind of a reputation.

Many boys feel their reputation for manliness is on the line when it's time to have an erection. Anxiety about this is enough to keep one from happening.

Just about all men, at one time or another, have been unable to get or keep an erection. It is very common and absolutely normal, and becomes a problem only when you start worrying about it.

Usually it's your mind and feelings, not your body, that causes problems with erections. You may have trouble getting or keeping an erection *if:* you aren't in the mood for sex; there's no privacy; you fear getting a girl pregnant or getting or giving an STD; you feel embarrassed or shy about sex; you are nervous at being with a new person; you're not sure whether what you're doing is right. You need to listen to feelings like these and respect them: your body and mind might just not want you to be having sex at this point. Something needs to change so you will feel more relaxed.

Sometimes having trouble with an erection *once* will make you worry so much the next time that you won't get one then, either. There are also a few physical causes. *Drinking too much alcohol or using some kinds of drugs will usually keep you from getting erections.* In a few cases some disease or health condition will inhibit erections. If you never get erections, even when you are alone, it would probably be a good idea to see a doctor. But this is very rare.

The best thing to do is to try to take the pressure off. Boys are unfortunately taught to think about sex as a performance on which they are going to be judged. If you can let go of this, you might be less critical of yourself and more able just to flow with your body. Nate, eighteen, said:

I couldn't get it up the first few times we tried. After that, when we were together it was pretty tense between us, and we didn't talk about what happened. Finally I said, "Let's try again and not worry about whether we can do it or not. Let's just go slowly and try it." We had some trouble that next time, but by the third or fourth try we really started to get into it.

Talking with your partner helps. Most people will understand if you talk to them and explain what's going on, and will feel closer to you because you've shared something so personal with them. If you don't say anything, the person you are with might feel that it's her or his fault, or that you don't find her or him attractive.

It especially helps if you and your girlfriend can put *less emphasis on actual intercourse* for a while. If you are finding other ways to satisfy each other, then there's not so much pressure on you to get your penis into her vagina. Older men can teach us something about this. In their sixties and seventies and eighties, men get fewer erections. They learn, if they haven't known it before, that intercourse is far from the only way of making love, and orgasm isn't the only thing that feels good.

Coming Too Quickly. The other problem that boys worry about is reaching orgasm quicker than they want to. This happens to guys all the time, especially when they are young or with a new partner. Fred, who is gay, said:

I was so excited the first time I had sex with a guy that I came just taking my pants off. He hadn't even touched me yet.

Martin, seventeen, told us:

Sometimes when I haven't seen my girlfriend in a week or two and we start going at it, I shoot off before I even get inside her.

The boys in a discussion group in Boston got laughing about "endurance records like screwing for six hours." Stories like these set up an expectation that a "real man" has perfect control over when he comes, and can last for hours. This expectation can make you feel lousy if you come in two minutes. But coming "too fast" is a matter of what is too fast for you or your partner. Sex is not an endurance test.

Coming quickly, like problems with erection, is often triggered by something in your head. (See above for some feelings that might be causing it.) Also, if a boy tends to climax very fast when he masturbates, it can take practice to be able to slow down when he is with a partner.

If you are having intercourse with a girl and want to last longer, you can stop thrusting for a few moments when you feel yourself getting very aroused. If the girl is on top and controlling the movement, you can ask her to stop for a minute or to move more slowly. Sometimes just breaking the rhythm a little or changing positions can forestall orgasm but still keep the stimulation going.

A second way to stall orgasm is described by this high school senior from Providence:

All I have to do to stop myself from coming right away is to force myself to think about something totally unsexy—like baseball or my job or something like that. My cousin told me about that, and the first couple of times I tried it I just about lost my erection altogether, but pretty soon I got the hang of it. Just when I feel myself getting to the edge of out of control I switch into a different gear and think about something else—just for a few seconds, but that's usually enough to slow me down.

Since this method involves thinking about things totally unrelated to lovemaking, it's not a good habit to get into. You might prefer the first method, which allows you to stay focused on the situation you are in.

A third way to keep yourself from coming too soon during intercourse is to have an orgasm through other kinds of lovemaking before you have intercourse. You can spend a lot of time stimulating each other, and if you feel the urge to climax, do it. Wait to have intercourse until you feel aroused again, and this time if you penetrate you will probably be able to hold off your second orgasm for quite some time.

Learning to control your climax in these ways will probably make sex better for you and your partner. It can be nice if intercourse lasts for a while, so you can both feel each other's building excitement. A girl usually enjoys a longer period of getting aroused before she is ready to climax (see above), and many boys say that the longer they last, the better their own orgasm feels.

Sometimes you won't want to "control" anything: it might feel great just to let the buildup take over your body and spill over into an orgasm when you're not expecting it. Then afterward you can find other ways to help satisfy your partner. Lovemaking doesn't have to be the same every time.

Pain with lovemaking. If your penis hurts during any kind of sex play, you may have a simple infection or an STD, and need to see a doctor. If it hurts you during or after intercourse, you *may* be allergic to the particular brand of birth control cream or to the lubricating fluid on the condom you used. In this case, try changing your products but, of course, keep using birth control.

EXPLORING SEX WITH SOMEONE OF YOUR OWN SEX (HOMOSEXUALITY)

A NOTE TO READERS WHO ARE
MAINLY INTERESTED IN RELATIONSHIPS
WITH THE OTHER SEX

Perhaps you have at some point felt romantic about or attracted to someone of your own sex. Many people do. Lots of people have homosexual ("same sex") fantasies or dreams (see p. 78). Many people have one or a few homosexual experiences—anything from kissing to making love—maybe with a special friend in their childhood or teenage years, or when they are adults.

Quite a number of people, about 10 percent, are *mainly* attracted to people of their own sex. Their deepest and most emotionally satisfying relationships for part or all of

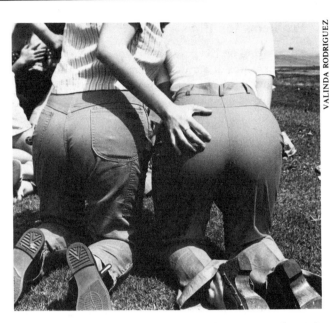

their lives are homosexual. That's a large group of people who feel that way: one in ten of our friends, relatives, teachers, doctors, ministers, priests, rabbis, bank tellers, nurses, plumbers, entertainers, athletes.

Homosexual men are often called *gay* and homosexual women are called *lesbians,* while homosexual people in general are often referred to as gay. In this section, teenagers who have mostly gay and lesbian feelings and experiences will talk about their lives. First, however, we will talk about teenagers who consider themselves heterosexual ("other sex," often called *straight*), because many straight teenagers also have occasional same-sex feelings and experiences.

If you have ever had a crush on someone of your own sex or felt excited by homosexual thoughts about someone, chances are that it felt nice in some ways, but a little frightening, too. "What does this mean?" people ask themselves. "Am I sick?" We have this response because our society has such a fear of homosexuality. We are taught that two people of the same sex loving each other in a romantic and sexual way is bad, sick, sinful, weird. We learn insulting words for homosexuals: fag, dyke, queer, butch, fairy, pervert. Many jokes make fun of gay people. We hear scary rumors that homosexuals "seduce" children, when in fact most of the people who bother children sexually are "straight" men. It is hard to accept, much less enjoy, same-sex feelings or homosexual friends, when we have been taught all these negative things.

We learn, wrongly, that if you have even one homosexual feeling or experience, that means you are "gay." This isn't true. We're also taught that a person is either all heterosexual or all homosexual, and for life. This isn't true either, but it makes us afraid of any same-sex feelings we might have.

Most people are neither "all straight" or "all gay." It

helps to picture a line with "gay" on one side and "straight" on the other.

Gay		Straight
Homosexual	———————	Heterosexual

There are people all along the line. Maybe a boy will have a passionate affair with a girl in his senior year in high school and find out when he gets to college that he mainly loves men. A girl may make love with her best girlfriend for a year or so while dating boys all the time, and later have a long married life with a man. Or someone will go into a one-sex environment—a prison, the armed services, a single-sex school—and find his or her emotions and natural sexual urges coming out toward the people closest by. Each of these people would be somewhere in the middle of the gay–straight line.

At either end of the line are the people who feel they are exclusively gay or straight. More people would be on the "straight" end—but many would be on the gay end and lots in between, too. Looking at a line like this can help those of us who fear that a fantasy or a kiss or even making love with someone of our own sex means that we are "gay." Maybe we will find ourselves at different points along the line at different times in our life.

You may never have a single homosexual thought or fantasy. That's fine. There's no point in trying to feel anything that doesn't come naturally to *you,* but if you think you are "more gay" than not, it is important for you to know you are not alone.

You may believe that same-sex feelings and experiences are wrong—for *anyone*—and may just not be able to accept the idea of homosexuality. As Robert put it:

Look, I think it's weird for two guys to French-kiss each other or to screw. Being in love is for men and women, and any other way is unnatural. I read all this stuff about being open-minded, but you have to draw the line somewhere.

And Miriam:

I live in a city where there are gay couples walking around. The men are OK, but when I see two women arm in arm looking lovingly into each other's eyes, I go to the other side of the street. I don't know, I just can't handle it.

John told us:

This friend I play basketball with a couple of nights a week told me he's gay—you know, he digs guys. He didn't come on to me or anything, just told me. But I freaked out, man. Here I've been playing ball with this guy who's a queer. He wants to stay friends, but I say for now it's out of the question.

Finding out that a friend has had gay experiences may make you feel fearful or uneasy, especially since you have been taught that same-sex loving is bad. You may worry that your friend will try to seduce you, although this rarely happens. In the teenage years, too, a person is asking deep questions like "Who am I, separate from my family?" and "What kind of person am I becoming? What am I going to do with my life?" When so much of your identity is in transition, and when sex in general is such a confusing mix of urges, feelings, needs and worries, feeling sure of your sexual identity may seem especially important. It can be a hard time to be "open" to same-sex feelings or to a friend who has them. Unfortunately, this can make life harder for anyone in your school who has homosexual feelings and experiences.

Fear of gayness hurts straight people, too. Fear of seeming to be gay puts a lot of people on guard about themselves. Boys, especially, talked to us about being afraid that people would think they were gay if they weren't always trying to get sex. As Roy put it:

If I'm not in bed with some chick on the second date, they're going to think I'm a fag or something.

Boys said they were afraid of being called gay if they had a more "feminine" body or hobbies, or if they showed that they had close, loving ties with another boy. Girls felt more free to have affectionate friendships with other girls, but not past a certain point. Marion said:

There were these two girls in seventh grade who were real close. I mean they really loved each other. We used to call them lesies behind their back, but I don't know if they were.

Some girls, too, worry they'll be suspected of being lesbians if they have a masculine build or a deep voice or a hairier body than their friends.

Fear of gayness, then, makes people suspect anything in their personality that seems to be more like that of the opposite sex. Boys may try not to seem soft or graceful or sensitive, and girls may try not to seem assertive or tough or strong. Being on guard in this way keeps people from being their whole selves. We who are writing this book hope that gradually there will be less fear of homosexuality in our society.

Fear and prejudice go away quickest when you can meet some open homosexuals and know them as people. Jerry, sixteen, is in a teen rap group with a boy named Ed, who is openly gay. Jerry said:

When Ed first said he was gay I thought, Let me out of here! But I knew the guy, we were friends already, I knew what he did in his spare time, what kinds of fights he had with his mother, what kind of movies he dug. I mean, he's a person. So by now his being gay is just something else I know about him. I never thought I'd hear myself saying that.

The rest of this chapter may be a way for you to "meet" some gay and lesbian teenagers indirectly, and dispel some of the myths that contribute to the fear and discrimination against gay people.

Do I have to call myself one thing or the other? There's some pressure these days to "decide" whether you are straight or gay. The main pressure, of course, is toward deciding you are straight. But many teenagers with one or two homosexual experiences feel they should say they are gay. For some this is correct. For many, however, there are years of loving and living ahead, before they know what their real preference is. You may never want to say you are finally or exclusively gay or straight, anyway. Some people believe that an openness to loving, sexual relationships with both sexes (called bisexuality) is our true nature. It's a good idea to resist the pressures and *decide in your own time.* There's no need to label yourself at this time in your life or to make choices before you're ready.

The rest of this chapter is based on conversations with many teenagers who identify themselves as gay or lesbian at this point—that is, their sexual feelings and romantic, loving relationships mainly involve people of their own sex.

Growing Up

If we can remember back to our childhood, it's quite common for kids to have lots of different kinds of sexual feelings and experiences. Some of our early sex play may have been with girls, some with boys, and some with both girls and boys (see pp. 63 and 64 for a discussion of this). Unless we were caught and punished, or somehow hurt, most kids enjoy this kind of sex play and exploration. It usually feels good (and sometimes exciting) to have someone touch our body, or to touch someone else's body. Here's what a young woman from the Midwest remembers:

> I can remember experimenting with sex as early as age four. It made no difference to me whether it was a boy or a girl. That went on for years.

And an eighteen-year-old guy recalls:

> I used to have sex with my best friends, who were guys, all the time. This was until I was fourteen or so. And I never thought it was wrong or anything like that.

We may find ourselves getting close to people of our same sex. It's natural to feel attached to certain friends. A fifteen-year-old boy from the South said:

> I remember when I was in the eighth grade and I got really attached to a friend at school. When he moved away, I remember being really upset and crying over it. I guess I must have been in love with him, in whatever way I could as a thirteen-year-old.

A nineteen-year-old girl from the West Coast said:

> I moved in with a girl that I had met at the job I was working at. We used to both buy each other presents, you know, once a week at payday. It was a kind of goofy type of thing. I'd give her a little stuffed bunny, because she was a thumper and I was koala bear, and she'd give me a bear or a card with a bear on it. It was like she was my sister, you know, and we'd write each other poems about how much we loved each other. Sometimes I wondered about that, but it felt OK, it felt good.

These close friendships, and even love, may or may not include feeling sexually attracted.

Sometimes we may have quite intense sexual feelings of being excited and turned on to people of our own sex. A guy from the East Coast recalls:

> In junior high, I was actively interested in sex with other guys, almost any guy. I remember sweating it out in gym class thinking, God, if I get a hard-on in the locker room, everyone will have a field day with me.

For some, a close friendship gradually and naturally leads into being sexual together.

A sixteen-year-old girl from New England said:

> I was with my friend, just the two of us together. We were kind of partying and had drunk a little too much. We were listening to a record and she started to stagger and I caught her, and she held me and we started slow-dancing together. She started kissing me. And through it I kept thinking, What's wrong with this, you know, it feels good, I love to kiss.

So it's pretty common for people to have homosexual attractions, feelings and maybe even experiences during childhood and early adolescence. This doesn't actually predict whether we will choose homosexual relationships later on. It's a part of learning about our sexuality.

Becoming Aware of Homosexual Feelings

Adolescence is the time that many people who are mainly attracted to people of their same sex begin to notice it. For some that self-awareness and understanding is a natural and positive thing. A seventeen-year-old girl describes it this way:

> I never went through a thing like, "These feelings I have are gay feelings, so I better go talk to somebody like a shrink about them." I always thought that it was natural. I just followed my feelings and went along with them, and everything was fine. I never had any head problems about them.

An eighteen-year-old guy from the East recalled:

> When I realized that I was gay I was about fourteen. I was dating a girl—really, the only girl that has ever

been in my life—and I was with this guy. There was some conflict there. You know, I liked them both. But then I realized that I was more attracted to the guy. Every weekend I'd go over to his place, and his parents weren't around very much. We'd go horseback riding in the woods. We really had a great relationship, including sex.

For others, this discovery can be difficult and even painful. For instance, this fifteen-year-old boy from the Northwest remembers:

When I was growing up and I realized that I had emotions for other men, I didn't know that that was anything different. But then I started to hear words like ''faggot'' and ''queer'' and I began to have second thoughts and questions about my feelings.

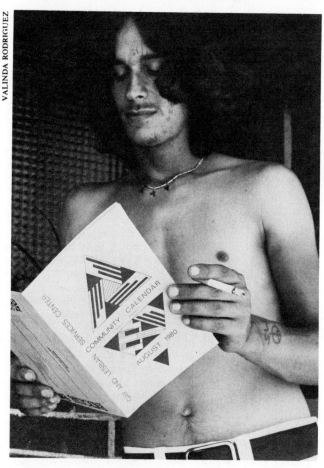

Another boy stated it this way:

I was messing around with boys—you know, like two buddies experimenting with something. It was really no big thing. By the time I was twelve, though, I began to get a social awareness that you can't continue to enjoy these feelings with people of your own sex, because it just doesn't fit in with our society.

Where sex is concerned, lots of people have very definite attitudes about what is right or wrong. If our behavior

or feelings don't fit with their attitudes, they may begin to call us names, or laugh at us or put us down. We begin to notice that when two people are loving or caring for each other—on billboards, in magazines, on TV and in the movies—it's always a man and a woman. It's never two women or two men together. We begin to get the idea that homosexual feelings are not OK in our society. A nineteen-year-old guy from California put it this way:

In high school, I had a girlfriend. I got tired of her, but I still couldn't bring myself to be ''one of them.'' At school when someone calls you a ''faggot'' it not only means homosexual. It also means sissy or something like that. And I knew I wasn't no sissy!

As a girl from high school in the Northeast said, ''Being called a 'fag' means you are some kind of nerd.''

Because we have so little information about homosexuality and so few models of gay relationships, most of us grow up with dreams and expectations for the future that are based on heterosexual lives—like falling in love with someone of the other sex, getting married and having a family. Discovering that you are mainly attracted to people of your own sex can initially give you a sense of disappointment and loss. But gay people fall in love too, many stay together for a long time, and many gay people are mothers and fathers. More and more gay *and* straight people are building alternative emotional-support networks in order to live lives that are not based on the traditional nuclear family.

Denying and Hiding the Feelings. Some people may try to deny that they have any homosexual feelings and attractions. A seventeen-year-old girl from the South said:

Well, at first, when I was just kissing other girls, it wasn't hard for me to face up to kissing, but I wouldn't admit I was gay or bisexual or anything like that. I just said it was fun, and it just happened to be with a girl. But so what? There was no such word as gay or homosexual in my life. Later, as I got involved with more sexual activity with girls, I thought, Now maybe I'm bisexual or something, but that's it. I'm not a lesbian! Oh no, not me!

An eighteen-year-old guy from Illinois remembers how he tried to deny his feelings and attractions:

By the time I was twelve, I realized that men were a part of my sexual fantasies. I liked guys, you know? And once, around that same time, out of the clear blue sky, someone said to me ''Hey, man, if you don't watch it you're going to be a homosexual.'' And I said to myself, Nah, not me. That's the last thing I'll ever be. I'll never be a homosexual. So from about the age of twelve to sixteen I squashed those feelings whenever they came to me.

Some people who have strong homosexual feelings try to date people of the other sex and pretend to be interested

VALINDA RODRIGUEZ

in them as sexual partners. Usually there is pressure from parents and friends to do this, and some teenagers told us that even they themselves thought this might help them to change. A sixteen-year-old boy from the West Coast said:

> In a straight person's mind, getting a homosexual guy in bed with a girl is going to be all he needs to make a miraculous change into being a heterosexual. It's funny. Some people think that the only reason that you're gay is because you had a bad experience with a woman. Like a woman laughed at you or something. So they think that all you need is a good experience to turn you straight.

A seventeen-year-old girl said:

> I had a boyfriend long after I knew that I was feeling these feelings towards other girls. I knew that I really didn't get anything out of being with a boy. The sex was OK, but emotionally there was always this wall that was never there with the girls I was attracted to. I kept seeing him because I thought maybe things would change.

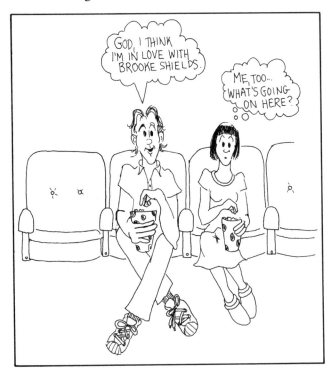

Another guy recalled:

> I would try to talk to all these girls and we would pick up girls in the show. I had no problems having sexual thoughts or erections over girls. But what really bothered me was that the more I pressed myself on them, the less success and satisfaction I got. I began to get a lot of anxiety over that. Pretty soon I couldn't get an erection over girls and my fantasies became totally male.

You don't want to deny your feelings and attractions, even if they happen to be toward people of your own sex. Yet you have to be aware that there are people who will consider you bad or sick because you have them. For instance, gay people are sometimes called names like "dyke" or "bull-dyke" or "faggot" or maybe "queer" or "fairy." People use these names to hurt others. These names and labels are based on "stereotypes"—that is, false generalizations about who people are. Stereotypes lump people together because of one quality they all share, and are almost always wrong. They ignore the fact that, whatever our sexual preference, each of us is unique and different. To say "all homosexuals are . . ." ignores a person's individuality. Stereotypes are nearly always negative and destructive, and they help to keep people ignorant and afraid of homosexuality.

These negative, hurtful names and stereotypes cause problems for people who have homosexual feelings because they get the message that their feelings are bad or wrong. A seventeen-year-old girl put it this way:

> When you first find out that you're gay, it's a real shocking experience for a lot of people. Like, I called myself sick. It was like I was even mentally disturbed.

Another guy in high school in Michigan recalled this:

> I had more enjoyment with guys than I did with girls, and it just confirmed what I had already been thinking. I cried about it a lot. I said to myself, You're a homosexual. And I didn't want to be, not then anyhow. I called myself all sorts of names: You're a fag, you're a freak. Where was my belief in God? Where was my future with a wife and kids? All this was going through my mind at that time.

Three members of a young lesbians support group in Providence talked about having to hide their feelings:

> Molly (nineteen): In junior high I would look at girls' bodies and they'd be aware of it, so I'd look down at the floor and try to control it. I did a lot of strange things to cover up my impulses. In the locker room I'd take a shower way down at the other end away from everyone else to make it clear I wasn't looking.

> Alice (twenty): I got so I avoided touching my friends, I was so afraid my feelings would show. One time a friend asked me to zip up her dress and I remember my hand shaking.

> Beth (eighteen): When a rumor leaked out in tenth grade that I was gay, this group of girls would tease me by coming up and hugging me all the time, and I'd have to push them away and say, "Oh, gross!" It was awful.

> Alice: What makes me so angry is that I held the feelings down for so long that now when I get with someone I love I can't just relax and touch her. There's this tightness inside me.

One of the reasons why some teenagers feel they have to deny or hide their homosexual feelings is that they may not know many other people who feel the way they do. An eighteen-year-old girl from the Midwest said:

I knew one gay guy in junior high, but in high school I didn't know anyone else who was gay, especially any lesbians. It was pretty lonely. Gradually, I got to know more gay kids in school, but not a lot. Sometimes it takes a while for people to decide that they're gay, and some people just aren't ready to come out.

And a seventeen-year-old guy remembers, rather painfully:

For me, it was a real lonely experience. I could never show the real me, especially that part of me, to anyone because I felt that would mean that no one would want to be with me. I was sure that if I told them about my homosexual feelings, no one would care about me. The loneliness was awful.

Or the only homosexual people they do know act very differently from them. A fifteen-year-old boy from New York remarked:

I felt like the homosexual stuff I knew about was dirty, negative, too painful for me to want to get mixed up in. You know, dirty old men who grabbed you and did things to you. Or very effeminate guys. I grew up in a very proper town, so I couldn't find anybody else my age who was feeling like me but didn't want to have to act like a "fem" (effeminate or like a woman). I wasn't a "fem" and I definitely was not a dirty old man!

This boy couldn't identify with the only gay people he thought he had seen. He probably saw many other gays in his community and just didn't know it, because for the most part you can't tell if people are gay or straight just by looking at them.

A more effeminate seventeen-year-old reported being lonely, too:

The only other gay guys I knew in my high school were both jocks—real macho, on the football team and all that. I was clearly not as masculine as they were. In fact, I look more like the stereotype many people have of homosexuals. It's one thing to be gay and macho, and another to be gay and effeminate. I felt really isolated.

A seventeen-year-old guy who now lives in the Northwest remembers:

I grew up in a big city in the East where there were lots of gangs. Like my brother is in a gang. So I used to watch all these gangs beat up people, beat up fags. I used to watch. I even watched someone get beat up so much he was bleeding all over. One guy even was murdered. And I was just watching, deep down inside knowing that I was a gay, but I would say to myself, "They're fags. I'm not." Finally I couldn't stand just

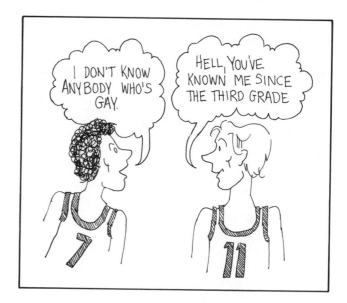

sitting back and watching these gangs beat up on gays. One time I started beating up some of the gang members. And I told the gay guys to stay out of my neighborhood because it was too dangerous for them there.

A seventeen-year-old girl from Ohio said:

I remember one incident, with some good friends of mine. There were four girls and about ten guys. We were all fooling around together. Then the guys started talking about gays and putting them down. They didn't know at the time that I was an active lesbian. I got really upset and I just came out and started putting them down right back to them. I told them that they had *no* right to put down homosexuals, homosexual acts, the homosexual life-style, anything. Not unless they have actually been around homosexuals and have actually gotten to know what their life-style is like. I told them to think twice before they talk and make fun, hurtfully, of other people. Because they are going to be insulting a lot of people. And they all looked at me really strange. But they never said another word about homosexuals. That incident really opened me up. Although it hurt at the time, it was a positive thing for me.

Standing up against these kinds of insults and violence can be scary, but for a gay person it can be a way of expressing pride, and for both gay and straight people it can be a way of standing up for what you believe.

Coming Out

The process of feeling more open about yourself and gaining strength and pride as a gay person is known as the "coming out" process. For many people this can involve many stages—admitting to yourself you're gay, coming to know other lesbians or gay men, telling your friends or family, marching in a demonstration for gay rights, joining a gay organization or social group. The process of coming out means leaving some of your old feelings behind—giving up feelings of shame, guilt or self-hatred. It means coming to have a good sense of yourself and standing up to people who may not react positively to the fact that you're openly gay.

For some people it is an important step to be able to define themselves as "lesbians" or as "gay males." They feel that using these words helps them identify themselves by openly stating their true feelings—that they are boys who love boys and girls who love girls. This is important for gay people, because many have spent a long time hiding and denying this part of their identities.

Some people have a difficult time finding one word to name their sexuality. This may be because they are not yet fully aware of their feelings and attractions. It may be because they are attracted sometimes to girls and sometimes to boys. Some people may not want to consider themselves homosexual, heterosexual or bisexual. Others may want to wait until they've had enough real experience to know what they enjoy and what kinds of relationships are meaningful to them.

There is no way for anyone to tell you how you can determine if you are gay or straight or both or neither. Time and experience, reading books from the suggestions on p. 130, talking with trustworthy people in your life—all these can help you to define yourself. *No one should be pressured to place himself or herself in any category of sexuality.*

Coming Out to Yourself.   This is the first step. An eighteen-year-old girl from New England said:

> In a lot of different senses, before I came out to myself, I wasn't honest with myself. I didn't trust myself really or respect myself in many different areas. And when you first come out, it's like you're telling yourself something you don't want to believe. "You kissed that girl, didn't you? It felt good, didn't it? So what's wrong with it?" You finally begin to relate to yourself. After that it's like the rest of your life opens up and you stop blocking things. You start asking yourself, "Hey, what's going on?" It's made me a lot more honest with myself.

A sixteen-year-old boy from the East said:

> After I came out to myself I kept finding pieces from my past that made more sense. A lot of my actions when I was younger became clearer. Like, I'd always kind of wondered why I never wanted to go out with girls, and now I knew.

Some teens told us that admitting they had homosexual feelings and attractions helped them discover that they did have sexual feelings after all. A seventeen-year-old girl from the Southwest said:

> When I was with men, I thought I was not sexual at all. I thought that I didn't like sex. I always seemed frustrated, and I didn't know why. And it was embarrassing to tell my friends. They would say, "Gosh, I haven't seen you go out with anyone for eight months, you know? What's the problem?" And I would say, "Well, I can take or leave sex." I would always say that. Matter of fact, when I got my first gay lover, I told her the same thing, "I can take or leave sex." But then, after the first time we made love I loved it. I loved sex.

A twenty-three-year-old young woman looked back:

> For years I had been holding my sensuality down as hard as I could, because I was so scared my lesbian feelings would take me over. A month after I said to myself OK, I'm a lesbian, and had my first female lover, I suddenly started to go dancing a whole lot, to take bubble baths, swim nude at night, wear soft slinky shirts.

This nineteen-year-old California guy described the rewards of coming out to himself:

> Finally, just about when I was graduating from high school, I looked at myself and just accepted the fact that I was gay. I looked in the mirror and said, not "You're a homosexual," but "I'm a homosexual." And from that point on I could admit to myself who I was, and that made me a man in my own feelings. It's funny, because a lot of people think that being a homosexual robs a guy of his manhood. But for me, admitting my own homosexuality gave me my manhood.

Coming Out to Others.   Sometimes when you first realize that you are gay, you may want to shout it from the rooftops and let everyone know about this exciting self-discovery. But it's important to take the time that you need to get ready gradually to tell your friends and family. It can be painful to have a secret like this from the people who know and love you, but it is more painful to do it too fast. Don't let anyone or any situation push you into coming out before you're feeling strong enough and good enough about your identity to be ready to deal with people's reactions.

Only you can decide when the right time is to tell the people who are important to you. If you are in a period of being very angry at your parents, it can be tempting to "come out" just as a kind of rebellion. Occasionally teenagers do this even when they are not sure they are gay. This isn't a very good idea. Coming out can bring some big changes in your life, and it's best to take your time about it.

Usually it's good to begin by telling people who know you and like you and will, you hope, accept you. You may want to test the situation by telling a close friend first and then using that person to support you as you tell the others. Remember that not everyone knows what homosexuality is all about, and most people have been taught that it is bad. You'll have to be ready to deal with a lot of questions, and with reactions of confusion and perhaps hostility. A nineteen-year-old girl from the West Coast related this experience:

Most of my friends that I've told have accepted· it, and me, more or less. It's funny, the only person that has ever turned completely against me was my closest friend. We were best friends for the first seventeen years of my life. Actually, she was the first person I had sex with, when I was seven years old. Anyhow, she's the only person that has turned away from me for good. You have to be careful because it's easy to get hurt.

A seventeen-year-old from Wyoming had this experience:

After people at school found out that I was gay, a lot of them kind of kept a distance from me. I think they were scared that I was going to do something to them. You know, the old fears about gay people attacking you and that junk. I guess that was one of the reasons why I didn't come out sooner, because I was afraid that they would be scared of me. It's stupid and crazy, but a lot of people feel that way.

If you want to keep the people you've told as friends you may have to be willing to work through their feelings with them. You may also decide that a friend who can't eventually accept your homosexuality isn't such a good friend after all. Angry and hurt by this, a sixteen-year-old boy from a city high school wrote to us: "Friends, that is, people I *thought* were friends, turned full-fire against me, but used other reasons for their constant verbal attacks."

Something that may help in telling others is to remember that they may have lots of false stereotypes and need information that you can give to them. You can tell your friends that you're not going to attack them or try to seduce them. You can explain to your parents that although some of their expectations and hopes for you are disappointed, other hopes (like happiness, self-acceptance and pride) can be fulfilled. You can also remind your friends and family that you haven't changed at all from who you were yesterday. A fifteen-year-old girl from Missouri said:

When I told my sister, she cried, and then she started calling me names and telling me I was sick. I told her, "Damn it, I haven't changed! I'm still your sister. I'm still the same person I was. Have I changed physically, besides growing up? Have I changed in any other sense? And if so, have I changed for the better or worse?" She said, "You've changed for the better from the last time I saw you." And then I said, "Only other news is that I'm gay, and it hasn't made me any different, has it? Has it changed your or my relationship?" And she said, "No, not really." And I said, finally, "It's just my sexuality preference. That's it, that's all. It's my life preference. It doesn't change me as a person, personality-wise. It just

changes my life-style a little. And I'm happy. You should be happy that I'm happy."

And an eighteen-year-old guy from the East Coast remembered:

I was telling a friend and she said, "I can understand how you can have close male friends, but to be sexual with them, that's sick!" I said, "It's sick when a guy isn't attracted to women and won't face up to loving men. That's what sick. It's not sick when you face up to who you really are."

Coming Out to Family. Because parents and family are an important part of everyone's life, there may come a time when you really want to tell them who you are and how you feel. A sixteen-year-old girl from the East recalled:

My mother said, "You didn't need to tell me. I knew it all the time." But I wanted to tell her, because it was coming from me. I *needed* to tell her, even if she already knew.

Your family members *may* already know. They may have felt awkward about bringing it up, and perhaps relieved to have it out in the open. A fifteen-year-old boy from Oregon remembered this situation with his father:

The term "gay" or "faggot" never came up in my house. But my father got a hint that I was gay because he heard one of my friends talking about being gay. One night he took me out to dinner and he told me about all the girls he's had, and then he told me about all the guys he's had. That was a real shock for me! He was trying to get around to asking me if I was gay. He never really did come right out and ask me, but I'm pretty sure he knew and knows now.

And a sixteen-year-old boy from Michigan had this experience with his family:

My sister was the first one I told. Really, she asked me. I think she suspected it for a long time, and she finally asked me straight out. And I told her. She accepted it without any hassle. Then about two weeks later my mom asked me if I was gay and I told her too. She started crying and we sat around and talked. She wanted to know if she had been too domineering or something like that. We ended the conversation hugging each other and saying that everything will turn out OK. My mom told my dad, and he was real understanding too. But he kept thinking and hoping that I would change, and he kept influencing me to see girls.

In many cases, coming out to parents is more painful than this. Some parents may react with extreme anger, blame and hostility. Even after they have time to get used to the idea, some parents don't seem to move toward accepting your gayness—or at least making peace with it. This may feel as if they are not accepting *you*.

Some parents may become extra strict and try to keep you from seeing any gay or bisexual friends. They may be so angry and blaming that family life gets impossible for everyone. A seventeen-year-old told us:

> When I told my folks that I was a lesbian, they totally freaked out. It was so against their religion, their lifestyle and friends, that they just couldn't deal with it. I'm not living at home anymore and I hardly ever talk with them. I hope after a while they'll mellow out about it.

This girl went to live with a friend's parents in a nearby town. If this kind of alternative is available, it can help cool down a hot family situation. But some gay teens, like some straight teens in other kinds of family battles, end up leaving home on their own, hoping to find a more accepting place somewhere. Unfortunately, our world is such that it is pretty dangerous for a young teenager, especially a young gay or lesbian teenager, to move to a new city with no resources. Several big cities have begun to realize that ''gay runaways'' are a growing homeless and vulnerable population.

If you or a friend feel so much anger and rejection from your family that you wonder how long you can last living at home, the section ''Feeling Bad, Feeling Better'' may be of some help to you in thinking of steps to take short of leaving home. It's not so much your problem alone as a *family* problem, and maybe your family can get some help.

Your parents may want to send you to a psychiatrist or psychotherapist, believing that emotional problems have made you think you are gay. Working with a good therapist is sometimes a great help in sorting out feelings and problems (see p. 143) as long as the therapist listens to what *you* want and to how *you* see things. But therapy does *not* work to ''cure'' a person of being gay if that's the preference he or she feels most strongly.

Parents. A teenager's coming out can be a difficult and challenging experience for parents, too. A forty-year-old St. Louis mother of three told us:

> When our oldest son, Ted, told us he was gay, it was a very hard thing for my husband and me to handle. First we blamed ourselves because we thought that we had made some mistake or something. We also felt a lot of strong, kind of crazy feelings toward Ted: we were angry, disappointed and felt sorry for him. It was a real difficult time for all of us, and we began to worry about our other kids.

Parents who react against their child's ''coming out'' are often thinking of the stereotypes of what gay people are. They may need to learn more before they can open their minds. They may also fear being ''blamed'' by society, which often blames parents if their children turn out to be unusual or nonconformist. Parents may feel they have done something ''wrong'' in bringing them up. They may

worry about how their friends or their own parents will react, or feel disappointed because they hoped for grandchildren. They may worry that being gay will make you drift away from them.

Parents may be upset because they know that some people will try to make life harder for you because you are gay. They see that you may have trouble getting jobs or housing, for instance, because of discrimination against gays. They may worry that you are trapping yourself into an identity that you won't be able to get out of if you want to later.

Some of these are deep and legitimate concerns, and parents need time to work them through. There can be some very loving feelings behind the upset, as this father shows:

> I disapproved of my daughter's lesbianism not because I had any moral problems with it but because I felt it would make her life too difficult. My overwhelming concern, though, was to let her see that none of this had anything to do with my love and continuing support for her. I was terribly afraid that because I was so hurt and upset I would push her away from me and jeopardize our relationship.

It is a great relief on all sides if parents come to accept their son's or daughter's gayness. A father from Los Angeles said:

> My wife and I were really shocked at first when our son told us about his homosexuality. I felt betrayed and angry, and we had some ugly fights. But he finally convinced us that he was happy and pretty well adjusted. He kept saying to us, ''Do you want me to lie to you, to pretend that I'm someone I really am not to you?'' So after a year or so we finally began to accept his being gay.

Some parents find assistance and support in special groups or organizations for parents and friends of gay and lesbian people. Parents of Gays groups are now active in most major U.S. cities and many smaller ones. These groups offer a chance to meet other parents who are wrestling with similar feelings and problems, and to learn new information about what homosexuality is and isn't. A mother reported:

> I think we were mostly worried about our daughter's happiness, about her life. We thought all lesbians were big, fat, mean truck drivers. The Parents of Gays group taught us that homosexual people are as varied and individual as the rest of us, and let me tell you what a difference that made!

Many of the groups also work toward ending discrimination against gay and lesbian people, as the parents find themselves getting angrier and angrier at the injustices that make their children's lives more difficult. Interested parents and friends of gay and lesbian people can contact Parents and Friends of Gays, P.O. Box 24528, Los Angeles, CA 90024 (213-472-8952), for information and local assistance.

Meeting Other People

Gay and bisexual teenagers need to meet other people like them for friendship and support, but this can be difficult. Sometimes, however, coming out brings new friends where you didn't expect them, as this sixteen-year-old boy discovered:

> I met this kid in my school who was bisexual and seemed really insecure about it. I told him that I had a lot of feelings about guys and that I looked at guys' bodies in the locker room, too. He saw that he wasn't the only person having these feelings. It feels good to have an ally, because our school is a tough place for gays.

Sometimes lesbians meet each other through shared political work in the women's movement. Many gay people meet through organizations, clubs or gay rap groups. Going to one of these may be scary at first. One boy told us:

> After I knew I was probably gay I tried to go to this gay group in a church in the city, but I was so shy that all I could get myself to do was to walk around and around the building.

A seventeen-year-old girl who joined a gay youth group in New York said:

> The group was great for me. I met other gay kids and they weren't outrageous or awful—they were just like the kids at school. It was like a Y program: we hung out, played sports, talked a lot, had dances. I met my first girlfriend in the group.

An eighteen-year-old girl from the Midwest said:

> I remember what an incredible feeling I had when I went to my first rap group meeting at the gay community center. I couldn't believe that there were so many people who had the same kinds of feelings that I had. It was a fantastic relief. Some were like me, and others were very different from me. So I felt that I could just be myself and be accepted.

Calling a local hot line, or possibly a local social service agency, may be a way of finding such a group.

Gay bars are sometimes more problematic than clubs or organizations, but often are among the only places to find openly gay people. Many teens find their way into gay bars despite being under the drinking age. Bars have been a lifeline for lesbian and gay people, but the gay-bar scene can be rough, especially for males, and especially for someone young and inexperienced.

One way that gay men meet each other is through something called "cruising." This involves making eye contact with someone—usually a stranger—on the street or in a

---

ODE TO COMMITTEE FOR GAY YOUTH

The group is a very large part of my life
    It means so much to me
It means helping and caring, trusting and guiding
    and responsibility
It means meeting new people, making new friends
    trying to show people I care
For the world is not kind to my Brothers and
    Sisters
    I'd rather see them OUT HERE than out there
For we all need each other, or at least I need you
    to help me through each day
We're like links in a chain, with that one special
    bond
    we're young, we're proud . . . and we're GAY.

                    —George Smith

---

park or store that is popular with gay men. People who connect in this way may have a conversation, flirt with each other, go for a walk, go dancing. Some end up having sex. They may become friends, or never see each other again. Some people make the contact mainly for sex, but for others it is simply the best way to meet other gay men who might become friends or lovers.

Cruising can be fun, but there are dangers to it too. The people you meet through a bar or cruising may be a good deal older and more experienced than you—this can be great, but it can sometimes bring pressure to do things you aren't ready for. The people you meet may be more into drinking or drugs than you want. Some may think you have come for sex, when maybe all you wanted was to meet a few friendly people.

Unfortunately, there are some people—gay and straight—who have violence in mind, so *it can be dangerous to get sexually involved with a stranger*. (This is also true for straight teenage girls in the pickup scene with older guys.) As one twenty-five-year-old gay man said, "Be sure to take your entrance into gay social circles *at your own speed*!"

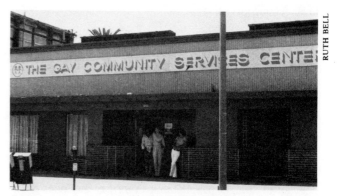

Some cities have community centers where gay people can meet.

A seventeen-year-old boy from Chicago told us this about cruising:

> After I realized that gay men cruised in part of the park near my house, I started going there a lot to get some fresh air and some fun. One evening this good-looking guy in his twenties started talking to me, and I could see he wanted to go further. But something about him didn't sit right with me, so I went on my way. Later I heard that undercover cops had arrested nine people in the park that night!

In "entrapment," a policeman who is out of uniform will approach someone and try to get him to do something against the law—this could be talking about going home to have sex, or having sex in a public place, or even making a move that could be interpreted to mean that is what you intend to do. If the gay man does any of these things, he finds himself arrested. Victims of entrapment are often young. Although many people believe that police ought to keep out of personal affairs and focus on combating violent crimes, many cities still have a "vice" squad that hassles gay men in this way.

Sex

Most homosexual sex is like heterosexual sex: kissing, fondling, rolling around with someone you like or love and are attracted to, telling each other what is exciting to you. "Exploring Sex with Someone Else" (p. 84) talks about things that gay and lesbian as well as straight couples do—except, of course, the section on heterosexual intercourse. (Even for straight couples, male-female intercourse isn't the *only* way of "making love.")

People sometimes wonder what it is that homosexuals "do." A young lesbian said to us about sex, "I thought there'd be something that girls did together that I didn't know about."

Lesbians make love in lots of ways. Sometimes one will caress the other's clitoris and vagina (see p. 25) with her hand or tongue, or they might lie together and press their bodies against each other. There are many other possibilities. As one girl said:

> It feels natural. I don't try to do it "right," I just feel this flood of affection and excitement and I somehow know how I want to touch her.

Gay men, too, have many ways of making love. One may caress the other's penis with his hand or his mouth. Or one may put his penis in the other's anus. (This is called anal sex. Heterosexual couples sometimes do it, too.)

One teenage boy said:

> A lot of straight people think every gay guy does every gay sex act, including anal intercourse. That's not true. I've only done it once. What my lover and I do

depends on what we're both wanting and feeling at the time.

Knowing your limits, talking about sex, learning how, taking responsibility—all these are just as important in gay relationships as in straight ones. See the discussion of these in the previous chapter. Also see Chapter VII for information on sexually transmitted diseases (VD).

Issues in Homosexual Relationships

Perhaps the single most important thing in any kind of relationship is communication: expressing our feelings and needs to our friend or partner, and listening to the feelings and needs of the other person. Having a partner of the same sex doesn't guarantee that the relationship will be easy or that communication will be automatic.

One of the problems gay and lesbian teenagers talked about was initiating: asking a person out, suggesting certain activities, or maybe making the first sexual move. This can be scary, because the other person may say no or, worse yet, reject you for even asking. It can be particularly awkward at first for girls, as this eighteen-year-old from New England recalled:

> When I met Paula I knew I liked her, but I had always waited for the guy to ask me out. I wasn't used to calling someone up and saying, "Hey, what'cha doing Saturday night?" She wasn't either so we waited around for weeks. We agreed later it was good for us to learn to make the first move.

Initiating can be difficult for guys too, according to this nineteen-year-old from the South:

> I thought that it would be kind of rough being single and gay. I was scared of it. I thought, Me go into a gay bar? By myself? But when I finally got myself together and got up the courage, I walked into the bar and I saw people I knew. It was easier than I thought, but it's hard for me to pretend I'm comfortable when I'm not. I can look at a guy—it's called "cruising" when you check someone out—but I'm shy when it comes to actually approaching someone and saying, "Hi, how are you? Want to dance?"

Initiating the moves toward sex can feel even more risky. A twenty-year-old from Texas recalled her first lesbian relationship:

> My lover was really horny. She wanted sex on a daily basis. So for a while I didn't have to say much. But then there would be certain days that I wanted it and she would be taking time off. It was hard at first to flirt with her and let her know that I wanted sex because I had never done this before. With men, it was always, "OK, I'll lay here and let him do it to me." It was never something that I really wanted. I must admit I was embarrassed to face up to the fact that I was horny too. The first time I asked for it was hard.

But now sometimes it's even fun—especially when I'm successful.

Another common issue in both homosexual and heterosexual relationships is what kind of commitment or length of time you want with the other person. One stereotype is that homosexuals are sex-crazed animals who jump from bed to bed. That's not true. Some people, both heterosexually and homosexually attracted, enjoy one-night stands. A seventeen-year-old girl who didn't want to restrict herself to just one person said:

> With my first relationship, my lover kept telling me that she wanted me just for herself. And I said to her, "Look, you know, I just tasted the honey, you could say. Give me a chance to see what this thing is all about. I don't want to be tied down. I want to be single, at least for a while."

Others of us may prefer one relationship at a time, perhaps long-term relationships. This sixteen-year-old guy from Utah said:

> I don't like one-night stands. Guys who go to the bars, they're usually looking for things like that. One-night, maybe one-week relationships. They usually don't go for long-term anything. I like to have somebody there for a while. I don't like to say "Let's go home" and then the next morning say "Bye-bye, see you later." I like to get to know the person. Get to feel them, get to relate to them more.

And a nineteen-year-old woman from the East Coast who has had and enjoyed both short-term and long-term relationships said:

> It's different in gay life, at least for me. I may sleep with a woman for three nights in a row, or I may have three different partners for three nights. But it's never just a screw or a lay for me. I always have to feel good about a person I'm with, and not feel abused or used. Each time I've been with a woman sexually, I've felt like I've made love to her, and I've felt like I've had love made to me.

Roles. If you become involved in a homosexual relationship, you may find that the main challenge is the same as it is an any kind of relationship: how to become close and intimate with another person while being true and honest with yourself. One of the most common things that interfere with this is playing roles. Women in our society, for instance, are told that they should be passive and quiet, pretty and sexy (but not sexual), like to cook and sew and stay home with the children. Men are told to be strong and aggressive, to get a lot of sex but not show feelings, to go out and work and make a lot of money and be very successful.

In heterosexual relationships these roles rob both the woman and the man of half their humanness. These kinds of roles sometimes happen in homosexual relationships, too, but because you both grew up being taught the *same* role, usually something has to give and you have to become more flexible about who does what.

There is an old stereotype of homosexual relationships that one person always plays the masculine role (sometimes called the "butch" role) and the other the feminine role (often called the "fem" role). This is less and less true. An eighteen-year-old girl from the West Coast recalled:

> When I first came out, my lover was very "butch" as the phrase goes, and I was more feminine. The role was kind of male-female type traditional in the gay life. But then I realized that I don't like roles. I like women who are more butch in the sense that they like to hike and do outdoors kinds of things. But although I may dress feminine sometimes, I love to work on cars and mechanical kinds of things. I don't consider myself a butch or fem. I'm versatile. Every woman is. Actually, everybody is. It's just that some people pick a role, you know?

No matter what kind of people we are attracted to, all of us want to feel good about ourselves and proud of ourselves. We want to like and respect ourselves, as well as the people we choose to be with. This healthy self-respect and pride is the foundation of good relationships—whether homosexual or heterosexual—and good relationships can help to nurture these feelings of respect and pride.

A seventeen-year-old guy from Wisconsin put it this way:

> I'm doing really good for myself. I smile a lot more since I've been gay, since I've come out. The definition of "gay" is being happy, and they sure picked a perfect word to describe it. Because I do, I feel very happy.

A sixteen-year-old girl from the Midwest said this about herself:

> I've always been proud that I wasn't embarrassed about being a lesbian. Because people would ask me, "Well, aren't you embarrassed or ashamed about it?" And I would say, "No, I'm not." I always enjoyed being able to open up other people's minds about it. Being different for me was a way of teaching people to respect others and to open their minds.

V SEX AGAINST YOUR WILL

RAPE

When someone forces you to have sex against your will, that is called rape. Even though it involves a sexual act, rape is *not* lovemaking. Rape is an act of force and hostility and violence and humiliation. Rape violates a person's sexuality and a person's humanity. People who have been raped describe it as a horrible and frightening experience.

Most of us think of rape as a surprise attack on a woman that happens in dark alleys or parks, or on isolated streets late at night. Some rape happens like that. But according to the police, over half of all reported rapes happen between people who know each other or who have seen each other or met before. These rapes happen on dates, in people's homes, at parties, and in daylight as well as at night. The phrase used to describe being raped by someone you know is *acquaintance rape*. Many rapes involving teens are acquaintance rape.

Acquaintance rape is like an acting out of the worst stereotyped images of men and women in our society. The man is "supposed" to be aggressive and dominant, to be sexually powerful and demanding. The woman, on the other hand, is "supposed"to be coy and shy and passive, to lead men on but not let them get "too far." Boys have been taught *not* to believe girls when they say no, and they learn to pressure girls to give in, in order to maintain their "macho" image. A sixteen-year-old boy told us:

> A lot of times boys think that girls are expecting them to make the advance, so they do it because they think the girls will think they're creeps if they don't. Even if the girl's saying no, they feel like they have to.

Being pressured—or pressuring someone else—mentally or emotionally, or physically, into having sex is something most of us have experienced (see p. 92). Sometimes sexual pressure turns into a kind of rape. Lenora described an experience, not of actual rape but of feeling enormous sexual pressure and intimidation:

> I was on this date and we were with another couple, and we were in the back seat and this guy was trying to put my hand down his pants and I was thinking, Shit, I don't believe this. I don't want to do this. He wants me to beat him off and I'm thinking I want to be inconspicuous. I don't want the people in the front seat to know what's going on and meanwhile I'm trying to fight this guy off and he keeps trying to stick my hand down his pants.

Sometimes it's pretty obvious, as fourteen-year-old Gloria told us:

> I was so drunk the first time it happened. I was thirteen and I didn't know what to expect at all. The guy took advantage of me. I was so drunk I couldn't walk and he took me back to his house. Afterwards I was scared to death. It hurt and I was so drunk I said, "What is this? Am I dying or what?"

Guys who get involved in acquaintance rape situations are generally acting out the idea that a "real man" goes for all he can get, without regard for what the woman wants or feels. They may feel pressure from friends or from the media about "scoring" or "getting" a woman. They may feel hostile or angry toward women. It is hard to generalize because each person's reasons for raping and each acquaintance rape situation are very different.

How Do You Know If You Have Been Raped?

This may sound like a silly question, but there is a lot of confusion and misunderstanding about rape, particularly acquaintance rape. You know it's rape if someone grabs you from behind or breaks into your house and attacks you. But so many situations are less clear than that. A good definition to follow is this: if you *feel* violated, if you feel that someone did something to you sexually *against your will,* then you have been raped. In an acquaintance rape situation, a girl may have said yes to certain things but at some point has started saying no. If the guy successfully pressures her to have sex anyway, through verbal or physical force, then a rape has taken place.

What is sad about an acquaintaince rape situation is that many times it can be avoided if the people involved would communicate their needs and their limits to each other. Since girls have been taught to "lead guys on," they have to begin to learn to give straightforward messages. Boys have to learn to believe what girls are saying. It is important to say yes *only* when you mean yes; and to really mean no when you say no. A sixteen-year-old girl from Los Angeles talked about the situation she once found herself in:

> I was at this party once and I was getting pretty drunk and making out with this guy I didn't know. We were really getting into it. And then he expected that I would just do it with him. I got pretty scared and I had to push him away. I yelled at him, "No way!"

Giving clear messages *before* the situation gets too far along will help avoid the panic that this girl experienced. But even if you haven't given clear messages, the other person has no right to rape you. Getting raped is *never* fair punishment for being stupid or not giving clear messages. It is important for girls to look at their role in the situation and how they helped to set it up. But it is also important not to assume the responsibility for being raped. Remember, you may be guilty of miscommunication and bad judgment, but that's all.

Myths about Rape

One of the problems with doing something about rape is that there are so many misunderstandings and myths about it in our society. Looking at these myths to separate fact from fantasy is the first step in understanding this difficult subject. Here are some of the most common myths about rape:

Myth: "Most Women Secretly Want to Be Raped." All of us at some point or another in our lives have fantasies of being "taken" sexually, or being swept off our feet in a moment of passion. For girls and for boys the fantasies are somewhat different, but the idea of being forced, or forcing someone else, into sex is very common. There is an important difference, however, between fantasy and actual rape. You control your fantasies. They can be a sexual turn-on, but they are not reality. We can think about being held or "taken" and the thought is sexually exciting. In reality, though, rape is not sexually satisfying. It is an act of force and sometimes violence, over which you have *no control.*

Because fantasy rape and real rape are so confused in our minds, you often hear both males and females making jokes, or even saying seriously that girls secretly want to be raped. But that isn't true. A fifteen-year-old girl from Los Angeles described the following "real rape" situation:

> I once went to a party with a friend of a friend. It was all the way on the other side of town and I didn't know where I was. I got really wasted. Somebody slipped a Quaalude in my beer and I couldn't even move. So I went into the bedroom and lay down. Some guy came in and saw that I was totally out of it. He came over and ripped off my clothes and raped me. When I would try to scream, he would cover my mouth. Nobody could hear me because the stereo was so loud. It was horrible. Finally this guy's brother heard me screaming and came in there and beat up his brother. After that I couldn't go out with a guy at all. It took me about a year to get to where I could trust any guy. I still have bad dreams about it. I wake up screaming. I didn't tell anyone about it for a year.

This is just one of the many rape experiences girls have told us about. It helps us see clearly how frightening rape is. *No woman wants to be raped,* despite what movies or popular stories or soap operas tell us.

Myth: "If a Woman Gets Raped, Then It Is Really Her Fault." Another common myth about rape is that it is really the woman's fault. If she got raped, then there must have been something in what she did or how she looked or acted that caused the rape. Partly this myth comes from the idea that in sexual situations women are responsible for saying no. So if a woman got raped, then she must not have been saying no loud enough. In the case of rape by a stranger, this is just not true. Research has shown that the way a woman dresses or acts or behaves has very little to do with whether or not she is raped. In acquaintance rape situations, it is somewhat different, because clear messages may help prevent rape situations from developing (see p. 125). But a woman doesn't "cause" herself to be raped. The rapist causes the rape. Flirting or wearing tight pants or low-cut blouses cannot "make" men rape you.

Myth: "Most Women Enjoy Being Raped." We live in a society that increasingly links sex and violence. And it is often made to appear that the most exciting sex, the "sexiest" sex, is sex mixed with violence or the threat of violence. Advertising and movies and record-album covers show sex and violence all wrapped up together. Fashion advertising uses themes of whipping or beating women as they display the latest clothes. Record albums have covers of women chained or stabbed or tortured. And for years, movies have used the "fantasy rape" scene, where the woman is threatened and starts out resisting, but soon melts under the man's power and charm. Scenes like these foster the myth that women like to experience violent sex. In the movie, *Gone With the Wind,* Rhett Butler carries Scarlett O'Hara up the stairs, kicking and screaming. Then the scene cuts to the next morning as Scarlett wakes up—happy and satisfied.

No one enjoys pain. But advertising, records and the media make it seem possible that people do. And, sadly, many people in our society today actually believe that women enjoy being sexually abused or raped.

The reality of violence toward women is very different from that. Fourteen-year-old Susan told us:

> I was walking home from a friend's house early in the evening. I was one block from my house when these two older guys I had never seen before jumped out and chased me and caught me. Then they both raped me on the sidewalk. I felt like I was dying. They beat me, and then afterward they beat me until I would thank them. Then they left. I sat there on the sidewalk for a while. Then I got up and walked home. I didn't tell anyone about it for a long time.

Myth: ''Women Rape Men Just as Men Rape Women.'' This is a common misunderstanding about rape, and it happens because people so often confuse the words ''rape'' and ''sex.'' One way for boys to understand how rape is not sex is to think about being raped by another man and forced to submit to sexual acts against your will (forced oral sex and forced anal sex). Cases of men raping other men do happen in our society, and a woman could brutalize another woman. But because of our culture, and because of the traditional roles of men and women, by far the majority of all kinds of sexual assaults are committed by men against women.

In most states, for it to be legally considered rape, a man must put his penis in a woman's vagina against her will. Therefore, by law, only a man can rape a woman. There are other laws that make it a crime to sexually force someone in ways other than intercourse: sodomy, forced oral sex, and sexual battery. Think about this: a girl has a gun at a boy's head and she says, ''Have sex with me or I'll kill you.'' In that kind of situation, is a boy going to be turned on? Not likely. Real rape *always* involves violence or the threat of violence. It is not a sexual turn-on, and a boy is not going to be excited enough to maintain an erection in a rape situation. When boys say that they want to be raped, what they really are saying is that they want to be ''fantasy-raped'' (taken sexually) by a woman.

Who Is a Rapist?

It is very difficult to define the kind of man who rapes. Most studies are done on men in prison who are called chronic rapists—men who rape over and over again. These studies show that most men who rape are not crazy or even mentally ill. Rather, rapists appear to be ''normal'' by society's standards. What seems common to all rapists, however (and this includes men who get involved in

acquaintance rape situations), is that they have a lack of self-confidence and self-understanding. Many rapists come from families where they were beaten or humiliated or sexually abused as children.

Also, people who rape generally have poor communication skills. They do not know how to communicate what they want or need from a situation. And perhaps most important, men who rape cannot see women as human beings. They see women only as sex objects or ''cunts'' or ''whores.''

It is also important to understand that the desire for sex is not why men rape. Many rapists have sex available to them through their girlfriends or wives. Generally, men report that they rape for the feeling of dominance over, and intimidation of, another person. It's as if they were using rape as a way to make themselves feel more powerful. Rape is an act of power and hostility, not of sexual desire.

Who Is Likely to Get Raped?

All kinds of women have been raped: young, old, rich, poor, pretty, plain, college students, professionals, working women and women on welfare. The old myth that only ''bad'' girls, prostitutes or girls from poor families get raped isn't true. Anyone can get raped. What police say, however, is that in stranger rape situations, rapists are looking for women who seem like victims, who seem passive and easily persuaded or intimidated. Your body language when you are walking down the street is especially important. In acquaintance rape situations, a girl has a greater chance of being raped when she does not give direct messages about what she expects from a sexual situation and what her limits are.

In any potential rape situation, probably the most important thing to remember is to *stay alert*. Be clear about what you do want and what you don't want. And be assertive about getting out of a situation that seems strange or threatening to you. This doesn't mean that you should never talk to strangers or never get involved with people you have just met. We all take risks, and part of the fun of life is meeting new people and getting involved in new situations. It does mean, however, that you stay aware of what is happening, that you trust your own judgment about situations, and that you know and communicate your own limits.

In both acquaintance rape and stranger rape, teenagers told us that some situations are more dangerous than others. Here's what a group of teens suggested:

—Don't walk late at night alone or on poorly lit streets or through parks or alleys.
—If you feel that someone is following you, cross the street and walk on the other side.
—Don't get drunk or stoned in situations where you don't know anyone or have no way of getting home.

—*Be direct* about what you do want and don't want from any situation.

—Don't hitchhike! No matter how many times you have been lucky, it is important to know that many boys and girls have been sexually assaulted and murdered when they were thumbing rides.

—Take a self-defense workshop on rape prevention. Learning what you can do with your body will help increase your self-confidence in a potential rape situation.

If someone does try to assault you, probably the most important weapon you have for self-defense is your own intuition, your own gut feeling of what you should and shouldn't do. Trust yourself. There is no one right way to act in a potential rape situation. Some women have fought and screamed their way out of a rape; some women have made human contact with their attacker and talked their way out of being attacked; some women have been saved because they vomited or became—or acted—ill. What you will do depends on the type of person you are and the particular kind of situation you find yourself in. Sometimes there's just no way out.

If You Have Been Raped

The most important thing to do for yourself if you have been raped is to *get help*. Many girls want to go home, take a shower, and try to forget the whole incident. The girls who described their rapes on p. 128 didn't tell anyone else about it for a year or more. But immediately after a rape you need both support and comfort and prompt medical attention.

The best place to go for medical treatment is a hospital emergency room. If you call the police first, they will probably take you there. If there is a rape crisis center in your community, call them.* Many centers will send someone out to wherever you are to take you to an emergency room and to give you support. Also, call a girlfriend, your sister or brother, parents or boyfriend. You need all the support you can get at this time. Remember: *Being raped wasn't your fault.* This may help you get over the embarrassment or fear of telling someone.

At the hospital you will be checked over for injuries. Even if you don't feel hurt, it is possible that you have internal injuries and you should be examined. You will also be given pregnancy and VD tests. At the emergency room, trained staff will gather evidence in case you decide to prosecute the rapist—that is, go to trial to convict him of the crime of rape.

Gathering of evidence involves taking samples of your

*Most cities have rape crisis centers or rape hot lines listed in the phone book (under Rape). If there is no rape crisis center in your community, call the community mental health center nearest you or call Planned Parenthood or a local women's clinic. Some colleges and universities offer rape assistance; call the student center.

hair and saliva, and getting swabs from your vagina and possibly rectum. Generally this does not hurt, but it must be done by specifically trained people in order for you to use this evidence in a trial. If you are absolutely sure that you will not want to prosecute, you can refuse to have this procedure, but we advise doing it because you may change your mind in the future.

Taking care of your medical needs is only part of what you must do. You also must take care of your emotional needs. Rape is a very frightening and traumatic experience. You may feel embarrassed or humiliated or furious or revengeful or ashamed or dirty or anxious or frightened, or all of these things. There is no one "right" way to feel, and your feelings will change over time.

You may also feel guilty, as many girls do. After a rape experience, a woman may say to herself, "If only I hadn't done this," or "If only I hadn't gotten drunk," or "If only I hadn't gotten into that car." This is a natural reaction to a rape experience, and it is important to keep in mind that rape is not the victim's fault. Remember, no matter what you did, *rape is never a just punishment for it.*

After the initial upset, many girls experience feelings of extreme anger, even rage. These feelings are completely appropriate reactions to rape. A seventeen-year-old girl from the West wrote a poem expressing her feelings of helplessness and anger:

> I have killed you a
> thousand times inside.
> I have gotten my revenge safely.
> I have seen the good
> in people,
> and the bad,
> but I can see no
> good in you.
> There are animals
> that are more human than you.
> Have you once thought
> back and regretted
> a thing?
> Probably not.
> I have killed you a
> thousand times inside.
> But you haven't died
> in my mind.
> It is a fine scar
> you have left on me;
> inside and out.
> I have killed you a
> thousand times inside.
> Please die.

One very important kind of help you can give yourself to work through your anger and other emotions is to *start talking about the rape* with sympathetic friends or family as soon as possible. Keeping your experience inside yourself, or trying to pretend it didn't happen is too much of a burden and may feel like a great weight inside of you. Talking to people will help you move through your pain and bad feelings.

If you don't feel comfortable talking to friends or family, a rape crisis center or rape hot line has people available who are trained to help you talk about your experience. They can also help you make decisions about talking to your parents or others who are close to you. Remember, parents, friends and lovers will all have their own reactions to your experience. Sometimes they, too, will need to see a counselor, because people who love you may have an emotional reaction to your rape.

One thing that many rape victims say is that it is very helpful to talk to someone who has also been through a rape experience. Sharing experiences helps people feel not so alone and isolated and lets them see that the emotions they are going through are similar to the emotions that others experience. One sixteen-year-old told us how important a group for rape victims was to her:

> A long time after I had been raped I got into this group with other women who were also rape victims. Until then I had hardly talked to anyone about the rape. Talking to the other women gave me a great sense of release. I got a lot of support to see that I was not responsible for what had happened. Now I help other women who come into the group talk about their experience and work through their feelings.

Deciding Whether to Prosecute. Deciding whether or not to prosecute someone who has raped you can be very difficult. Maybe you know the person, or maybe you are afraid of hurting someone or of getting hurt again yourself. Sometimes people who work with rape victims encourage women to prosecute because they feel that it is one of the few ways of doing something about the problem of rape in our society. Reporting and prosecuting a rape can also be a way of dealing with your own feelings of guilt and anger. Your friends and family will give you advice, but in the end, you will need to make your own decision.

It is best to call the police immediately following the rape incident. Your ability to remember the details of the experience is best at this time, and it is more likely that the police will be able to use the information you give them to locate the rapist. Even if you don't prosecute immediately, the law says that you can report a rape for up to three years after the incident has occurred. Here is what Cindy told us about her decision to prosecute:

> About two years after I was raped I finally decided to report the guys who raped me. Before that I was too afraid and didn't want to go through the hassle. I also thought nothing would come of it. Going down to the police station was really scary. I had to give descriptions of the guys who raped me and I had to tell the story in detail. It was really hard to do, but I'm glad I did it.

If the rapist is caught and the court agrees, you can prosecute. The court process is not easy to go through and you will need support. If you wait a long time to report the rape to the police, it is unlikely that it will be possible to prosecute in court. Still, the information you've given to the police may be useful if the rapist has also attacked other women. Rapists usually continue to rape.

After It's All Over. For most people, rape is a horrifying experience. You can help avoid or prevent a rape from happening to you by using your good judgment, taking commonsense precautions (see p. 126), and being assertive about what you want and don't want from sexual situations.

But sometimes, even if you are conscientious and careful, you can end up getting raped. If this does happen to you, or to someone you know, probably the most important thing to remember is that old saying "Life goes on." You have many years to live; you will have many more experiences, both good and bad. And the wonder of human beings is their ability to absorb really terrible experiences, to grow through those experiences, and eventually to move beyond them.

INCEST

It's an ugly fact that there are people who will force sex on others. It is a misuse of power, and an abuse of sex and sexuality. One of the scariest and most upsetting situations occurs when a relative forces sex on you—anything from touching you to unwanted sexy kisses to oral sex to intercourse. The word used to describe sex that happens in a family is incest. It happens to children who are very young, as well as to teenagers.

The most common type of incest is between brother and sister, while they are growing up. This may not be harmful or upsetting to children, especially if they don't continue as they get older. It is more like experimenting with sex with your brother or sister before you begin to have sexual relations with other people. What *is* harmful, however, is to have sexual contact with an older family member. Almost always, that person will be a man: father, stepfather, grandfather, uncle, big brother or cousin. Victims of incest are mostly girls. When boys are molested, it is usually by their fathers or by a male relative. Incest between mothers and sons or mothers and daughters is not very common, but it does happen occasionally.

Incest is not necessarily a violent attack like rape. Instead, it is more like persuasion—an older person pressuring a younger person to do something sexual. An older family member has tremendous power over you, because of both physical strength and his position in the family. There is very little that most young people can do to resist this type of pressure. But even so, most incest victims feel that they "caused" the incest, that somehow they said yes because they didn't fight or resist their father or relative. And incest can be a pleasurable experience for young children—being rubbed or touched physically. Often the incest can go on for many years. The person initiating the incest is unwilling or unable because of his sickness to take responsibility for stopping it. So the victim, through guilt and shame, assumes all of the responsibility in his or her mind.

Incest is something that many people, particularly incest victims, find very hard to talk about. For victims, their experiences are the cause of much shame and humiliation and anger. Like victims of rape, incest victims carry with them a tremendous sense of guilt, sometimes for many years. Some carry it with them forever.

The most important way to do something about the problem of incest—in fact, almost the *only* way to do something about the problem—is to *tell someone*. Opening up about the incest to someone you trust, *and* to someone who will believe you, is the first step in solving the problem.

Telling someone can be very, very hard. You have to face the anger or hurt or sense of betrayal from your parent or relative. Sometimes relatives, especially mothers, don't want to believe that it's happening. So they may tell you that you caused the incest or make you feel like a liar. If that happens, it is important not to give up. Find someone who will listen to and believe you (an older sister or brother, grandmother or aunt, or a friend of your parents, a relative, a teacher, a counselor or someone from the rape hot line). You need to keep reminding yourself that it is *your*

right not to be touched sexually by *anyone* when you don't want to be.

As long as the incest is a secret, there is no way that you alone can change the situation. When the problem is out in the open, however, not buried in the closet as a deep dark family secret, then everyone—the person committing the incest, the victim and the other family members—can begin to help change the situation.

Incest is a "curable" sickness. Though it is a criminal offense, most of the time when incest is reported, the person is not sent to jail but usually is ordered by the judge to get psychiatric help. Trained counselors will also work with the other members of the family to help them talk out their feelings.

Getting help is essential. If you are a victim or if you know someone who is a victim, encourage him or her to talk to someone. However frightening or painful, beginning to open up about your experience is the most important way to do something about the problem. Here are some places you can call for help:

—Local rape crisis center or hot line
—Community mental health center
—Planned Parenthood or women's health center
—YWCA
—Women's center

AUTHORS' NOTE: We would like to thank the following people for their help with this chapter: Cathy Barber, Susan Forward, Grace Hardgrove, Rebecca Magdaleno, Paul Potter.

RECOMMENDED READING

Autin, Al, and Hefner, Keith, eds. *Growing Up Gay*. Youth Liberation Press, Inc., 2007 Washtenaw Ave., Ann Arbor, Michigan 48104. Send $1.75 to order. Excellent collection of essays on gay youth issues, mostly written by gay youth.

Barbach, Lonnie Garfield. *For Yourself: The Fulfillment of Female Sexuality*. Garden City, N.Y.: Anchor Press, 1976. A book for women about getting to know their bodies better.

Boston Women's Health Book Collective. *Our Bodies, Ourselves*. New York: Simon & Schuster, 1976.

Changes: You and Your Body. Pamphlet. Order from CHOICE, 1501 Cherry Street, Philadelphia, PA 19102.

Comfort, Alex and Jane. *The Facts of Love*. New York: Crown Publishers, 1979. Good discussion, beautiful illustrations. Mainly for younger teens and preteens.

Eagan, Andrea Boroff. *Why Am I So Miserable If These Are The Best Years of My Life?* New York: Pyramid Books, 1976. A guide for teenage girls. Has a section on legal rights.

Gordon, Sol. *You*. New York: Quadrangle, 1978. There are lots of books by Sol Gordon that you may want to look at. This is one to check first.

Hass, Aaron. *Teenage Sexuality*. New York: Macmillan, 1979. Sociological survey of teenage sexual practices.

Julty, Sam. *Men's Bodies, Men's Selves*. New York: Dell, 1979.

Kelly, Gary F. *Learning about Sex: The Contemporary Guide for Young Adults*. Woodbury, N.Y.: Barron's Educational Series, Inc., 1978. Informative, nonsexist book for older teens. Cited by American Library Association as one of the Best Books for Young Adults in 1978.

McCary, James L. *Human Sexuality*. New York: Van Nostrand Reinhold, 1978. Excellent, maybe the best, textbook on the subject. Used in many college courses.

McCoy, Kathy, and Wibbelsman, Charles, M.D. *The Teenage Body Book*. New York: Simon & Schuster, 1978. Very helpful in answering lots of questions. We don't agree with the section on plastic surgery.

Pomeroy, Wardell. *Boys and Sex* and *Girls and Sex*. New York: Delacorte Press, 1968, 1969, respectively. Two books with clear and basic information about body changes and sexuality.

Silverstein, Dr. Charles. *A Family Matter: A Parents' Guide to Homosexuality*. New York: McGraw-Hill, 1977. Good overview for parents and for people who aren't gay.

Zilbergeld, Bernie, and Ullman, John. *Male Sexuality: A Guide to Sexual Fulfillment*. Boston: Little, Brown, 1978. Sensitive discussion of male issues, especially with regard to sexuality.

All of the books listed above are nonfiction books. There is a libraryful of fiction for teenagers, such as the books written by Judy Blume and Sandra Scoppetone. Here is a list of a few titles that have been recommended to us that deal with teenage sexuality:

Diary of Anne Frank

Good Times, Bad Times, by James Kirkwood

Happy Endings Are All Alike, by Sandra Scoppettone

I'll Get There; It Better Be Worth the Trip, by John Donovan

Can You Sue Your Parents for Malpractice?, by Paula Danziger

TAKING CARE OF
YOURSELF

VI EMOTIONAL HEALTH CARE

VALINDA RODRIGUEZ

Feeling Bad, Feeling Better

From time to time everyone has feelings they wish they didn't have. Even babies. When a baby is hungry or cold or uncomfortable, he or she cries for help. Most people, young and old, have developed their own ways to cope with troublesome feelings and problems and to ask for help. In this chapter, we'll talk about some of those feelings, and describe the methods some people use to help themselves get through them.

Writing about and reading about depressing, painful feelings aren't much more fun than the feelings themselves. Many people, maybe even most people, are afraid of mental or emotional "problems" because they seem so mysterious. We tend to be afraid of things we don't understand. Somehow it's easier to deal with a physical ailment like a stomachache or a broken leg. Emotions aren't as easily mended.

It's our hope that reading what other people have to say will help you understand that if you have confusing or upsetting feelings, you're not alone. We hope that as you read you'll be able to get some ideas about how to help yourself, how to ask for help, and also how to help your friends if they seem to have problems. More than that, we hope this chapter will make emotional "ailments" seem less mysterious.

Troublesome Feelings and Problems

Most teenagers feel a jumble of crazy, beautiful, frightening, mixed-up emotions. A lot of people have several different feelings at the same time about the same things. For example, you might both love and hate your parents or school or yourself, or you might be both excited and scared that pretty soon you'll be out on your own. One minute you may feel a particular way, and then a minute later you may find yourself feeling the opposite way. This can be tiring and confusing. And under these circumstances, making a decision can be next to impossible.

One side effect may be an upsetting moodiness. You may withdraw from people or lash out at them, pick fights, cry uncontrollably, or laugh at nothing and everything. Jim-Bob, a fourteen-year-old from Missouri, said:

I think when your moods change the way mine do it's weird, because it's like, what's real? It's not outside things, it's all inside stuff. If you don't even have a hold on the inside, how are you going to know what's real on the outside? That scares me.

Many of the teenagers we met said they are particularly affected by special occasions, such as birthdays, holidays, parties or anniversaries of important events. Even when the occasion is one they've been looking forward to for weeks or even months, they said when the day actually arrives they break into tears or start fights with their parents or lock themselves in their room. The teen years can be times of great expectations and great disappointments. Everything can seem to have special importance. Caryn told us about her eighteenth birthday:

My parents took me and my sister to a hotel on the weekend of my eighteenth birthday. It was really nice, but I was feeling lonely because my boyfriend was back home and I missed him. My parents kept expecting me to be really glad that we were there, so I felt like I had a lot of pressure on me to act happy. On the morning of my birthday I just felt miserable. I came down to breakfast grouchy, and it was horrible for everybody. At lunch my mother had arranged with the head waiter to bring a big birthday cake to the table, but somehow he had forgotten all about it, so no cake came, and when my mother explained what happened I burst into tears and ran up to the room. I cried the whole day. The next day my father told me I was the most selfish person he'd ever met.

Part of Caryn's unhappiness on her birthday may have been caused by the mixed feelings about getting older that Laurel describes:

> About a month before my seventeenth birthday I went through a lot of pain. I cried and felt depressed, like one of those dark clouds was over my head. It was as if I'd just faced reality. I felt like I was getting old. Like all of a sudden you're supposed to be grown-up, but you're still just a kid. I realized I'd never be sixteen again or fifteen or fourteen.

Getting older is a mixed bag. Many people have told us they have a hard time accepting their birthdays, because getting older means leaving childhood farther and farther behind. On the one hand, that's great because it means more freedom and more independence. On the other hand, it means taking on more responsibility.

Sometimes moods seem to be caused by nothing at all. Just a look on your mother's face can set you off, or a sad song on the radio, or the dog whining to go out or be petted. Whatever starts it, when it hits you it just seems to take over. Fifteen-year-old Mathew described the feeling this way:

> You feel like everything's crashing down on you. Everything's happening to you. Everyone else has fine lives. Everything bad only happens to you. You're the unlucky one. You can't hide from it. There's no escape.

The teenage years are a time of transition. You're not really an adult yet, but you're not a child anymore either. It's a time when most people feel a little shaky about their ability to handle themselves in the world. Problems and decisions often feel overwhelming. When the people around you treat you with respect and seem to understand that you're dealing with some important issues, that can ease the pain. When they don't take you seriously, that can make things worse. In Detroit, Beth told us:

> Problems that teenagers have are real. They aren't phony or unimportant. Your first crush, the first time you fall in love, deciding whether to go to college, looking for a job—hey, that's real stuff and parents should take it seriously. I know some parents say, "Oh, that's nothing. At least you don't have to worry about putting food on the table." But when you're going through a problem, I don't care who you are, it's real to you. It hurts you, and if parents make us feel like our problems aren't worth anything, then we grow up thinking our feelings don't matter. It's like *you* don't matter.

Most people say that at one time or another problems just get to feel too heavy. Some of the teenagers we met said at those times all they want to do is go to bed and get taken care of. Luke lives in Arizona. He told us:

> I get in these moods sometimes when I feel so depressed. Inside myself I know I could get out of

them, but I don't always want to. Sometimes I just like to give in and act like a depressed little kid who whines and cries and pulls the covers up over his head. I want my mom to come in and take care of me.

Fifteen-year-old Terri said:

> If I'm depressed, I'll go home and I'll just lie there. I don't do anything or say anything, I just lie there and stare at the ceiling. I don't enjoy it, but it's too much trouble to do anything else.

It's pretty natural to feel the way Luke and Terri are describing once in a while. But if it happens often, and if your depression lasts a long time—more than a couple of weeks—it's a good idea to try to write down what you're feeling or find someone to talk to. (On p. 136 some teenagers talk about different ways they've discovered for themselves to get out of depressed moods.)

Taking Out Feelings

Often the feelings inside a person are so confusing and so strong that they can't stand doing nothing—they have to do something. When action comes from negative feelings, it usually turns out to be negative or destructive action.

Some of the teenagers we met direct their negative actions against themselves. They take out their feelings on themselves by not getting enough sleep or by overeating or undereating, by pushing themselves to the point of exhaustion, by using drugs and/or alcohol to try to forget what's on their mind. Seventeen-year-old Shelly said:

> For me, food is like drugs are for other people. When I'm feeling bad I'll eat and eat and eat, thinking that will make me feel better. But if you could see some of the things I stuff myself with, you'd know it's not out of the pleasure of eating. It's out of frustration. My friend throws up when she's nervous. I eat.

Julie, a sixteen-year-old Midwesterner, took out her depression on herself even more directly. Julie remembered:

> Even when I was little, I've gone through times of, you know, not liking myself. And I still go through them. I have this bad way of handling it, which is to hit myself. You know, punch myself. I remember a time when I was with a group of people and I was having this bad feeling and I just kept punching myself on the leg and then I stopped because I hadn't realized what I was doing. It was just my instant reaction to how I felt, and right after I did it I was saying, "Oh, my God!" I couldn't believe I'd actually done that in front of people.

Fifteen-year-old Warren remembered his ninth-grade year:

> After my dad moved out I went steadily downhill for about two months. I just about quit going to school.

I was drunk and stoned every single day. And finally one of my teachers caught me and said, ''You're not going to make it out of junior high if you don't start shaping up.'' And I really wanted to graduate with my class, so I started going back to school.

Warren told us he was reacting to his mother and dad's separation, but a lot of other teens told us they don't seem to have any real problem to pin it on. They just have a heavy kind of feeling that lingers on.

As we've said over and over in this book, it helps to get your feelings out. Maybe you're feeling sad about something. Sadness needs to be expressed—crying is a great release. Billy, a fifteen-year-old who helped us with this book, told us:

I think you should talk to people when you're sad. I do. Sad is a real heavy thing. Like one of my friends died, and a bunch of us guys who knew him all got together and we just sat there and cried and talked about him. It was good.

You might be sad because you broke up with your boyfriend or girlfriend, or because you failed a test and will have to take a class over again. Maybe your mom and dad are fighting or you feel they don't love you anymore. Whatever is causing your sadness, if you talk about it or write about it or paint a picture about it, you may feel a lot better.

Anger is the same. Holding it in can turn your anger into rage. The tighter you hold it in, the more it's going to want to come out.

Lots of people are afraid to express anger because they worry about hurting others, or more often, they worry about the reaction others will have to their anger. Some lit-

tle kids who get angry get hit or put in their room. If you were always punished for expressing anger, you may not have developed any successful ways of dealing with your angry feelings. If you were always told not to get so angry, you may have learned to hold your feelings in. Or maybe you try to hold your feelings in and just can't, so you end up lashing out wildly at whoever's nearby.

Anger is a very natural feeling. You don't have to be afraid of it. But you don't want to let the way you express your anger hurt yourself or someone else. It's not OK to hold in your anger so tightly that you develop some physical illness or bad headaches or nervous twitches. It's not OK to mistreat yourself because you're angry. It's also not OK to go around fighting with people or acting violently toward them because you feel that you've been misunderstood or unfairly accused of something or mistreated by someone else.

Talk about your anger. Tell a counselor or your best friend or your parents. Hit a punching bag. Run around the block a couple of times. Ride your bike up a hill. Better still, tell the person who made you angry that you're feeling that way and explain why. Bonnie said that's what she's learned to do:

I don't get angry much, but if I do I just look myself in the mirror and say, ''Now, why are you angry? This is so dumb. Figure out what's bothering you.'' Usually I can calm myself down that way and I feel better. But when somebody triggers me off and I get pissed right then and there I just flat-out tell them. I don't hold it in at all. I just tell them.

It's easy enough for us to say ''Talk about your feelings,'' but actually doing that is another matter completely. Lots of people feel scared by their feelings and are afraid that talking about them will make them feel worse. Others worry that no one will want to listen. Alice, a thirteen-year-old from California, said:

I don't like to lay my problems out, even to my close friends, because for some reason I just figure that they don't want to hear about me.

And fifteen-year-old Morgan said:

A lot of people don't want to admit their feelings even to themselves because they're afraid that their problems will scare their friends away. I usually think, Well, if they knew I felt that way they'd think I was weird.

Sometimes people work pretty hard to cover up their feelings by putting on a show of toughness or sweetness or coolness that no one can crack. That's called a defense. It's a way of defending against the real ups and downs and confusion that most of us feel at various times.

We think people have a right to work through their confusion. We think people have a right to know that they

---

BRUSSELS SPROUTS*

I'm like a tightened fist. Holding
back all my anger. Trying to stay closed
and trying not to open and explode
with anger. I can't hold my leaves
closed any longer. I'm exploding.

My leaves are opening. I feel like
a rocketship that just took off
for Mars. My outside leaves are green,
but my innerself is yellow with fur.

Now that I have been rid of my
anger, I can return to the field
and start all over again.

—Anonymous

*The authors have tried to contact the poet, but we have not been able to reach him/her. If he/she sees this poem, we hope he/she will contact us.

ARTICHOKE

I build up my protection,
　　layer after layer
I put sharp points where their
　　fingers will pluck my pieces off.
Really what I'm hiding most
　　is my heart.
　　　　　　　　So tender it is.

Still they eat me.
　　It must be hard
　　I must admit.
Every layer they peel right off.
　　Ha! Ha!
　　the outsides too hard!
The teeth scoop out my tender inside anyway.
　　So much work for so little food.
Ohhh my h e
　　　　　　a
　　　　　　　r
　　　　　　　　t

　　so soft and silky
The prickles didn't stop them.
　　Nothing can.
　　Nothing will.

　　　　　　　　—Diane Hurley

---

aren't weird or sick or dumb for feeling anger or sadness or fear. If we spend years defending ourselves against those feelings, they only get buried deeper and deeper inside and find their way to the surface later on when we're least expecting them. Then they may come out without our being able to control them—sometimes in sickness, sometimes in rage, sometimes in deep depression. If we can, it's better to recognize our feelings at the time we're feeling them, and to do something about them then.

Trying to Ask for Help

People who look or act depressed all the time, people who are always getting into trouble, people who get drunk or stoned out of their minds every day are often asking for help in their own way. Nineteen-year-old Gina, a first-year college student from New York, remembered:

> When my mother found a stolen watch in my drawer, she threatened to take me to juvenile hall. All she wanted to know was where I got it. She never once tried to talk to me and find out what was going on with me. I felt like I was a bad person. Her talking to me that way just confirmed it for me. It was like she was saying to me, "You do bad things, so you are bad and you should be punished." All I really wanted was for her to tell me she loved me anyway, and that I was good, not bad.

Gina wasn't able to say that to her mother until years later. Even then it was hard because Gina's mother thought Gina

was accusing her of being a bad mother. They had to argue awhile before they were able to understand that all they each wanted was to be loved and appreciated by the other.

Zeke, a tenth-grader from Michigan, told us that he really wanted to talk to someone too, but he didn't know how. He was getting drunk and falling asleep in class, but no one seemed to notice. He said:

> One day I wrote this poem in class:
>
> > I'm not a big stoner
> > You must agree
> > But can't someone help me?
> > I don't like what I see.
> >
> > I've only gone from beer, pot, to speed,
> > But can't you do something?
> > Help me. Please
>
> I showed the poem to my health teacher and I remember she just looked at me and said, "Why don't you go talk to your counselor? She'll help you." That was good because I did go see my counselor. When I got to her office, I just put the poem down on her desk in front of her and I burst out crying. I must have cried for about forty-five minutes straight. I couldn't stop. I had never cried for *me* for as long as I could remember. But I just sat there and I cried my eyes out.

Zeke told us that that experience in the counselor's office was the beginning of a change. The counselor invited him to join a group of other people who were going through hard times, and Zeke said that was a great eye-opener for him. He found out he wasn't the only one with problems, and that made it easier for him to talk about them.

OTHER STRUGGLES

As a teenager, in many ways you are a beginner, facing certain adult experiences and problems for the first time. To cope with new situations, you need as much understanding, guidance and encouragement as you can get. That's especially true when you make mistakes—and you're bound to make many, since everybody does.

A lot of people have trouble dealing with mistakes. As sixteen-year-old Diana said:

> Sometimes you just get to the point where you say, I hate myself. How could I have done that? How stupid! Or you say, I'll never be able to do anything right.

If your parents have their own difficulty handling mistakes, they may not be very helpful to you when you most need their understanding. Jack, a fifteen-year-old from Wyoming, said:

> My father's really good at fixing things. So when we're working together, he expects me to be as good

as he is. Well, that isn't right. I don't know as much as he does about it. He calls me a dummy and sometimes that makes me feel like I *am* a dummy.

Eighteen-year-old Maria told us:

My mother's always downgrading my little brother. He can't ever do anything right as far as she's concerned. But I think if she keeps doing that, he'll never be able to do anything.

You're going to be trying a lot of new things during your teens. Sometimes you'll have great success and other times you'll fail miserably. That happens to everyone. It can be hard to hold on to your self-esteem during all those ups and downs if the important adults around you, such as your parents and teachers, are putting you down. You need encouragement now. If you can't find it at home, it's a good idea to find some other helpful, supportive adult to talk to and learn from. Churches and temples often have youth leaders on their staffs. Community centers or programs at a local park may have adults who work with teens. Maybe there's an understanding counselor or teacher at your school. This is the time when you deserve to hear some good things about yourself. This is the time when someone should be building up your self-confidence. Maybe you can do that yourself, but many people benefit from some outside support.

As you deal more and more with the "real world" outside home, you're bound to have some negative experiences. They can be a rude awakening, especially for people who are used to being protected by their parents. Don't be too quick to blame yourself for these failures. Teenagers, in general, are not treated with the fairness or respect given to older people. Fifteen-year-old Cindy told us:

I went down to apply for this job at a store near where I live. I was real excited about it because the pay was pretty good and it was within walking distance. Well, I had the interview and the guy told me I got the job. It was Wednesday and he told me to start on Monday. So Monday comes and I go down to work, and the guy comes to the door and tells me, "Oh sorry, we hired somebody else." Since I'd lied about my age I didn't think I could fight it, but I bet the whole thing was that somebody white applied and they'd rather give her the job than a black kid.

If something like that happens to you, you may be able to fight it, but you will probably need legal assistance. If your family has a lawyer, contact him or her. Otherwise call the NAACP or the American Civil Liberties Union. There is a branch of each of these in every state. Most big cities have chapters. Look in the phone book or call Information (411). If they can't help you, they will refer you to someone who can.

More often the problems you run into will not be things

you want to fight legally but will be just the kind of frustrating experiences that happen to all of us, no matter what our age. Sometimes, though, because you are a teenager, people don't take you quite as seriously as they would an older person. That is completely unfair, but it happens. Burke, a seventeen-year-old from New York, told us about this experience:

My family always used to go to this fancy restaurant whenever there was something to celebrate. So I decided to take my girlfriend there on our anniversary. We got all dressed up and we had enough money. Well, I couldn't believe what happened. The head waiter, who was always so nice to me when I was with my folks, just completely ignored me and my girlfriend. Finally he gave us the worst table in the whole place and the service was just as bad. I felt like a jerk, but I knew that if I made a scene, that would be worse, so I just put up with it.

FEELING POWERLESS

The kind of experiences Burke and Cindy had can make you feel powerless. In fact, the whole process of becoming independent is laced with times when you'll feel insecure and inadequate. Herbert, a senior from Michigan, told us about his fears:

I'm still living at home so I still feel protected from that great unknown out there. But when I finish school it will be up to me. I look at it and it all looks so hard, like a rat race. I mean, who has any real meaning to their lives? There are going to be wars, and murders, and famine and everything else whether I like it or not. It makes me feel like I don't have any control over my life. Who wants to be part of that?

We heard many teenagers express Herbert's fears. They wonder whether the whole thing is worth it. Often that's a

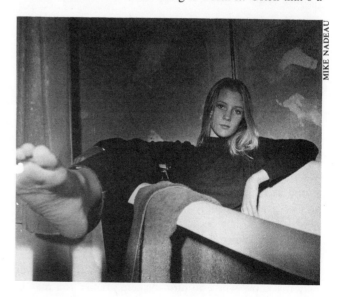

MIKE NADEAU

way to express the very reasonable uncertainty people feel when they have to face something they don't know much about. Fifteen-year-old Vicki put it this way:

> I think I use my family as a crutch. They really help me out a lot, but sometimes I just feel like breaking away from the crutch. I just want to be on my own. But when I think about that, it scares me. I think how lonely I'll feel. I worry that I won't be able to make it. I don't even know where to begin.

And Dennis, who lives in Oregon, told us:

> I used to run away sometimes because I'd think, Oh wow, this is really going to be a relief. No more nagging, no more hassles. And then I'd get out there on my own and I'd feel empty, like there was just this big void.

Some teens are lucky enough to know that their parents and families will be there to help them even after they move out. Other people can't be sure of that. Many teens we interviewed said they know they're going to have to make it by themselves. Warren, a fifteen-year-old from Wisconsin, described his sense of aloneness:

> My mother started picking on me and my older brother started yelling at me and we had this big fight. It was snowing out and about twenty degrees, but I went outside to get away and my mother locked the door on me. I was dressed in just a T-shirt and I didn't have anywhere to go. I was just crying and crying and I was freezing.

Violet told us her story in California:

> I used to get hit for stuff I didn't do, and that was the worst. I feel a lot of resentment for that. I don't think I'll ever forgive them for that. My father used to beat me until I'd confess to doing the thing, even if I didn't do it. He never believed me when I would tell him I didn't do it.

Warren and Violet had already left home when we talked with them. Marlene, a sixteen-year-old from Vermont, was trying to find a place for herself when we met her on the street in Boston. She said:

> My stepfather tried to rape me, so I told my mom because I thought she would be on my side. After all, I'm her daughter. I come first. But she got mad. She wanted to give me a lie-detector test.

Warren, Violet and Marlene have been pushed into independence before they feel ready for it. They're just as scared as Herbert and Vicki, but they don't have the support of a loving family. They are suffering, not because they are bad, but because their parents have emotional problems that keep them from being able to come through for their children.

If you're experiencing similar problems at home, you may not know where to turn for help. While you may be sympathetic toward your parents, and while you may love them deeply, you must also protect yourself and take care of yourself. There are some places that will help you if you call. We have listed them in the box opposite.

Sometimes, for some people, the feelings and problems they have are more than they can bear. They can't find their way out of the negative circle by talking or thinking things through. Attempts to distract themselves from the feelings—by going to the movies, playing sports, reading a book, helping other people with their problems, writing about the situation, drawing a picture—aren't working. Sixteen-year-old Tai has had that experience. She said:

> I just couldn't write anymore. My feelings were beyond writing. I couldn't even explain how I felt and I just stopped writing completely. It got pointless after a while. If I wrote down how I felt that *day*, it would take the whole book.

If that's ever happened to you, maybe you began to think that no one wants to listen to your pain. If you can't stand being alone with it anymore, you may find yourself boxed in. You would rather feel nothing than feel the pain.

It's still a mystery why thoughts of suicide and death seem easier to consider for some people and not for others. Probably each of us has thought at one time or another, Oh God, I wish I were dead. Most of the time that statement just means we wish for relief, for less pain and conflict

---

DESPERATE TIMES

I'm a blighted flower.
A parrot too old to talk.
An unfinished meal.
An overfed deer.
A childhood without toys.
A boat with no sea to be sailing away.
A tamed lion.
A castrated rabbit.
A curtain that never flings open to bare the stage.
A boring fairy-tale.
A housewife with a Women's Lib T-shirt.
A child's garbaged picture.
All the neatly nailed butterflies in the museum
    under the dusty glass.
A scary dream.
An expired fire of someone's heart.

I'm all I dislike.
I'm all there is in the world to hate.
I'm a left-over and a left-out.
So what a cruel irony it takes
To try to comfort me in my everyday grief
To soothe me, to make peace with me
And then, as a rule, to leave me.

—Anonymous

WHERE TO CALL FOR HELP

Help is available for teenagers in trouble. Help is also available for teenagers who have run away from home and feel lost and alone. Reach out by calling one or more of these numbers. Someone will help you.

National Runaway Switchboard: 1-800-621-4000

This is mainly a service for runaways. They will be able to help you find a place to stay. It is a toll-free number. You don't pay for the call. They won't hassle you.

Runaway Hot Line: 1-800-231-6946

From Texas   1-800-392-3352
From Alaska
    Hawaii   1-800-231-6762

This is another runaway service, which is set up to help teens who have left home.

United Way Information and Referral Services:

Most large cities have a United Way office. Look in the phone book. Ask for their Information and Referral phone number. Tell them what your problem is and what kind of help you are looking for.

County Department of Public Social Services:

This number will be listed in the phone book under the name of your county. There are many services listed, so if you have a specific problem like child abuse, alcoholism or drug abuse, look under those headings.

Free Clinics:

If there is a Free Clinic in your area, they may also provide counseling services. Call them or stop by.

Mental Health Clinics:

Most local mental health centers will offer teenager services. Look in the Yellow Pages under Health Services or in the white pages under the County services.

Local Police:

Your police department may provide special services to help teenagers. Call them. You don't have to give your name if you don't want to.

Churches, Temples:

Your church or temple may have a Youth Director on staff. He or she would be a very good person to call for help.

Local Radio Stations:

Stations that broadcast mainly to teenagers often have lists of teen services. If there is a talk show that deals with teenage problems, that would be the best number to call. You don't have to be on the air. When you call, tell them you don't want to be on the air, you want some help.

Doctors:

If you have a doctor, he or she may be able to help you or refer you to someone who will be able to help you.

---

than we're feeling at *that* particular moment. Rarely does it mean we want to feel nothing *forever*. We really wish we could tune out for a little while and then tune back in when the problem we've been wrestling with is solved. In some ways it may be a feeling of wanting to be a child again, of wanting to crawl into Mom's or Dad's lap and have them make it all better.

It's pretty natural, when confronted with a situation that seems painful no matter which way you turn, to take a leap into fantasy as a way of escape. Thoughts of death at such a time can be a kind of escape into fantasy. Death can become equated with peace and quiet, harmony and serenity, a desert island in the sun, a featherbed, something muted, soft, silent, still.

But if you can get through the pain of the moment, you will probably find that the intensity of your feelings subsides and you'll feel a lot better, a lot more hopeful, a lot more optimistic. Sometimes it's even hard to remember how bad you felt just yesterday or even just a few hours ago. Crystal, a high school senior from Indiana, described her own powerful feelings:

I always wonder how people can even consider suicide. I've gone through some pretty rough times and that's the one thing I've never considered. I feel as if I'd be hurting myself, but hurting other people even more. It's like I always have these dreams that I'm dying or that I'm dead and crying at my own funeral and I'm sad because I'm going to miss everybody and I'll never see anybody again. By imagining that, I just don't feel like I could ever do it. I think you can do so much in the world to better it, I just can't see anybody thinking of killing themselves.

Just as people develop strategies to deal with or divert themselves from depressing or painful thoughts, people also develop techniques for changing or escaping suicidal thoughts.

A variation on the imagine-your-own-funeral scene is to say, "Imagine how bad they'll feel after I'm gone." This scene has more of the quality of revenge about it. Your death becomes a punishment to those who have hurt you. But the pleasure of the revenge is much more effective in the fantasy than in the reality, because, in reality, of course, the dead person is not around to enjoy the guilt, remorse and sorrow of those he's left behind.

What really gets stirred up in these fantasies of loss and revenge are a lot of strong feelings about being alive, not about being dead. These feelings about the people in your life are usually about how you'd like things to be different. The real trouble comes when you give up hope of things ever being better. With great anguish, Barbara, a seventeen-year-old from the Northeast, described a time when she had felt that way:

> Sometimes you just get to the point where you don't really care how anyone else feels. You just want to get the hell out. You just want to escape. You feel the world is so cruel. When I felt that way, I didn't think about other people. I just thought about how much I wanted to get out, to get out of living. It's such a big pain in the ass. You feel like there's no other way out except death.

We talked to many teenagers who felt this desperate and this sad after a breakup with their boyfriend or girlfriend. Beginning to rely on someone outside your family for love and support is a powerful experience. When things are going well, it can make you feel great, and it can add to your feeling of independence. But when the relationship isn't working, you can feel *more* alone, more vulnerable and dependent than you did before. It's very hard to lose someone you've loved, even if you've known that person only for a short while. You can experience intense feelings of loss when someone dies, when they break up with you, when they're angry and seem to withdraw their love.

Roger, a sixteen-year-old Iowan, stopped just short of making a suicide attempt after a particularly angry family fight. He felt abandoned by his family. Roger said:

> I went near the bridge and I was going to jump off. God must have helped me. He told me, a voice told me, to call up my best friend, Dan. It was about twelve-thirty at night, but he came over running and he hugged me and he said, "Roger, don't!" I slept over at his house and I didn't go home for about a week.

Roger did a very wise thing: he called up his best friend, even though it was the middle of the night. He gave himself the chance to get help, the chance to reconsider his momentary desire to kill himself.

Sometimes you don't call out for help—as Roger did—or, if you do, there's no one around to hear you, or sometimes the help comes later. Ginger, seventeen and from

New York, did try to kill herself—she cut her wrists. Luckily, the cuts were not too deep, so that she was only badly hurt. But afterwards Ginger still felt terribly depressed. She describes her turning point:

> A guy at school spotted my wrists at the beginning of class and said, "Don't ever do that again." And just before we left, he said to me, "Take good care of yourself." And that's what started me right there. I said to myself, "He's right, man. You're all you got. You may not be the most beautiful chick in the world, but you don't need that shit." So when that one boy said that, bingo, it just shot to my head. "Yeah, that's what you gotta do. You gotta take care of yourself."

Peter, a sophomore from Maryland, didn't talk about what bothered him until *after* he had tried to kill himself:

> I never used to talk about my problems. I had to feel terrible before I'd talk to anyone. Two years ago, I tried to kill myself. I was in this hospital for two weeks, and when I got out they put me in outpatient therapy. That's where I met my therapist. That's when I started talking.

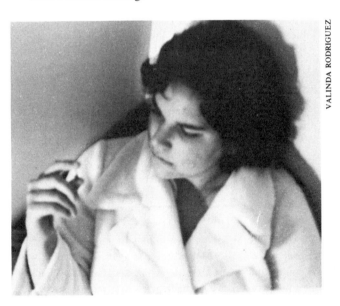

VALINDA RODRIGUEZ

When you're feeling so unhappy that thoughts of suicide don't scare you, you'll probably find, as Peter did, that talking about your feelings will help relieve them. People consider suicide when they think living is too painful. But there *are* people who really do care. You may have a friend or a relative who loves you and will listen to what's troubling you. Or you may choose to speak with someone you don't know. Some people prefer that.

If you need *immediate* help, there are 24-hour suicide prevention hot lines in nearly every big city. Call the operator and ask for the number. If you don't live in a big city, you can call the emergency room of your local hospital or the police. During the day you can also call your church or temple or even the local health clinic. Tell the person who answers that you want to talk to someone about feeling depressed. This is important: if you or someone you know is in danger of committing suicide, *get help*. Take the time to let the feelings cool down. Take the time to reconsider. *Death is permanent. Feelings pass.*

TO TALK OR NOT TO TALK

All through this chapter we've suggested that you talk about your feelings and problems with other people. Many teenagers we met said they talk over those things with their friends. Others said they have an older sister or brother they talk to. A few people said they discuss upsetting concerns with their parents. Jeanie, a fourteen-year-old girl we met in New Orleans, said:

Lately my mouth has been running a lot. I've been telling everyone what's been going on. I just have to get it out. It's been bottled up for fourteen years, so it's about time to let go of some of it. Sometimes I want to know, How come I just can't shut up? But I have a feeling when I get it all out, I'll be able to shut up.

There are lots of people to talk with: friends, family members, teachers, coaches, ministers or rabbis, neighbors, club leaders. Anyone who cares about you and will listen to you and whose good sense you trust.

Patsy, a sixteen-year-old from Chicago, has to be in a wheelchair, so she's in a special program at school. She said:

The reason I can feel so open about talking about my feelings is thanks to the teachers here at this school. They've been like a second family to me. They're always there when you have a problem and they'll talk to you. Maybe it's lucky to be disabled to be able to have teachers like that. They're always there for you. They'll talk about anything with you.

Probably the strongest argument for letting someone else know how you're feeling is that they may have a different perspective than you do. Precisely because they aren't you, they might be able to see something about your situation or feeling that you can't see because you're too close to it.

Have you ever felt really stuck? Been in a dilemma that you can't figure out? You think through the problem step by step, but every time you do this, you arrive at the same dead end? Feeling stuck is one of the best indicators that it's time to involve someone else in what's bothering you.

In addition to giving you a new perspective, talking to someone else about what troubles you can just be a relief. You can get those troubles off your chest; not feel so alone as when you keep them all to yourself; you can get support and maybe even some concrete suggestions for changing things and some help in carrying out those suggestions.

Finding Someone to Talk To

What qualities or characteristics might a person have that would make him or her a helpful person to talk to? What questions do people ask themselves when they're looking for a helper? The list is a long one. We've found

---

SUICIDE PREVENTION HOT LINE

Most cities have suicide prevention hot lines that can be called twenty-four hours a day. Their number is listed in the phone book under Suicide or Suicide Prevention. In some areas the group that runs the hot line is called the Samaritans, so you might try looking under Samaritans also. Call them before you do anything. They will help. IF THE LINE IS BUSY, *KEEP TRYING*.

WARNING SIGNS

1. A big change in eating or sleeping habits.
2. Suddenly not caring for prized possessions—giving away favorite records, a pet, clothing.
3. A loss of interest in friends.
4. A long and deep depression over a breakup or the death of a beloved person.
5. A great change in school grades.
6. Feeling hopeless or full of self-hate.
7. Feeling constantly restless or hyperactive.
8. Actually making a suicide attempt.

DANGER SIGNS

1. They say they intend to hurt themselves.
2. They have a plan for how to do it.
3. They have in their possession pills or a weapon of some kind.
4. There is evidence they have already hurt themselves.
5. The person is dazed or unconscious.

IN AN EMERGENCY, CONTACT ANY OF THE FOLLOWING:

1. Your local police.
2. An adult you trust.
3. An ambulance service in your town.
4. The emergency room of a local hospital.

DO NOT LEAVE THE PERSON ALONE!

that friends will have more of some of the qualities, while parents will have more of others and counselors still others. If you're looking for someone to talk to, you'll have to decide which characteristics are the most important to you. You may find someone you really like who has qualities very different from the ones you thought would be important. It's good to remain flexible, but, most important, it's good to be true to your intuitions. A counselor may have the best credentials in the world and the nicest office you've ever seen, but if you don't like or aren't comfortable with her or him, it's not going to work. Your own feelings are more important than the degrees on the wall or the furniture in the room. If everyone you know—except you—loves to confide in one particular friend or favorite teacher, don't be swayed—stick to your guns, and find a person of your *own* choosing to talk to.

Here's a list of the questions many people found important to ask themselves when they were looking for someone to talk to. Some of these may be important to you; others may not. Pick and choose from this list in making up your own. Remember that it takes time to get to know

someone. You may have some very quick impressions of your listener. Other qualities may take longer to become clear. Give yourself the time.

—What do you know about your listener? If it's a friend, you may know lots. If it's a counselor, you may know relatively little. Are there facts, such as age, sex, training or life experiences, that seem important to you to know about someone you'll be talking with? "Factual" information may not be what matters to you as much as how it *feels* to talk together.

—What expectations does each of you have about talking together? Are they similar? Different? Adjustable?

—Does your listener feel he or she can be of help? It would be hard to begin talking to someone who felt pessimistic about you or about the effectiveness of talking about problems.

—*Do you feel respected?*

—Do you and your helper seem to feel pretty comfortable together verbally *and* nonverbally? If not, then your words may sound easy while your bodies seem stiff, formal or unfriendly.

—Who decides what will be talked about and who does most of the talking? If you can't get a word in edgewise, or have to follow someone else's program, the time spent together won't be very helpful.

—Does your listener make assumptions about who you are without your having provided any information? If you correct his or her misimpressions about you, are your corrections accepted as true or are they argued with? Is your helper judgmental?

—Does she or he try to solve your problems for you or try to talk you out of what you've said you're feeling?

—Is it possible for you to express the full range of your feelings—anger, sadness, joy, depression—or are some of your feelings more acceptable to your helper than others? *Does he or she seem to be afraid of your feelings?*

—*Do you get the sense that you're being understood?* One way a good listener can let you know she or he has understood you is by rephrasing what you've said in such a way that you have the feeling, Yes, that's just what I'm feeling, but I hadn't thought of describing it that way. Often the benefit of this rephrasing is to give you a new angle on or even new words for what you've been struggling with inside your own head. Getting a new perspective can clarify or reveal a conflict that has been hidden from view before. Once you can see a conflict it's easier to figure out how you want to handle it.

—Are you in charge of the pace? If the talking feels too personal, too fast, are your desires to slow it down respected?

—Through time, can you feel yourself grow a little more open and trusting? Does it become a little easier to talk about difficult, painful or shameful feelings? Do you feel that the trust and respect between you will keep growing?

SUICIDE
MYTHS AND FACTS

Myth: People who talk about suicide don't kill themselves.

Fact: Eight out of ten people who commit suicide tell someone that they're thinking about hurting themselves before they actually do it.

Myth: Only certain types of people commit suicide.

Fact: All types of people commit suicide—male and female, young and old, rich and poor, country people and city people. It happens in every racial, ethnic and religious group.

Myth: Suicide among kids is decreasing.

Fact: The suicide rate for young people has tripled in the last ten years.

Myth: When a person talks about suicide, change the subject and try to get his or her mind off it.

Fact: Take them seriously. Listen carefully to what they are saying. Give them a chance to express their feelings. Let them know you are concerned. And help them get help.

Myth: Most people who kill themselves really want to die.

Fact: Most people who kill themselves are confused about whether or not they want to die. Suicide is often intended as a cry for help.

Here's a brief checklist:

—Do you feel that your talks are helping?
—With the help of your listener, can *you* look pretty openly and honestly at your feelings?
—Do you feel free to really *feel* them right there when you're together?
—Is it OK to cry? Laugh? Rage?
—Do you *understand* more about your feelings and concerns?
—Are you able to *deal* more effectively with those feelings and concerns? Are you able either to *accept* them or to *change* them?

One thing you may not be able to decide in advance is how long you will want to talk to someone. You may feel like really settling in, letting the relationship build, taking your time. Or you may feel like talking with someone just once or twice about a very specific concern of yours. The choice should be up to you.

THE PROFESSIONAL HELPER

Another part of the choice is whether you want to talk with someone who has professional training in helping people with their problems—a therapist or counselor—instead of a friend, teacher or parent.

Cynthia explained why she felt more comfortable talking with someone on the "outside." She said:

You don't have to worry about what the therapist really thinks of you. You can say anything you want. But with your friends, you have to deal with their reactions.

Jason, an eighteen-year-old New Englander, gave us his impression of therapists:

They don't have a whole lot of preconceived opinions. They remember the things you said, and since they're objective, they can put it all together and just make it clearer. Talking to someone outside yourself helps. It brings you down to earth. You're not alone.

This "outside" professional help might be found through the guidance counselor at school or through a local medical or mental health clinic, a hospital or a free clinic or teen center, if your town or city has one. Often, there is a hot-line telephone number you can call to find out where you can go for good counseling. It's important to know that what you say to a professional helper is confidential. He or she will not reveal what you say to anyone else. This assurance is harder to come by with friends or relatives.

Money may be an issue. A counseling service may be provided free through your school, your parents' health plan or a local free clinic or youth center. Otherwise, talking to a trained helper will probably cost money. Some professionals work on what is called a sliding fee scale:

their fee depends on how much money you have or earn. If you have no money their fee might be very low or nothing at all. Other professionals do not have a sliding scale. So if you've picked someone who charges a full fee, you may have to get an after-school job to help pay the cost, or ask your parents for help or try to get a small loan or pay off your bill over time. In any case, fee is an important subject to discuss if your helper charges for her or his services.

Generally speaking, a therapist with professional training would have a degree in counseling, social work or psychology. Medical doctors who have special training in psychology are called psychiatrists. If you're interested in what training your helper has had, you should feel free to ask.

We talked to many people who found it very hard to consider going to see a professional counselor. They felt that you had to be sick or weird or weak. It's as if asking for help means you're a sissy or you're crazy or desperate, rather than that you're doing something responsible—taking care of yourself or being good to yourself. Maggie, a seventeen-year-old from Seattle, said she used to think people who went to see therapists were "crazy": "I mean *I* don't have any deep problems that I have to talk about, and besides, *he* can't help me." Patricia, an Illinois senior, told us what her fantasy of therapy was all about:

I've always pictured that they'd be picking my mind and I don't want that. I don't want anyone picking at my thoughts. I really feel that my feelings are no one else's business unless I want to share them—and I usually don't.

Robert, sixteen and from Chicago, said:

Sometimes you feel like you're the only one who feels that way. It's embarrassing. It's hard to open up to somebody who's not opening up to you.

Mark stated his objections this way:

I just can't see going to a therapist. It's difficult because you know that you're paying him to listen to you, to analyze you. With a friend, you're just talking nonchalantly.

We talked to some people who felt very positive about seeking help but who got very negative judgmental reaction from their parents or friends. One boy, Hugh, from the Midwest, said:

My father told me, "Well, I had a lot of problems when I was your age too, but I managed to work them out on my own. I never had to see anyone."

Teresa, a fifteen-year-old from New Hampshire, told us:

I have a friend whose mother has had a lot of problems, and now she's having problems. But she can't tell her mother because her mother would never go to anyone for her depression. She just would never do it. She would say, "You should have the strength within yourself to solve it."

Anita summed up the thoughts of many people we spoke with when she said:

People say, "Do you have a psychological problem? You must be crazy." You get insulted if somebody says you need to see a psychiatrist. It's your thoughts, it's you that they're looking at. It's not just your arm or something like that. It's because you have something wrong with your thinking.

Obstacles and Expectations

Sometimes the road to finding a good helper has been so long and so rough—from deciding to look (that is, managing your own feelings, your parents' and those of the people around you about seeking help) to actually looking (getting names and making appointments), to figuring out how to pay for the help, if there is a fee, and, finally, to arriving at the exact day and time—that by the time you actually get help, either the need may have passed or, even more likely, your expectations will be so high that no person or single encounter could ever live up to them. Mary Alice *knew* she had huge expectations about the help she'd get:

For years, I always wanted to see a psychiatrist. I had this vision that once I got into this psychiatrist's office all these feelings inside that I had would be able to come out. I imagined this scene in my head of all these things I'd say to the psychiatrist and then maybe I'd cry or something. Like the psychiatrist would be the mother I felt I'd never had, hugging me and loving me, loving me for who I was and not caring about things that I thought were bad about me.

Having fantasies of a perfect helper or a perfect encounter can make the beginning pretty disappointing. Michele, who had worked hard to find herself a therapist, described her feelings on the day of her first appointment:

I went to this guy, but by that time I was just on a really tense point. It was like, "OK, so now you've finally got it so that you're going to have a therapist," and "Now the appointment is finally made." By the time I actually had that first appointment I *needed* help immediately. But that didn't happen. Because what was supposed to happen the first day, y' know? He said, "I'm Doctor So-and-So and this is what we'll be doing here." And that night was the first time I ever hurt myself physically because it had just kept building up and building up. I couldn't take it any longer.

Once Michele got to know her therapist better, she was able to tell him when she was needing more immediate help, or when she was sad or angry or disappointed. You may not even realize, as Michele didn't, that you have so many hopes and dreams about the help you're waiting to get until *after* the first appointment or two. It might help to anticipate the possible letdown. Be kind to yourself and your helper. *Give both of you time to develop a relationship before judging it.*

Don't Judge a Book by Its Cover. We heard a lot of complaints from young people who had seen therapists who they felt were closed off and distant. Sometimes it may be hard to tell the difference between a therapist who's quiet but tuned in and one who's quiet and tuned out. A therapist who talks a lot, even one who talks about herself or himself, may not be more helpful to you than someone more reserved. Sometimes talkative therapists are just filling up time because they're nervous and don't know what else to do. A real helper is someone who helps *you* to do the work of exploring, expressing and dealing with *your* feelings. If a therapist tries to manage your feelings for you or is constantly telling you what *they* did or would do in a similar situation or uses *your* time for *their* problems, then *that's not good therapy.* It's not good friendship either. An outgoing style doesn't necessarily mean that there's caring, compassion and objectivity behind it. It takes time to know someone. A person is not always what you've imagined them to be by their looks or their manner. Learning whom you can really trust—someone who genuinely has your best interest in mind—is very, very important.

However it comes about, it's essential that you feel *some* connection to your helper eventually. We talked to people who never felt that connection. Most of them had the good sense to stop seeing that person after a while. Janey, a fifteen-year-old from the East Coast, had a vivid story to tell:

The guy I had was a total jerk. I'd try and open up to him and I'd make myself do it. Then I'd ask him a question about *him*self, like, "Are you married?" or something and he'd say, "Why are you asking me that question?" It's like, "Well, gee, Mr. Freudian psychiatrist, I know you're taught that you're supposed to be this way, but why can't you also be a *person* and react to me as a real person, because that's what I'm also curious about." It's kind of like, here I am, I have this fake relationship with this person I'm supposed to be totally opening up to and it doesn't work. This psychiatrist was like that. I don't know how many are. I feel that to do some real work with a psychiatrist, you have to like them and feel like they like you or else it just won't work.

That Janey's psychiatrist wouldn't answer her questions may be less important than *how* he refused, or the fact that, basically, she didn't feel that they liked each other.

Will, a seventeen-year-old from Maryland, told us that

his assumptions about how it was supposed to be had changed over time. He let go of some of the more superficial expectations, like what his therapist should look like, and clarified for himself some of the more important ones:

> I had to get used to him because he didn't look at all like what I thought a therapist would look like. He didn't wear a pinstripe suit. He didn't wear glasses. He didn't have a beard. He had longish hair. At first I didn't feel comfortable with him at all. But he was honest. It's important that it be someone who isn't going to make you feel strange; someone who will open up a bit to you too. Also, it takes a long time to trust someone. That's important to know.

Across the country, Melissa shared the experience she had with a child psychologist. Like Will's, her experience changed over time:

> At first I didn't like it too much. I thought I was just boring her, just laying my problems on her. I'd go in every week and say the same thing. It just started to get monotonous. So I said, "Aren't I boring you every time?" And she said, "No, no." And finally we started really talking to each other. I liked it more then. I really enjoyed it. I honestly can say that I really started to care about her and love her, and I think that was nice.

The Group. Several of the people we talked to had had experience with group therapy—that is, more than one person seeing a therapist at the same time. Sometimes they knew the other people—friends or acquaintances from the same school or same town—but sometimes they were strangers.

One benefit of a group is that there are as many angles on a single problem as there are people in the room. That can mean a lot of extra help when the group focuses on *your* problems. You may feel really understood and supported by members of your group. Sometimes there is one or more people in your group whom you can really identify with. Listening to what they say about their lives can help you think more clearly about your own. A therapy group can even become like a second home or a tight group of friends.

Sixteen-year-old Jeanette told us her guidance counselor at school suggested that she join a therapy group:

> I started going once a week. I met these other kids in the group who also wanted to straighten up their act. They didn't just have problems with drugs and alcohol, they had problems with their families, with parents. There were a couple of gay kids in it. Everyone was there because they felt like they couldn't deal with what was happening in their lives by themselves. Everybody was asking for help. I had faith in that group. And it really helped me.

Christine described the group of teens she belonged to at her high school in Nebraska:

> We have a group at school where we meet once a week and we talk about a bunch of different things. Like love and sex and friends and marriage. You know, like what you think about, what you want.

Rachel went to see a social worker with a girl from her neighborhood with whom she was always getting into fights. In the presence of an objective person, the girls could say things to each other that they wouldn't have dared to say in private. Here's what Rachel told us:

> This girl was just much bigger than me and I was scared to tell her to stop picking on me. So when I'd see her in the neighborhood, I'd say, "Sure, Linda, I agree with you; you're absolutely right, and stuff like that. But when we were with the social worker, well, I felt braver to tell her what I really thought. Then I might say, "Y'know, Linda, I'm not satisfied with your personality. I think you ought to stop picking on me." It wasn't my idea to see Linda like that. It was the social worker's. But it sure helped!

Ron also had the experience of hearing or saying things in a group that he never would have in private. Ron's experience was with his father:

> My father's a really closed person. We never could talk about much together. For a while, we went to this therapist, just him and me. We didn't say that much to each other, but I learned a lot about my father because he talked about how it was when he was my age and how he felt. They just weren't the kinds of things he'd ever get around to saying in front of the fireplace at home. I understood him a lot better after that. I even respected him more.

Katy went to see a therapist with her whole family:

> My whole family had to go—my parents, my brother, my two sisters and me. My parents would do all the talking. They'd argue with each other and everything. The counselor would say to us, "Do you have anything to say?" We'd always say, "No," but we were listening. I'm sure my parents said things to each other they'd never said before. At home they'd always seemed afraid to talk things over. Even though us kids didn't say anything, I think that time helped our whole family communicate better.

Making It Better

While talking to a professional helper is one very good way to help yourself, there are lots of other ways. You may be surprised by the creativity and usefulness of your own and your friends' ideas about how to help yourselves. We talked to many people around the country who were full of good suggestions. We'd like to share some of these with you now.

Family Support. Having the basic love and trust of your parents doesn't mean they will automatically agree with everything you say and approve of everything you do.

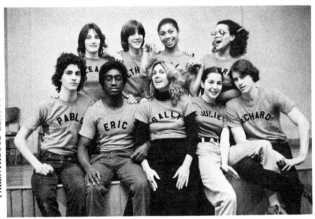

Youth Expression Theater, a teen drama group (with their leader, *center*)

But it does make possible discussions in which each of you can express and stand behind your particular ideas and decisions, and it may also help you to feel good about yourself even when other people are being critical or unsupportive. You can take from the outside your family's love for you and put it inside.

Friends. Many people told us that the good feelings their friends had for them were very important in helping them through rough times. Maybe friends take over the function that family had when we were younger: they love us even when the rest of the world doesn't; they love us when we can't love ourselves. Here are just a few of the comments we heard. Kerri, a sixteen-year-old girl from Cape Cod, said:

When you find somebody that accepts you, who likes you the way you are, you say to yourself, Well, something must be good about me.

Sara, from the South, remembered:

When I started seeing Steven, having somebody love me because of who I was, that definitely put on the final touch, as you might say, in confidence about myself.

Talking to a friend, by telephone or in person, can be a great way to get out of a bad mood, work through a tough problem, share a sad or mad feeling or just to feel understood and supported. Some people told us that they talk to their pets because they can say everything that's troubling them without fear of judgment, criticism or unlooked-for advice. They know the response will be unqualified affection, and that's what most of us want when we're unsure.

Several other people told us that when they helped someone else, they ended up feeling better about themselves. Charlene said:

If I help a friend and a friend is grateful, that's the best thing—especially when I know I've been really sincere.

Sixteen-year-old Robby also had that reaction:

When you do a good deed, as they call it, you sort of feel really good inside. You know you can respect yourself because you've helped someone else. No personal gain was necessary. It's like being all shined up again.

One way to help yourself and to help others is to start or join a self-help group. (People get together for lots of different reasons.) You don't have to wait for a professional to lead the way. The reason could be as general as just wanting to have a group of peers to talk to or as specific as wanting people with the same experience—such as divorcing parents, drug dependence, being black, female, male or gay—to share what they personally have learned. Just among the people you know, there is a wealth of experience and knowledge. Why not take advantage of it?

More Good Ideas. Here are some more ways that individuals have developed to help themselves through rough emotional times.

Bill, a boy from Utah, described his experience of examining his own feelings:

Last summer I went through this really bad time. Every night I'd just sort of crawl into myself and I'd think the whole night about what I hated about myself and how I was going to change it. I *really* got to know myself. I got to know the things I didn't like, and by knowing the things you don't like, you can start to change them and then you can become a person you like. That's what happened to me.

Les, a fifteen-year-old boy, likes to express his feelings outwardly:

If I have a really bad day, I usually go out in the backyard and scream or yell just to relieve myself.

Jonathan prefers to keep some of his feelings to himself, especially the angry ones. He feels he can work them through better that way:

My mom and dad have to guess if I'm upset. I don't like to talk about what's pissing me off. I hate it when people come up and say, "Oh, Jonathan, what's the matter? What's wrong?" I think being pissed is a time when it's good to be left alone with it, till you get over it yourself.

But with other feelings, he wanted to be able to share them. He said:

Feeling sad is different. I think you should talk to people when you're sad. It's good to be able to cry.

Many people told us it made them feel better to cry, by themselves or with people they feel close to. Getting feelings *out* can be a great relief. It can help get you started again.

Another way of helping yourself to think through a

problem or a troubled feeling is to write it out. Some people are very organized about their writing. They keep a daily diary and faithfully record the important aspects of each day. Other people write only when something moves them in a powerful or particular way. Some people put all their writing in one book that they keep to themselves; no one else is allowed to read it.

ALONE WOLF

A lone wolf with no companion
The sun shining reflecting off the snow
makes his fur seem glossy, thick, soft and warm.
And his eyes show wisdom and wildness,
but kindness, loneliness and sadness.
Isn't he something like me.
He is strong, cunning, skillful
But merciful and gentle.
He faces the elements
that would make him mighty
For he has no companion, no mate,
and no leader. He lives
but barely. But it is his wisdom
his kindness, his loneliness, his sadness,
his mercy and his gentleness that makes me
feel pity and love for him. I say again,
isn't he something like me.

—Chris King

Peggy, an eighteen-year-old from Maine, described what it's like for her to use her diary:

Sometimes, when something's really on my mind and I can't go to sleep because of it, because I keep thinking about it, I write in my diary. Then you can sort of clarify your thoughts, like, Well, this is what I'm thinking and I don't need to think about it anymore because it's written on paper. I don't have to worry about forgetting it. I can go to sleep now.

A seventeen-year-old boy from the West Coast said:

I keep a journal. I definitely think it helps me. It's a super release. It relieves tension and helps you get out exactly what you're feeling without having to feel embarrassed or anything like that. No one thinks you're weird because no one else is there to hear you. I write feelings, usually when I am depressed—feelings more than anything else.

Tammy wrote poems rather than entries in a diary. She said:

I write a lot of poems. When I get in this mood, I write poems and save them. Months later I go back and think, "Oh my God, when did I write this?" Or I try to remember what was happening at that moment that made me write that.

Other people told us they write short stories about the situations they themselves are experiencing. This gives them some distance or objectivity about whatever is troubling them. Writing out the situation helps them to think it all the way through. Some people doodle or draw pictures along with or instead of writing as a way of organizing their feelings.

Many people we talked with use a different method: doing nothing. Quiet time or time away from the troublesome situation helps them to get unstuck. They just change their surroundings, go to a different room, a different space. Or they flip through a magazine, listen to the radio, watch TV, go to the movies. Jimmy, a sixteen-year-old from the center of the country, gave us this description of his own experience:

I like to be alone. When I come home from school, I can't even study right away. I have to have a period of time when I can throw myself in the easy chair and just relax and get my head straight. Just a period of time where your body doesn't do anything and nothing's important. It's a time to relax and get everything back in order. It's almost like you get a second wind after it.

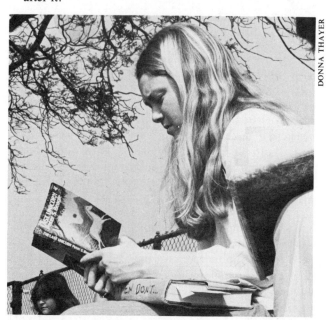

DONNA THAYER

Betty, seventeen, and from a town near the Canadian border, sometimes feels overwhelmed by all the things that need her attention:

Sometimes, when I have too much to do, I don't even want to do any of it. I can't deal with it. I just can't do it. I throw everything on the floor and go to bed. When I wake up, I have more to do, but then I can deal with it. I can do it.

Some people use physical activity as a way of temporarily stepping away from the situation that is troubling them. Fifteen-year-old George told us:

I try and run about five miles a day at least. It's im-

HELPFUL RESOURCES

The Yellow Pages: Here are some headings under which you can find special services—Ambulance, Alcoholism, Drug Abuse, Churches, Hospitals, Health Services, Clinics, Mental Health Services, Physicians, Psychologists, Psychotherapists, Social Workers, Social Services, Parks and Recreation Centers, Religious Organizations, Synagogues, Counseling Services.

Telephone operators: Dial 0 for operator assistance and 411 for Information about a particular phone number.

Police: The police are good resource people to ask about local services and to call if you have an emergency.

Newspapers: Especially small, local, alternative newspapers that devote themselves to information about a particular city or community. They usually have several pages listing self-help and professional-help organizations.

Hot lines: Nearly every area has special hot lines you can call if you're in trouble or want assistance or information. We have listed several general hot-line numbers in other sections of this book. Some hot lines: Drug Abuse hot line, Alcohol Abuse hot line, Birth Control Information hot line, Sex Information hot line, Suicide Prevention hot line, Runaway hot line, Child Abuse hot line, VD hot line, Rape hot line. If you want hot-line assistance call Information (411) and ask the operator to give you the phone number.

School guidance counselors: The guidance office is often one of the best places to go for information about resources and help.

---

possible to think about anything but what you're doing, and it takes a lot of pressure off your mind.

Playing team sports, running, swimming, doing gymnastics, tennis, boxing, jumping rope, yoga—all these are ways to put your concentration on your body and take it off your mind. Team sports are generally a good way to make friends, too, which gives you the opportunity to find someone to talk to about what's going on in your life.

And, of course, if your body is run-down, you're bound to feel worse than if you're in good shape. So exercise helps in that way too. So does a good diet—without too much sugar or junk food—and enough sleep.*

The most important thing to remember about emotional situations is that you don't have to be alone. When you lock yourself up in your own troubled world, it may feel as if there's no one who cares and no one who notices. That isn't the case. By reaching out, you can find someone to share your troubles with, and you may also find out that you're not the only one who feels the way you do. Most of us have upsetting, confusing and painful experiences at one time or another. We tend to think we're the only ones in the world who've had these experiences, but, of course, we're not. Try to put what's happening to you in that perspective—other people have been just where you are now. They've come through OK, and so will you. Try to imagine yourself a year from now, looking back at this hard time, but out of it, as you find yourself in some new and better situations.

*For example, if you don't eat enough foods containing vitamin B, it can lead to depression and/or nervousness. Be sure to eat whole grains and/or take B-complex supplements. B₆ is particularly helpful.

RECOMMENDED READING

Agee, James. *Death in the Family*. New York: Bantam Books, 1969. A boy's account of his father's death.

Angelou, Maya. *I Know Why the Caged Bird Sings*. New York: Bantam Books, 1971. A black young woman comes of age in the South.

Green, Hannah. *I Never Promised You a Rose Garden*. New York: Signet, 1964. A sixteen-year-old girl's frightening experience with mental illness.

Gunther, John. *Death Be Not Proud*. New York: Harper & Row, 1949. The author's memories of his son, who died at age seventeen.

Knowles, John. *A Separate Peace*. New York: Dell Publishing Co., 1962. A high school boy's introduction to competition, guilt and friendship.

Plath, Sylvia. *The Bell Jar*. New York: Bantam Books, 1972. A college girl's depression leads her closer and closer to suicide.

Salinger, J.D. *Catcher in the Rye*. New York: Bantam Books, 1964. An adolescent boy searches for his identity.

Scoppetone, Sandra. *The Late Great Me*. New York: Bantam Books, 1976. The story of a teenage alcoholic girl.

Valens, E.G. *The Other Side of the Mountain*. New York: Warner Books, 1977. A young woman athlete's heroic adjustment to a crippling accident.

Zindel, Paul. *Confessions of a Teenage Baboon* and *I Never Loved Your Mind*. Both books published by New York: Bantam Books, 1978. Humorous stories of teenage life.

Drugs and Alcohol —AND TAKING GOOD CARE OF YOURSELF

Many of you are faced every day with decisions about drugs and alcohol. Should I drink or do drugs at all? If I decide to use drugs or alcohol, how can I make sure that I don't mess myself up? What should I do if someone I care about—my brother or sister, a friend, a lover, or one of my parents—is heavily into drinking or doing drugs? Most of the people we talked to were concerned about these things and had plenty of questions.

Deciding about Drugs in a Chemical Society

In this society almost everyone uses drugs. Most of us use medicine to help us heal ourselves when we're sick. Beyond the use of drugs for health reasons, millions of people use different chemicals to change the way they feel about themselves or about the situations they face from day to day. People drink tea or coffee or soft drinks to get them started in the morning or to pick them up during the day. The caffeine and sugar in these drinks gives people a feeling of extra energy and a lift in mood. Tobacco helps some people to relax. And many people use alcohol because they like the feeling they get from that drug. People use all these drugs to change their state of consciousness—the way they think and feel—and to influence the way they relate to other people.

Because these chemicals have been in use for a long time, it is legal and socially acceptable to use them, at least for people above a certain age. This is true even though we know that some of these drugs, such as alcohol, can be quite harmful if used to excess, or even if, as in the case of tobacco, used at all. When we talked with teenagers about drugs and alcohol, they reminded us again and again that they didn't think it was fair that when authorities talk about ''the drug problem'' few of them mention these common drugs that so many people take for granted. That's why our discussion of drug use includes the legal drugs as well as the illegal ones.

Marijuana was by far the most common illegal drug that the people we talked to had tried. Many people today smoke marijuana regularly. Of course, people use lots of other kinds of drugs too—so many that it can be confusing when you try to figure out what these chemicals are and what effect they have. We have found that it's easier to talk about these drugs when we group them together into certain classes as we've done here.

You'll see in our discussion that we include many of the dangers associated with these drugs. Most of the teenagers we talked with said we should advise people to stay away from most drugs. We were surprised to hear them say that, since so many teens use drugs. They said, ''Sure, people use drugs. But a lot of people get messed up by drugs too.

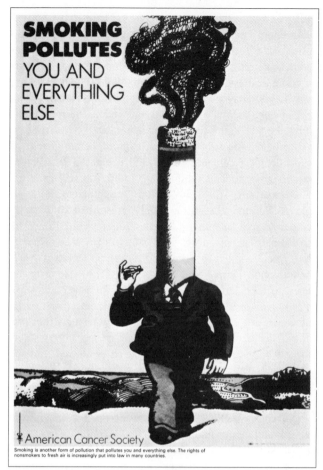

SMOKING POLLUTES YOU AND EVERYTHING ELSE

American Cancer Society

Smoking is another form of pollution that pollutes you and everything else. The rights of nonsmokers to fresh air is increasingly put into law in many countries.

THANKS TO THE AMERICAN CANCER SOCIETY AND THE WORLD HEALTH ORGANIZATION

We think people should know what they're getting themselves into.''

Alcohol is one of the most widely used and misunderstood drugs. People think it's a stimulant, but in fact it's a sedative whose effects on you vary depending on your mood and situation. It can make you laugh or cry, become sleepy or aggressive. Other effects include a lowering of inhibitions, a lessened ability to concentrate, and reduced coordination and reaction time. Even when taken in small amounts, alcohol seriously impairs driving ability, and no one should ever drive if he or she has been drinking.

People often get hangovers afterwards—they feel sick, weak, dizzy, and ache all over. Overdoses of alcohol can depress breathing, cause a loss of consciousness, coma or even death.

Many people become physically addicted to alcohol, and still others become psychologically addicted. These people, along with those whose frequent use of alcohol impairs their health or damages their family life or relationships or job performance, are said to suffer from alcoholism.

Stimulants (uppers) are drugs such as amphetamines (Dexedrine, Methedrine) known as speed, certain diet pills, and cocaine (known as coke). These drugs increase your energy and, for a short time, lower your appetite and give you a feeling of self-confidence. They also increase your heart rate, blood pressure and blood sugar. You may become restless, irritable and anxious. If you take high doses, you may go into panic, confusion, hallucinations, aggression, mental breakdown and serious heart irregularities. People can become dependent on these drugs, because when you stop the use of even moderate doses, you can become fatigued, drowsy and depressed, and have a strong desire to take another dose to lift yourself up.

Depressants (downers) include tranquilizers (an example is Valium, the most widely prescribed drug in the country) and sleeping pills (barbiturates and drugs like Quaaludes). These drugs may calm your nerves or temporarily help you get to sleep, and make you feel as if you've had alcohol. People become "tolerant" to these drugs and need to take larger and larger doses to make themselves sleep. However, they don't become tolerant to the danger of these drugs, and taking larger and larger doses may cause death. People who are high on barbiturates have trouble thinking clearly, their speech is slurred and they cannot concentrate. They become emotional, irritable, suspicious. They may even become paranoid, depressed or suicidal.

Narcotics include morphine, codeine, heroin and pills with brand names like Percodan and Dilaudid. These drugs are used as pain-killers by doctors, and they may produce a feeling of peace and quiet in certain people. However, many people experience nausea, dizziness, mood changes and a feeling of being "burned out," without any desire for sex or food. People become tolerant to these drugs and have to increase the dosage to get the same effects. They also become physically dependent on the drug and experience withdrawal symptoms when they don't get enough. People end up taking these drugs for the "high" and then continue taking them to avoid the painful withdrawal symptoms.

Hallucinogens include LSD, mescaline, peyote buttons, certain mushrooms, and PCP (angel dust). These drugs produce unusual changes in the way people perceive things. Their physical effects on the body include an increase in blood pressure, rapid beating of the heart, tremor, nausea, muscle weakness, a rise in body temperature, sweating, headache, insomnia, decreased appetite and, occasionally, convulsions. The effects of these drugs on the mind are not predictable, and different people at different times will have different reactions. Some people say they have important insights when they are on these drugs. Other people report experiences of panic, fear, hallucinations and depressions, as if they were having some kind of mental breakdown. Drugs like LSD occasionally trigger a long mental breakdown that can last for many months, and it is impossible to predict who will respond to them in this

way. PCP (angel dust), one of the drugs in this group, affects the spinal cord and the brain, and produces disorders in your thinking, hallucinations, temporary paralysis and a feeling of being removed from your surroundings. People have stopped breathing and their kidneys have failed on PCP. Convulsions, raised blood pressure and memory loss are fairly common. In fact, the effects of this drug are very much like the severe mental disease called schizophrenia.

Marijuana and hashish are the drugs most used by the people we talked to. The effects seem to include a dreamy state, a change in the sense of time, a feeling of free-flowing ideas and of increased awareness. Some people say they enjoy things more when they are high on these drugs; other people say they have bad effects from the drugs including anxiety, difficulty in concentrating, loss of memory and unpleasant fantasies. Some people have described a feeling of panic, suspiciousness, headaches, nausea, dizziness, depression, and loss of control. Smoking marijuana, like smoking tobacco, carries with it the risk of cancer, emphysema, heart disease, etc. There is believed to be more tar, for example, in a marijuana cigarette than in a regular tobacco cigarette. The fact is that there is a lot of controversy about the effects of marijuana in long-term and short-term use. Some studies show that marijuana changes the hormone balance in a person's body

It is important to know what the different drugs are and what they do. But more important is how people use them in their lives (or choose not to use them). All of the drugs we mentioned, both legal and illegal, are strong chemicals that will have some effect on the body and on the way users relate to other people. None of these drugs is perfectly safe. There are people who choose to use these substances because they decide that, for them, they are worth the risks, or they think that if they are careful, they can use certain chemicals without suffering serious harm. Such people have a lot of confidence in their ability to control their use of alcohol or drugs. Kenny, fourteen, from Mississippi, told us:

> I can stop drinking anytime I want. I quit smoking cigarettes two years ago when I decided it was too expensive, not worth it. I'm not addicted to anything. If I don't have a joint in six months it doesn't make any difference. It's just nice to have a little trip now and then, a little vacation.

Some other people we interviewed told us that they had decided to avoid drugs and alcohol altogether. Amira, fifteen, said:

> I never touch alcohol. I feel that if I get drunk one night and don't remember anything the next day, then that's it, I just can't drink. So I don't.

Some people were concerned that people might use drugs

just because of peer pressure. Lincoln, seventeen, from Chicago, said:

> You have to know why it is you want it if you want it. Do you want to smoke reefer for yourself or just because everybody else is doing it? I've gotten to the point now that I just don't want to smoke, so if somebody offers me something I'll probably beat around the bush for a while and then finally I'll say, "Look, I just don't want to do it."

Shelley, thirteen, didn't like what she saw drugs were doing to her friends:

> They say they smoke dope or sometimes do speed to help them function or work better. But in a lot of ways it makes people more slow, makes them seem dumb. So I don't see why people would want to use it.

The one thing that all the people we talked with could agree about was that drugs and alcohol could be found everywhere. One person told us:

> Yeah, there are plenty of drugs here in school. You can buy anything you want here. A lot of kids come to class stoned and almost everyone drinks on the weekend.

That means that most teenagers are constantly faced with choices about whether or not to drink or do drugs and it's hard for them to get advice they can trust.

Basic Precautions—What Can Go Wrong

Physical Effects. None of these chemicals is totally safe, and some of them are very dangerous. We know for sure that alcohol and tobacco can cause a great deal of physical damage, especially when they are used in large quantities over a long period of time. We know that barbiturates and hard drugs like heroin and PCP have ruined people's lives both physically and mentally. *We believe people should stay away from these drugs.* Even in the case of marijuana, there are still many unanswered questions.

We do know that some combinations of drugs, such as alcohol plus downers, can mean serious trouble. People have died from mixing alcohol with downers. A number of the people we spoke with told us that PCP (angel dust, a drug sometimes sold as mescaline or THC or even cocaine) was a chemical that they avoided at all costs because it is so harmful. We also know that women who are pregnant should stay away from *all* the drugs we've mentioned, including alcohol.

Psychological Effects. People use drugs because the drugs change the way they think or feel. Some people get pleasure from drugs, some people get into trouble. Not everyone who uses drugs is an addict, but people often slip into being dependent on drugs without knowing it.

How do you know if you have a problem? One question you may ask is how often you use the drug. Emily, fifteen, told us:

> My boyfriend used to be addicted to marijuana. I didn't think that was possible, but he used to smoke every day, and he said he didn't like the way he felt when he wasn't stoned.

You may have a problem with alcohol or other drugs if you find yourself using them every time things go wrong. If you need a drink to face your problems, then you probably have a drinking problem. The same is true with other drugs. Valerie, a nineteen-year-old from Seattle, has been battling problems with drugs and alcohol for years. She told us:

> You know that something is wrong if you find that the drug or the drink means more to you than the other things in your life, like friends and lovers and family. If I could say anything to people, it would be that you have no guarantee that the person you party with is not an alcoholic or a drug addict, and you have no right to help that person kill themselves. You yourself may or may not be afflicted with the problem, but you can bet someone you know is, because one in ten

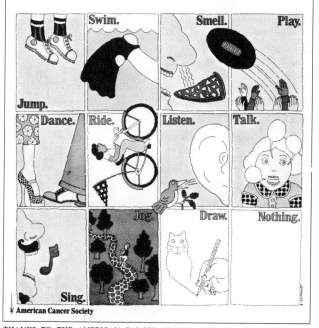

THANKS TO THE AMERICAN CANCER SOCIETY AND THE WORLD HEALTH ORGANIZATION is. It's not a matter of willpower with them, it's a sickness.

If you or someone you care about has a problem, you can probably get help by calling your nearest drug treatment center, mental health clinic or chapter of Alcoholics Anonymous. Your family doctor, guidance counselor, clergyperson, or just about anyone you can trust may also be able to help.

Overdoses, Withdrawal and Bad Trips. As a general rule, anytime someone doing drugs passes out or loses consciousness, he or she should be watched carefully. If you have any doubts about what is happening, get him or her to an emergency room as quickly as possible. Most hospitals will *not* contact the police if someone has a drug problem. Withdrawal from drugs (especially alcohol or other depressants) can be a serious business, too, so be sure to get medical care for anyone who is getting sick because he or she isn't taking the drugs that he or she is addicted to. Amarette, eighteen, gave us good advice on how to handle bad trips:

> I had a bad experience once with a joint treated with angel dust. I felt all these negative experiences in my head and I just wanted it to stop. You have to keep reminding yourself every minute that it's from the drug and it's not real and it's going to be over soon. That's real important. This is a trip and it's going to be over soon. It's not permanent. The trip's going to be over soon and I'm going to be just fine.

If you're with someone who is having a bad experience with drugs, it often helps to get that person to a quiet, safe place and to stay with the person until the drug wears off.

Quality Control. Since many of the drugs people use are not legal, you often don't know what you're getting when you buy or take these drugs. Chuck, seventeen, in Pennsylvania, put it this way:

> It's hard to test drugs because they're illegal. A lot of drugs are being handled by organized crime and they're not exactly into quality control. There's no USDA stamp, so you have to wing it. It's good to know who you're buying the drugs from, but even then you can get burned.

A sixteen-year-old girl told of an experience with ''bad'' marijuana:

> My boyfriend got some marijuana from a friend of his

at school and we took it at his house on Saturday night when his parents were out. I don't know what was in that stuff, but I had these wild, scary pictures in my head. I couldn't finish even one thought and I went into the next room to lie down. I thought I was screaming for my boyfriend but I wasn't even making a sound, and I ended up shaking so much I almost had to go to the hospital. That's the trouble. Somebody must have put something in that stuff we took, but we'll never know what.

Legal Problems. Another hassle connected with the use of illegal drugs stems from the fact that just having some of these chemicals in your possession is a crime. The drug laws vary from place to place, and the police are not consistent in the way they enforce these laws. Some of the people we spoke with were angry about these laws, which they saw as irrational and unfair, but as Scott, sixteen, put it:

> The laws are crazy, but what can I do, I can't even vote yet! So I try to be careful about what I do and try not to get caught.

Others we spoke with decided to stay away from drugs and to avoid alcohol until they reached the legal drinking age in their state simply because they didn't want to worry about getting busted. The laws in most states can be pretty tough on people who drink and drive. That's because drinking or doing downs or smoking marijuana while driving is really dangerous—these chemicals can seriously affect your reaction time and judgment.

The decisions that you make about drugs and alcohol may not be easy ones, but it's important that you make them carefully. If you find that you need more information to make these decisions, you may find these books a good place to start:

Edward Brecher, *Licit and Illicit Drugs* (Boston: Little, Brown & Co., 1972).
Lester Grinspoon, *Marijuana Reconsidered* (Cambridge: Harvard University Press, 1971).
Sandra Scoppettone, *The Late Great Me* (New York: Bantam Books, 1977).
Andrew Weil, *The Natural Mind* (Boston: Houghton Mifflin, 1972).

VII PHYSICAL HEALTH CARE

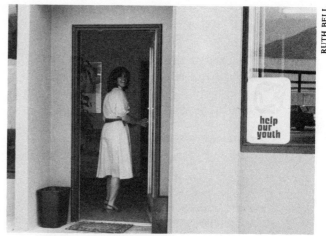

HOY Clinic, Arcadia, California. A clinic dedicated to serving teenagers in the community.

Going to the Doctor

One way to take care of yourself is to try to prevent medical problems by having a yearly physical examination. A regular medical checkup is especially important during the teenage years while your body is going through so many changes.

Where to Go for a Checkup

—Family doctor. Many of you will have a doctor you have been seeing since childhood. He or she will probably continue to serve you until you are sixteen or seventeen, if you choose to stay with him or her. Many pediatricians these days have special training in teenage health.
—Health maintenance organizations. Some families belong to health insurance groups. Check with your parents.
—Local health clinics. Some teenagers prefer to go to a local clinic for medical services. Look in the Yellow Pages under Clinics, Health Services or Medical Services. Ask friends for recommendations. Check with your school nurse and ask if he or she can recommend a clinic.
—Women's clinics or women's health centers. These provide complete services for women and girls. If there is a women's clinic in your city or town, call them to see if they also can provide treatment for males.
—Free clinics. Some areas have clinics that run solely on grants and donations. They do not charge anything for their services. If there is a free clinic in your area, that would be a good choice, since they are likely to treat many teenagers and they would therefore be set up to handle special teenage problems. Look in the Yellow Pages under Clinics.

Making an Appointment. You may want to talk to the people at different places before you decide where to go for your checkup. Call them and ask them about their services. Tell them your age.

Here is a list of some questions you may want to ask:

—Do they treat many teenagers?
—How many doctors do they have on their staff?
—How long have they been in operation?
—Are they affiliated with any hospitals?
—What do they charge for a complete physical exam?
—Do you need your parents' consent to be seen by a doctor?
—If you are a girl and would prefer to be seen by a female doctor, ask if they have one on the staff. Many places do.

You'll be able to determine by their answers and by their friendliness whether you want to go to that clinic. They should be courteous and respectful and answer all your questions.

Make an appointment for a time that is convenient for you. If there is a particular doctor you want to see, make your appointment for a time when that doctor is on duty. Once you make an appointment be sure to keep it. If you cannot keep it for some reason, be sure to phone the clinic or doctor's office to cancel your appointment.

Ask for directions to the place. Ask if you can get there by public transportation if you need to.

We advise you to bring a parent or a friend along with you to the appointment. It's nice to have company while you're waiting to see the doctor. If you prefer going alone, you may want to bring a book or some homework. There is usually a fifteen- to forty-five-minute wait. At some clinics there is a much longer wait.

A Typical Medical Examination

Lots of people put off going to the doctor because they are afraid of what the examination will be like. They worry about shots or other procedures that may hurt or be un-

---

CONSUMER'S RIGHTS

As a consumer of health care you have certain rights, regardless of your race, religion, age, sex or education. These are:

—The right to be treated with dignity and respect.
—The right to privacy and confidentiality.
—The right to have all procedures explained in language you understand.
—The right to have all your questions answered in language you understand.
—The right to know the meaning and implications of all forms you are asked to sign.
—The right to know the effectiveness, complications and possible side effects of all medications you are given.
—The right to know the results and meanings of all tests and examinations.
—The right to consent to or refuse any test, examination or treatment.
—The right to see your records and have them explained to you.

Doctors and health professionals are only human. They make mistakes. They may be very busy. They are not perfect. They can't read your mind. In order to get the best treatment possible, be sure to speak up when you don't understand something. Ask questions. Let the doctor know if what he or she is doing hurts you.

If you feel your rights have been violated, talk to the clinic director or to the nurse in charge of the office. If they aren't helpful, do not use their services in the future if you are able to go somewhere else. Tell your friends about your poor treatment. You and they may be able to get together and organize a list of good medical services in your area. You can boycott doctors and clinics that do not provide adequate services to teenagers.

If you have a serious complaint—for example, if you were physically mistreated or you were lied to or misled, or if you suspect that you are, or ever have been, the subject of a medical experiment and have questions about it, or if you feel any of your rights have been violated, you can write to the Institute for the Study of Medical Ethics, P.O. Box 17307, Los Angeles, CA 90017. Their phone number is 213-413-4997. Describe your mistreatment, and give them the name of the doctors and/or health workers who were at fault. Also include the name and the address of the place where you received the treatment.

---

comfortable. Some people don't like the idea of getting undressed in the examining room. Here we will explain what to expect from a typical exam in order to take some of the strangeness out of it and to help you to feel more comfortable.

Complete Medical History. An important part of any thorough exam is the medical history. This is a series of questions about your present and past health, and the health of members of your family. You will be asked what diseases you had as a child; what illnesses close members of your family have had; what, if any, special medical conditions you may have, such as diabetes, heart murmur, fainting spells, headaches, etc.; and what kinds of health problems run in your family, such as cancer, heart disease, diabetes, etc. The doctor will want to know if you have any allergies and whether you are allergic to any form of medication. It's also important for the doctor to know if you take any medication or drugs regularly.

Remember, according to the medical code of ethics and in some cases according to the law, the doctor must keep this information confidential.

In many clinics and doctor's offices a trained medical professional or the doctor will ask you about your medical history. In other places there will be a form for you to fill out. This will be a checklist naming various diseases and asking you to check which you've had and which you haven't had. *Only answer those questions you understand and know the answer to.* If you bring a parent along with you to the exam, he or she will be able to help you, especially with questions about your past health and the health of other members of the family.

If you have trouble reading the form or if you don't know what some words mean, *don't fill out that part.* Talk to the nurse, health worker or doctor and ask for an explanation of any part you don't understand. If the whole form is confusing to you, ask for help. You have a right and an obligation to yourself to have everything explained to you so you know what you are filling in.

Time to Talk to the Doctor. The examination should include as much time as you and the doctor need to discuss any problems or concerns you have about your development, your life, your feelings. Bring along a *list* of questions so you won't forget what you wanted to talk about. This time with the doctor should be private so that you can discuss things you might not want to talk about with someone else present. If a parent comes with you to the exam, you can arrange beforehand with your parent and the doctor to allow you this private time.

The doctor should discuss with you the process of development and explain to you why and how your body is changing. The doctor may discuss diet and health habits with you. Some doctors prescribe vitamins; others believe that if you are eating well, you don't need vitamins. That is still a controversial subject in medical circles. If you don't agree with your doctor's approach, feel free to ask him or her to explain the reasoning behind it.

One important part of the talk will be about sexuality. Since your body is becoming mature sexually and·you are going to be or are already capable of reproduction, the doctor should take this time to discuss birth control and sexually transmitted diseases with you—even if you have no intention of being sexually active with a partner for a long while. It's essential to know about birth control and VD prevention *before* you become sexually active. If the doctor doesn't bring these topics up, you should ask him or her any questions about sex you may have. If the doctor hedges, or seems embarrassed to talk with you about these things, you may choose to find another doctor for future checkups. *Find a doctor with whom you feel comfortable discussing sex.* For some teenagers, the doctor is the only reliable source of accurate sex information.

Be honest with the doctor about whether or not you are sexually active and what kinds of sexual activity you have experienced. It's for your own protection, because if you are having intercourse or oral sex you should be given tests for STD's during the exam. Also, girls who are sexually active should have Pap smears.

If you are having problems with drugs and/or alcohol and you want help, the doctor would be a good person to turn to for assistance. You will have to decide whether you trust the doctor enough to tell him or her your problem, but if you can open up about it, the doctor may be able to help you find a way out of the problem.

The doctor can be an important resource person. Even if your concerns aren't medical, the doctor will be able to put you in touch with other people who can help you.

The Physical Examination

After you've given your medical history and talked to the doctor, the physical part of the examination will usually take place—though sometimes the order is reversed.

Urine. You will be asked to go into the bathroom and urinate into a paper or plastic cup. Most people fill the cup about halfway and then let the rest of their urine run into the toilet. Girls hold the cup under them while they sit on the toilet. Your urine will be used for various tests to make sure your kidneys and bladder are functioning properly.

Measurements. Then you will go into the examining room and undress. You will be alone while you undress, and there will be a hospital gown or paper robe for you to put on. A medical professional will come in and take your blood pressure and measure your height and weight. If you've never had your blood pressure measured before, don't worry—it doesn't hurt. A pressure sleeve is wrapped around the upper part of your arm and pumped up to create

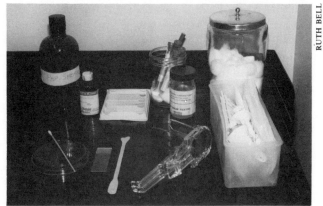
Equipment table in the examining room.

pressure. Then your pulse is measured as the pressure is relaxed.

Blood Test. Many exams include a blood test. A sample of your blood is taken from your arm with a needle. The nurse will make a tiny puncture in your vein and blood will flow into a small glass vial. Very little blood is taken. The initial puncture may sting, but the hurting should not last more than a few seconds. You can hold someone's hand if you are afraid.

Your blood will be tested to see if signs of any disease are present. Syphilis and hepatitis show up in the blood, as do many other diseases. There is also a blood test for pregnancy.

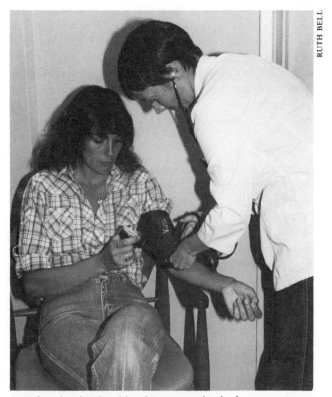
A patient having her blood pressure checked.

If you are terrified of needles, tell the doctor and he or she may decide to eliminate this part of the exam, unless it is needed for some specific reason.

Head Check. Your eyes, ears, nose, throat and teeth will be looked at and checked. The doctor or nurse may give you an eye test to check your vision. This usually involves reading from a chart placed about twenty feet from where you are asked to stand. Your hearing may be tested using a machine called an audiometer. You'll be asked to put on a pair of earphones and listen to sounds.

General Body Check. The doctor will look your body over, checking for swelling, rashes or anything else out of the ordinary. He or she will feel around your neck and under your arms and along your body looking for enlarged glands. This is the part of the exam during which the doctor may poke you a little here and there. He or she isn't trying to hurt you; it's just to check certain vital places on your body.

Your heart and lungs will be checked. The doctor takes your pulse and listens to your breathing with a stethoscope.

If you are having any pain or itching or other symptoms, this would be a good time to talk to the doctor about that. These are clues to help the doctor determine what, if anything, needs special attention.

Boy's Examination

The doctor will feel around your testicles, scrotum, and penis, checking for lumps and/or pain. Ask the doctor to show you how to check your own testicles for lumps (see p. 18). He or she may ask you questions about genital development and about whether you have ejaculated during masturbation or during your sleep. This is completely normal, and although it may seem embarrassing, answer honestly. It's a natural part of a boy's sexual development (see p. 14).

Rectal Exam. Sometimes the doctor will do a rectal examination—that is, feeling inside your anus to check for lumps or swelling or obstructions. First he or she will put on a thin rubber glove and lubricate his or her finger with some lubricating jelly. He or she will ask you to relax your bottom and then will gently insert the finger into your anus. One doctor told us the best way to relax is to take a deep breath and bear down, just as if you were trying to have a bowel movement, then breathe out and let your body go limp. If the doctor is gentle and you are relaxed, the rectal exam shouldn't hurt at all. If you are tight and nervous, it may feel uncomfortable. Be sure to tell the doctor if it hurts, so that he or she can slow down and be more gentle.

Sexual Functioning. The doctor should explain to you about the male role in pregnancy and about birth control.

You can ask him or her to show you how to put on a condom.

If you have had sexual intercourse or oral sex, you should have a test for syphilis and gonorrhea (see pp. 223 and 227).

Girl's Examination

The doctor will feel around your breasts, checking for lumps, swelling and/or pain. He or she will ask you questions about when your breasts started developing. Ask the doctor to teach you how to check your own breasts for lumps each month after your period (see p. 23).

The doctor will also look and feel around the groin area. He or she will examine the vulva, checking the urethra and the outside of the vagina. He or she will check to make sure there is enough of an opening in your hymen (see p. 26) to allow menstrual flow to escape easily. If you have a very small opening, the doctor may discuss with you ways to ease open the hymen yourself.

Menstruation. You and the doctor may have discussed menstruation during the "time to talk" part of the exam. Otherwise this is the appropriate time to talk about when your period first started, if it has, and how often it comes. The doctor will want to know how heavy your usual flow is, and how long each period lasts. Tell the doctor about any discomfort you may experience during or before your period.

If you haven't started your period yet, this visit can reassure you that everything is fine. Many girls don't start their periods until they are seventeen or eighteen. In our interviews we met several who didn't start their periods until they were nineteen.

The Internal (Pelvic) Examination. A girl's organs of reproduction are on the inside. Unlike a boy's penis and testicles, the uterus, ovaries and fallopian tubes cannot be seen or examined externally. In order to examine a girl's organs, the doctor must look and feel inside. The passageway to the internal organs is the vagina.

Doctors often choose to omit the internal exam with younger teenage girls unless there is a specific need for it, or unless the girl is already having sexual intercourse because many girls and women feel uncomfortable about having an internal exam. Many boys and men feel the same way when the doctor examines their genitals. Throughout this book we've recommended that you get to know your own genitals, that you look at them, touch them, and learn about their functions. If you haven't done so already, we hope you will read the chapter entitled "Changing Bodies," which will help you to discover and appreciate that part of yourself.

To do an internal exam the doctor will ask you to push yourself down to the end of the examining table with your buttocks just at the edge and your knees bent and spread

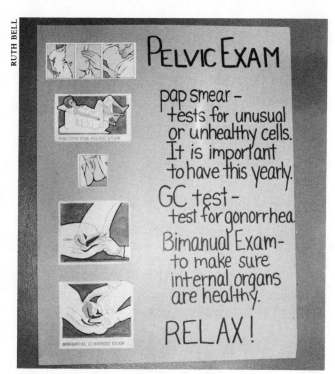

Sign in a teen clinic describing a pelvic exam.

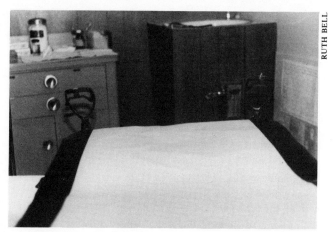

An examining table, with stirrups to put your feet in during an internal examination.

apart. Your feet will go into metal stirrups placed at the foot of the table.

It is an awkward position to be in, but doctors say it is the most convenient way for them to check you. Here is how eighteeen-year-old Mary described it:

> I think that position is really undignified. There's something about lying there on my back with my legs up and spread open that I just think is gross. But I try to psych myself up. I tell myself, ''This is OK. It's just normal. It's just a doctor. He does it all the time.'' I think about it that way and then it's OK for me.

There should be a female health professional present in the examining room while a male doctor is performing an internal examination on a girl or woman. If the doctor is a woman, no other person need be present.

The Speculum Exam.   Since the walls of the vagina are touching, the doctor wouldn't be able to see inside without holding open the two sides of the vagina. There is a special instrument, called a speculum (*speh*-cue-lum) made just for that purpose.

The speculum comes in both plastic and metal in several different sizes. There is a small size especially for young girls and for women who have small vaginal openings. The doctor inserts the speculum by holding the two branches of it together and easing them gently into your vagina. If it is a metal speculum, it should be warmed before insertion. Once the speculum is inside, the doctor opens it and presses down to lock it in place.

Putting in a speculum can be uncomfortable for you if the doctor is not gentle and/or if you are nervous and tensed up. Be sure to tell the doctor if he or she is hurting you. Ask him or her to give you a chance to relax.

The best way to relax the muscles in your pelvic area is to take a few deep breaths and blow all the air out after each one. Then take one deep breath and hold it. At the same time bear down on your pelvic area, just as you would if you were trying to move your bowels. Then breathe out slowly and relax your body totally. Let your mouth drop open. Relax your fingers and toes. Concentrate on opening your vagina.

Once the speculum is in place, your cervix and the inside of your vagina can be easily seen. Ask the doctor to hold a mirror in front of your vagina so that you can look too. It's fascinating to see what you (and all females) look

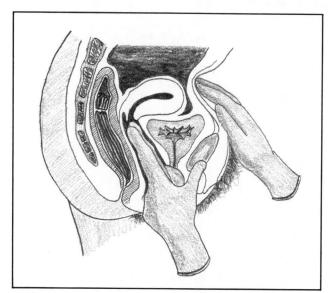

A doctor feeling your internal organs during a pelvic exam.

like inside. It helps you to understand how your body functions. (See p. 28 for a description of what you'll see.)

The doctor will be looking for redness or inflammation in the vagina which can be signs of infection. Normally the walls of the vagina are pinkish brown. He or she will also look for any unusual discharge and will check for cuts or tears or cysts on the cervix. He or she will also check the color of the cervix. It is normally pinkish or brownish pink, although there is a wide variation among different individuals. During pregnancy the cervix takes on a slightly bluish tint, so the color of the cervix can indicate a possible pregnancy.

The Pap Smear. The doctor will take a long Q-tip-like stick with cotton at the end and gently scrape some cell tissue from the cervix. Some doctors use a flat wooden stick that looks something like a tongue depressor.

The cell tissue will be sent to a laboratory to determine if there are any abnormal cells present. This is helpful in checking for precancerous conditions. You will be notified within a few days if any abnormalities appear in your test.*

The Pap smear, named after Dr. G. N. Papanicolaou, the physician who developed the test, should not hurt at all. However, as in everything else, some people are more careful than others. Let the doctor know if he or she hurts you.

Pap smears are recommended for girls eighteen and over or for girls, no matter what age, who are having sexual intercourse. You should have one once a year.† If you take the birth control pill, if you have genital herpes, or if you have many sexual partners, women's health advocates recommend having a Pap smear every six months. Be sure to have regular Pap smears if you are a DES daughter (see p. 18), meaning that your mother took the drug DES during her pregnancy with you.

If you are sexually active, at the same time the doctor does the Pap smear he or she should also take a sample of tissue to test for gonorrhea.

The Bi-Manual Vaginal Exam. After the doctor closes the speculum and eases it out of your vagina, he or she will want to examine your internal organs with his hands. He or she will put a thin rubber glove on one hand and lubricate one or two fingers of that hand with lubricating jelly. Gently he or she will insert the finger or fingers into your vagina while placing the other hand on your lower abdomen. In this way the doctor can feel the size, shape and position of your uterus, ovaries and tubes. He or she will be looking for unusual swelling, tenderness or

*See Boston Women's Health Book Collective, *Our Bodies, Ourselves* (New York: Simon & Schuster, 1976), pp. 143–46.

†The American Cancer Society has determined that women who have had three years of normal Pap smears need have a Pap smear only once every three years after that. Many doctors and women's health advocates disagree with that, and advise women to have yearly Pap smears.

growths. The doctor presses down in certain places. This can feel a little uncomfortable, but it usually doesn't hurt. Ask the doctor to explain what he or she is feeling for. Be sure to tell the doctor if you experience pain.

Try to relax during this exam by breathing slowly and deeply. Remember to keep your fingers and toes loose and let your mouth drop open.

The Rectal Exam. Sometimes the doctor can feel the organs better by inserting a finger into the anus (see p. 156 for an explanation of a rectal exam).

After the Examination

When the exam is over, the doctor will leave the room so that you can have privacy while you put on your clothes.

The health worker will explain to you if you should have another appointment soon, or whether you won't need to return for another year. If the doctor has medication to prescribe or if he or she wants to discuss some part of the exam with you, you will spend a few minutes after the exam talking with the doctor in his or her office.

If you are at a clinic, they may be able to fill prescriptions there. Otherwise, if you are given a prescription, take it to a pharmacy and the druggist will fill it for you.

If you have any questions or comments about the exam, feel free to speak up. You have a right to have your questions answered and your comments heard.

These final sections discuss birth control, pregnancy, and sexually transmitted diseases. They are full of information which will give you more control over your own life. People who have information about their bodies and their sexuality have more decision-making power than people who do not have such information. We advise those of you who are sexually active to learn as much as you can about how to protect yourselves from unwanted pregnancies and sexually transmitted diseases. If you are faced with an unplanned pregnancy, pp. 193–94 will help you understand what options are available to you.

Many of you who are reading this are not sexually active now. You may be thinking, I don't need to know about this stuff. Some of you may not plan to have sex with a partner for a long time. We hope you'll read these chapters soon anyway, even if you can't imagine having a sexual relationship for years to come. The information here is important to know *before* you have sex. Unwanted pregnancies can start the very first time a heterosexual couple has sexual intercourse, and sexually transmitted diseases can be passed even without intercourse.

Birth Control

There isn't any reason these days for you to get pregnant or get someone pregnant unless you're ready to and want to. Birth control methods, which can keep you from starting unwanted pregnancies, are available in drugstores, markets and health clinics throughout the country. But birth control won't help you if you don't *get it* and *use it*. This section will give you the information you need to do just that.

If birth control is that easy to obtain and use, why do so many people keep getting pregnant when they don't want to? A girl from Ohio who's a senior in high school said:

> One of my friends has been pregnant three times. Three times, can you believe it? Every time I talk to her she's complaining that she just got pregnant. But when I ask her why she doesn't use birth control, she says, because she doesn't think she'll get pregnant!

There are lots and lots of people like this girl's friend who are having sexual intercourse and not using birth control. Then when they get pregnant or get the girl they were with pregnant, they wonder how it could have happened to them. It was no accident.

Our bodies are designed to be able to start pregnancies. Once they pass through the changes of puberty, boys can produce sperm and girls can produce eggs. The two together are the basis for a new life. That's why if you are having sexual intercourse without using birth control, it is not an accident if you get pregnant. *It is an accident if you don't get pregnant.*

Some boys tell their partners, "Oh, don't worry, I won't stick it in all the way; we'll be safe." Or they say, "I'll pull out in time. Leave it to me." That's the way a lot of girls get pregnant.

Some girls tell their partners, "Don't worry, I can't get pregnant. I haven't started getting my period yet." Or they say, "Oh, I'm safe; it's the wrong time of the month for me to get pregnant." That's how a lot of pregnancies happen. A girl can get pregnant if she has intercourse standing up, upside down, or in the shower. She can get pregnant if she douches right afterwards or if she jumps up and down and runs around the block. She can get pregnant if she doesn't have an orgasm. It's even possible to get pregnant if the boy doesn't put his penis inside her vagina but leaves some sperm on her thighs or pubic hair. Sperm have been clever enough to find their way into the vagina by themselves under some circumstances.

Many people think they're safe because they're too young to start a pregnancy. That's one of the biggest mistakes of all. Here are some facts that show almost no one is "too young" to start a pregnancy:

—400,000 girls in the United States aged fourteen or younger get pregnant every year.

—A ten-year-old girl gave birth to twins in 1979.
—Two thirteen-year-old girls we interviewed got pregnant before they even had their first period.
—There is a report of a seven-year-old boy who fathered a baby.
—Boys as young as four years old have produced live sperm.
—A seventeen-year-old mother of two has had five pregnancies: two miscarriages, one abortion and two babies.
—Abortions have been performed on girls as young as ten and eleven.
—Each year in the United States *one million* teenage girls get pregnant.

Four out of every five girls who have intercourse without using birth control will become pregnant during the first year of their sexual activity. Four out of five. That doesn't give you much leeway. There are only two ways to make sure it doesn't happen to you or a girl you were with: one is not to have sexual intercourse; the other is to use a reliable method of birth control.

Be Prepared

The first and most important step toward protecting yourself is to have birth control around when you need it. As this sixteen-year-old Wisconsin boy said:

> I can't imagine stopping in the middle of the passion to get dressed again and go out to the store to buy a rubber. It would totally spoil the whole thing. You wouldn't be in the same mood when you got back. So you have to keep some rubbers with you. Then you're always prepared.

Birth control is available—all you have to do is get it. You don't have to be having intercourse, you don't even have to be dating someone to get birth control. Maybe you won't need it, but if you do, at least you'll have it.

It sounds simple enough, but that first step—getting birth control—is exactly where the problem comes in for many people.

Michele and Brian, two seventeen-year-olds who helped us with this book, explained:

> Brian: When you're still in high school, you have to deal with the whole guilt thing about "Oh, you're too young to be having sex." If you're only in junior high, it's even harder to deal with. So if you're not supposed to be doing it anyway, you can't really let yourself plan for it by getting birth control because that just adds to your guilt.

> Michele: That's right. You're taught that you shouldn't be doing it, so when you do it you have to tell yourself, Oh well, I couldn't help myself. I was

drunk. Or I was too stoned to know what I was doing. Or we just got carried away. That's why it's so hard to use birth control, because that would be admitting that you were thinking about what you were doing.

In this society we do give people, teenagers especially, a mixed message about sex. We say young people shouldn't be having sex, and we make them feel guilty for doing it or even wanting to do it. Then when the girls gets pregnant, we wonder why they weren't responsible enough to use birth control.

It would be much kinder if we taught people how to prepare for a sexual relationship. Not teaching people about sex doesn't stop them from having intercourse, it just increases their chances for starting unwanted pregnancies.

It's hard for most people to plan for sex by getting birth control in advance. It's especially hard for girls because many girls have been told that it's up to the boy to make the moves. The girl isn't supposed to prepare for it; she isn't even "supposed" to *think* about it. So a lot of girls leave it all up to the boy, letting him decide when, where and how it will happen. Patricia, a fourteen-year-old from a suburb near Cleveland, said:

> I think it's up to the boy. I feel like my boyfriend is sort of slowly leading us up to intercourse and I think I'll be able to say no. But if we do it, I think he ought to have birth control, especially at first. It's up to him because it's his idea in the first place.

Patricia isn't taking any responsibility because she doesn't think she's supposed to take any responsibility. But it's not fair to the boy to leave it all up to him, and more important, Patricia's the one who will get pregnant if her boyfriend doesn't come prepared. In fact, that's what happens to many girls who, like Patricia, leave the responsibility for sex entirely in the boy's hands. Cheryl was with her two-year-old baby when we met her. She said:

> Me and my boyfriend always talked about using birth control, and he kept saying he was going to get some rubbers, just in case. But he never actually got around to it. He kept putting it off and then we'd be screwing anyway. We were lucky for a couple of months, but then I got pregnant. I was only fifteen when it happened and I couldn't believe it. I thought I was going to die.

Talking about using birth control isn't the same as using it. Talking won't protect you against pregnancy.

Maybe you're willing to admit to yourself that intercourse is a possibility someday, but you're afraid that being prepared with birth control might blow your image with someone else. Maybe you think it will show the person you're with what's *really* on your mind. Boys have said that it was embarrassing to bring out a rubber for protection only to have their date say, "Oh, were you planning this all along?" Sixteen-year-old Peter, a junior from

Los Angeles, said when that happened to him he told his girlfriend:

> Hey, don't blame me for having a rubber. I thought you'd be glad not to have to worry about getting pregnant.

For girls the situation can be even more embarrassing, since, as we've said, many girls learn that they aren't supposed to give sex any thought until Prince Charming sweeps them away. That's why scenes like this one still happen:

> A guy I know was going out with this girl, someone he really liked and respected. One day after about two months together, they started making out and she said to him, "Well, do you have anything?" He was totally shocked and said "No." And so she said, "Well, I have some rubbers in my purse." Well, I thought that was great, because I think it's a terrific idea for girls to carry rubbers in their purses, just in case. But my friend said he just felt so stupid. It was his first time and he didn't really know what to do, but he was too embarrassed to tell her that he didn't really know how to use a rubber and he was too uptight to tell her that this would be his first time having sex. So he got angry and made up some excuse for not wanting to do it. He always figured if he ever did it, he would be the one to initiate it. He broke up with her soon after that.

The girl in this story probably would have been very supportive if the boy had been able to talk about what he was going through. One of the most important parts of a good relationship is trusting each other enough to talk about uncomfortable feelings. It's only natural to feel funny about having intercourse for the first time or for the first time with a new partner. Everyone feels that way. It's a problem, though, when embarrassment keeps you from using birth control. And it's a lot more embarrassing and a lot more serious to start a pregnancy.

The Myth about Sex

How are we going to learn about sex realistically when the movies we see and the magazines and books we read all teach us something very unreal? Certainly you never see a boy putting on a rubber in the movies. You never see a girl putting in her diaphragm. For that matter, you hardly ever see two people banging noses when they kiss, or squirming around to find a comfortable position, or getting up because they have to go to the bathroom. And gurgling stomachs—you never hear stomach gurgles during a love scene on the screen. Fantasy love scenes all work so perfectly and so romantically—and nobody has unwanted babies.

In real life it takes time to learn how to feel natural about sex—how to please each other, how to feel comfortable doing whatever you're doing. A lot of us think that we're automatically supposed to know what to do and how to do it. You think everyone else feels perfectly at ease and you're the only one who doesn't. Lucy, a seventeen-year-old girl from San Francisco, helps out at a birth control clinic near her home. She said:

When you're our age you want everything to be so romantic. Free and spontaneous. That's why so many kids tell me they don't use birth control—because that isn't spontaneous. I remember the first few times I had sex I didn't know what I was doing at all. The whole thing was anything but romantic or spontaneous. Birth control was just part of the craziness! I was trying to put in some foam and it got all over everything. I waited till the last minute to read the instructions, and there I was in the middle of everything trying to figure out how to use the stuff. It got all over my hand and everyplace else. It was embarrassing, sure, but it was also pretty funny. We spent a lot of time laughing about it.

Paul, a senior from Ohio, admitted that his first time was pretty embarrassing too:

I was about sixteen when my girlfriend and I had sex for the first time. It had been coming on for a few months, so I was all psyched up for it and I'd been carrying rubbers around—just in case. The trouble was, nobody ever told me *when* you were supposed to put the rubber on. So there I was trying to put that thing on, not knowing you were supposed to be hard before you could use it.

Of course, if someone had taught Paul how to use a rubber, or if he had been able to read about it, a lot of his troubles would have disappeared.

Talk about What You're Doing

Joanne, an eighteen-year-old from New York, told us:

I didn't use any birth control for a pretty long time because I was afraid of saying anything to the guys I was with. I was afraid to tell them how scared I was of getting pregnant. I was too scared to even let myself think about it. I would let these guys tell me, "Oh, don't worry, I'll take care of you. I won't get you pregnant." As if they had some magic. I was putting them ahead of *me* and letting them do it their way. I had absolutely no respect for myself or what I needed, which was to really feel safe.

Stuart, a senior from Detroit, said that since boys can't get pregnant, they can forget how important it is to protect against pregnancy. And they don't always know how much the girl they're with might be worrying about it. Stuart said:

Sometimes when you're getting ready to have sex, you don't have time to put on a rubber—even if you have one with you—because it happens so quick sometimes. You get into it so quick. But if you talk

first, or go a littler slower, take some time with each other—then you have a chance to think about using birth control.

Talk about what you're doing. After all, there you are in the most intimate physical relationship two people can be in. If you can't even talk to each other, maybe you shouldn't be there together in the first place. (See p. 105 for more about talking during sex.)

Having Respect for Yourself

Sally, a senior from Boston, said:

It seems really dumb to me nowadays to get pregnant if you don't want to. With all the precautions you could take, it just seems dumb. It's like you don't care about yourself a bit.

Using birth control is a way of caring about yourself. Some girls don't use it because they have the feeling that they're not really important, that only the guy they're with is important. It seems as if they're willing to take a chance with their own lives just to please the boy they're with. Fifteen-year-old Ginny said:

I think birth control is embarrassing. I wouldn't want to spoil the romance of being out with a really cool guy by talking about birth control.

And Estelle, a sixteen-year-old junior from Los Angeles, said:

There's this one dude I've had my eye on for a long time; if I could get a piece of him, man, I wouldn't bother with no birth control.

Why are these girls willing to take such risks? After all, *they're* the ones who are going to have to deal with the "mistake" pregnancy if it happens.

They may be afraid that the boy won't like them if they insist on using birth control. Maybe they're afraid the boy won't think they're worth the trouble. The truth is, if you don't respect yourself enough to protect yourself, you can't expect anyone else to respect you either. And in the long run, a girl would be silly to keep going out with a boy who didn't really respect her. She'd be putting herself down.

Mary Elizabeth, a senior from New Jersey, said that's exactly what she realized:

The first few times I had intercourse neither me or my boyfriend used birth control. I didn't want him to think that I didn't trust him, so I went that far—letting him tell me he wouldn't get me pregnant, and really sort of believing him. When I finally realized what was going on, how easy it would be to get pregnant this way, I said to myself, This is no way to be having a relationship—we're playing by a lie and I can't put my trust in a lie. So I broke up with him, and that was the best move I ever made.

Ellen, an eighteen-year-old college freshman from Montana, said:

> I think foam and condoms are a real good form of birth control, but I've met some guys who just refuse to use condoms. This one guy I went out with said, "No way." He said it just didn't feel the same for him. And so I said, "Tough." Now probably a couple of years ago I would have given in and let him talk me into doing it anyway, but I've had two abortions already and I'm not planning on ever having another one. I told him, "That's really nice; you're really into sharing this, aren't you?" I made him take me home right then and there and I never accepted another date with him. If he can't share in the responsibility, that's all for him.

Since girls are the ones who get pregnant, girls are usually the ones who eventually figure out that it's not worth taking chances. Many boys *are* aware of the problem too. A senior from Florida said:

> Before guys say no to rubbers they ought to really think about what would happen if they don't use them. If we got pregnant instead of girls, I bet we'd be more interested in using them.

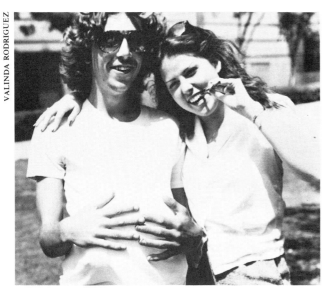

VALINDA RODRIGUEZ

Being pregnant isn't fun unless you want to be pregnant.

Many boys worry about how an unwanted pregnancy will affect their own lives. Seventeen-year-old Tim had this warning:

> I got my girl pregnant and now half my paycheck goes to her for child support. That's why I tell all my friends it ain't worth it. Use protection.

Leonard, a sixteen-year-old from Chicago whose fifteen-year-old sister got pregnant last year, told us:

> You know, I think birth control is both people's responsibility, but if they slip up or don't use it or

something, the boy can always skip town. The girl's not so lucky—ask my sister.

It takes a certain amount of maturity to realize that by not using birth control you might be ruining someone's life. You might be causing the girl you were with to go through changes that permanently affect her, and what's even worse, you might be starting the life of a child who comes into the world unwanted and resented. As fifteen-year-old Anthony said, it will be *your* child too:

> I think if a guy gets a girl pregnant it's his duty to stick by her, and if they decide to have the baby, then the girl especially needs him. Plus, the baby needs a father. But first of all, I think if they're willing to have sex with each other they should be willing to do something about birth control so the girl won't get pregnant in the first place.

Lots of boys check with the girl to find out what kind of birth control she uses *before* they go ahead and get romantic. Some boys keep rubbers on hand in case the girl isn't using anything else. And many of the boys we interviewed said they would rather not have intercourse at all yet, because the risk of pregnancy is too great. They said there are plenty of other ways to have sex without it (see Chapter IV, pp. 95–96).

> Whether you're male or female, using birth control is a way of protecting yourself. It is a way of caring about yourself. If you have plans for your future, you don't want an unwanted pregnancy to wreck those plans. Using birth control may take some time and some thought. It may even cause you some embarrassment. But using birth control will save your future for you.

BIRTH CONTROL

Many teenagers we met said, "Sure, I know about birth control, but I don't know where to get it. And even if I did, I'd be too embarrassed to go get some." A lot of people, no matter what their age, feel that way. Here's how some teens from different parts of the country expressed it:

> Allen, sixteen, from Michigan: I'd start laughing I'm sure. It would probably take me a half-hour to build up the courage just to go into the store.

> David, sixteen, from California: I can't stand to ask the guy in the drugstore for rubbers. He acts like he's my priest or something.

> Susan, fifteen, from Washington: I feel like everybody in the drugstore is watching me, and then I always think somebody'll go tell my mother.

> Ginger, sixteen, from Iowa: I would feel really embarrassed if I bumped into somebody I knew when I was going in or coming out of one of those clinics. Everybody knows what you're there for.

If you're feeling shy about the fact that you are or might be having a sexual relationship, then getting birth control can be embarrassing. But, of course, not using birth control can turn out to be much more embarrassing, since pregnancies are hard to hide. It would be easier if our society had a more realistic attitude about sex, and if people said, "Well, if teenagers are having sex, then they should use birth control, so let's make it simple for them to get and use it."

Some doctors and clinics are trying to help teenagers by making birth control available and easy to obtain. If you have a family doctor, you may want to test his or her attitude about sex and birth control by asking a general question like, "Do you think teens should use birth control?" or "Do you think it's OK for teenagers to have sex?" You'll be able to tell by the answers whether your doctor is someone who'll help you. Some parents have already discussed birth control with their teenager's doctor, and they have given their permission for the doctor to provide information and birth control service to their child.

In most towns and cities there are clinics that give birth control free of charge or at low cost to teenagers. Usually these clinics are set up to try to take some of the awkwardness out of the experience.

A lot of times, even after you get something to use for birth control, you have the problem of finding a place to keep it. This seems to be the reason a lot of people don't use birth control in the first place. A sixteen-year-old Chicago girl with a baby explained:

The only kind of birth control my mother told me about was, "Keep your dress down and your drawers up." I snuck out and got some birth control pills, but she went through my purse one day and found them. Maybe if my mother would have trusted me enough to tell me a little more about birth control and not get mad at me about it, I wouldn't have gotten pregnant. But it's too late now.

A seventeen-year-old Missouri girl, who had brought her baby in for a checkup to the clinic we were visiting, said:

I was scared to go to my mom when I needed birth control. My boyfriend used a rubber sometimes, but not always. He kept telling me to get on the pill, but I was scared my mother would find the pills if I got some. There isn't anyplace in my house to hide them because my mom goes through our drawers and even under the mattress when she cleans up. I was stupid, though, because one of the times my boyfriend didn't use a rubber I came up pregnant. So my mom found out the hard way.

The two girls we've just heard from were afraid that their parents would stop them from going out with their boyfriends if they knew they were having sex. So each one had intercourse without using birth control, and each got

pregnant. In the long run their families found out what they were doing anyway, but only after it was too late.

The second girl, Mary-Jo, said that after she got pregnant she and her mom had a long talk about using birth control, and now she's on the pill. Her mother also took Mary-Jo's younger sister in to the clinic for birth control, when she realized she was also having intercourse without protection.

Boys have the same kinds of experiences. One sophomore in California said:

I couldn't keep rubbers in my drawer—my mom would find them for sure.

> Some adults believe that they shouldn't tell teens about sex or birth control because that will only encourage them to try it. Actually, the opposite is true. Studies show that teens who have been given good sex education are *less* likely to get pregnant, *less* likely to get venereal disease, and *less* likely to have casual sex than teens who haven't been given good information. Also, teens who can be open with their parents about birth control are more likely to use it when the time comes.

A seventeen-year-old girl from California said:

I use my diaphragm every single time we have sex. If I didn't and I got pregnant, I couldn't ask my parents for help. They'd be so angry with me for being irresponsible. It would really be hard for me to admit that I was just being stupid and not taking care of myself.

Many teenagers and their parents have trouble talking to each other about a lot of things. It's as if it's the time when you could use the most communication that you have the least. Of course, talking about sex with your parents is probably the hardest subject of all, but it's worth trying. Most of the parents we interviewed said they hope their teenagers aren't getting into heavy sexual relationships too soon, before they are able to handle the emotional and physical consequences of sex. They are worried. But almost all of the parents we talked with said they would rather help their teens find and use birth control than have them take chances with pregnancy. A father of two teenage daughters, one seventeen and one fourteen, told us:

If my younger daughter came to me and said she wanted to get birth control, just to be prepared for some time in the future, you know, I probably would immediately think she was sleeping with someone, and I'd probably feel like giving her a lecture about her reputation and everything. I'd want to know why suddenly out of the blue this thing about birth control came up. But at the same time, I'd want her to have birth control if there was something going on. I wouldn't want her to be having sex without using birth control. I'd help her get some. But I guess I'd prefer that there wasn't anything going on!

FAMILY PLANNING CLINICS

In every state in the country there are clinics that give birth control free or sell it at low prices. To find the clinic nearest you, look in your local newspaper in the classified section for an advertisement, or look in the Yellow Pages of your phone book under Family Planning or Birth Control or Health Service. In some areas the local hospital provides family planning services in the form of birth control and pregnancy testing. Call the hospital to find out if you can get birth control there in the outpatient clinic.

There are many women's health centers and women's clinics throughout the country. These centers are generally very good sources of information and service. Though they focus on service to women, many of these centers will also provide condoms for men. If you know of such a clinic near you, that would be an excellent place to try. Call them first to find out their policies and how much they charge for their services.

Also, most states have Planned Parenthood clinics. You can look in the phone book under Planned Parenthood to see if there is one near you. If there is none in your town, try looking in the phone book of the largest city near you. The library will have that phone book. Many of the Planned Parenthood clinics can provide you with any kind of birth control you choose, and they generally work on a sliding scale, which means you pay what you can afford.

Another place to go for birth control, in some states, is to the county Department of Health. Health department clinics are listed in the white or blue pages of the phone book under the name of your county. Call first to find out if they provide birth control services, and ask if your visit will be kept confidential, if that is important to you. Some county clinics are better than others, depending on the politics of the area and the particular people working in the clinic.

If the county doesn't provide birth control services, the Department of Health may be able to direct you to a clinic that can help you.

How to Use the Clinic

The procedures in each clinic vary. Usually you call to make an appointment and then go in at a scheduled time. Some clinics have a special "drop-in" day so that people can come in without an appointment. Many clinics have a day each week set up specifically for teenagers. When you call the clinic, ask about drop-in days and teen days.

As you'll see when you read about the methods, most birth control is for girls to use. Condoms are the only effective birth control method for boys. But both males and females are encouraged to come to the clinic, because information about how and why to use birth control is important to both. Clinics often give condoms free.

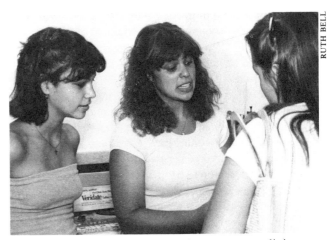

A teen advocate helping some patients at a teen clinic.

When you get to the clinic, you will probably be asked to sit in the waiting room until a counselor is ready to see you. In some clinics you meet with the counselor individually; in other clinics there are group information sessions. In either case, the counselor or group leader will explain about the different types of birth control and help you decide which type would be best for you to use. If you go to the clinic already knowing something about the different methods, you will be better able to make a real choice. Otherwise, you may find yourself being persuaded to use the kind of birth control that the clinic thinks would be best for you.

The pill, the IUD and the diaphragm must be prescribed by a doctor. If a girl decides to use one of these, she will be seen by a doctor. The doctor will examine her and explain how to use the method of

Parents and teenagers often have trouble discussing birth control because the parents don't want the teens to think they are in favor of teenage sexual relationships and the teens don't want to hear a lecture. Sometimes teens don't want to bring up the subject because they feel embarrassed or ashamed of what they're doing. Sometimes they just aren't thinking about having intercourse, so they don't want to mention it to their folks and maybe give them the idea that it's something they *are* considering. Some parents are very much against premarital or, at least, teenage sex, and they don't want to find out that their teenagers are engaging in it.

For these reasons and more, sex is a touchy subject. But since parents can help their teens overcome a lot of the guilt associated with sex, since they can support the teens who want to wait before having intercourse, and since they her choice. (In our discussion of the methods, we talk more about what to expect when you see the doctor.)

Before you leave the clinic you will be given the birth control you have chosen, and that's all there is to it. Sometimes the clinic gives birth control free of charge; sometimes they charge for their services. If they do charge, it is usually according to a sliding scale, which means according to how much you can afford to pay. When you phone for an appointment, ask them about cost.

Bringing a Friend

We recommend that you bring along someone you trust when you go to the clinic. It's nice to have someone to talk to while you're sitting in the waiting room. If you're nervous about going to get birth control, having a friend along may ease your anxiety.

If you are in a couple relationship, there are a lot of advantages to going together for birth control. You can ask to have a joint session with the counselor and/or doctor. That way you both learn about the different methods, and together you can make a decision about which kind to use. That way, too, you both understand the risks and the advantages and you both learn how to use the method properly. If you make the decision about birth control as a couple, you have a joint commitment to using it. That takes the burden off just one or the other of you.

Some teenagers have told us they would prefer to go alone for birth control. You may not want anyone to know you're going to the clinic, or you may just consider the whole experience a private one. The most important thing is to do what makes you feel the most comfortable. The people at the clinic will no doubt be friendly and helpful, since they believe that sexually active teenagers should use birth control.

If for some reason the people in the clinic are *not* friendly and if they do not treat you with respect and answer your questions carefully, you have every right to leave and seek help elsewhere. If there is no other clinic in your area, you have a right to voice a complaint with the manager of the clinic. Remember, you deserve to be treated with dignity and professionalism. You are acting responsibly by going to get birth control. You have nothing to be ashamed of.

can protect their children by informing them about birth control, the rewards of talking outweigh many times the desire to remain silent. Many parents we interviewed said they consider it their responsibility to advise their sons and daughters about sex and birth control, and they want to do so *before* their teenagers get involved in a sexual relationship.

You will make your own decision about whether or not

to talk to your parents about protection, just as you will make your own decision about whether or not to have sex. But even if you feel there's no way your parents would understand or if you're afraid to give them the opportunity to come through, *don't let that keep you from finding out about birth control yourself so you can protect yourself against an unwanted pregnancy.*

Birth Control and Sexual Liberation

Thanks to birth control, it is possible to have sexual relations without getting pregnant. But that is no reason to feel that you *have to* have sex whenever someone suggests it. *You have a responsibility to yourself to have intercourse only when you feel ready for it and when you choose to.*

Being able to say "No, I don't want to have sex with you" or "No, I don't feel like it right now" takes self-confidence. For males and females both, it's worth working on your ability and your willingness to say no without feeling guilty or scared or worried about what someone else will think.

The Methods

The rest of this section is devoted to a discussion of the different methods of birth control that are available today. We'll talk about each one separately except in the case of foam and condoms, which are most effective when used together. You'll probably discover that some methods sound better to you than others. Choose your method according to its effectiveness, its health risks, and whether you'll feel comfortable using it. Remember, birth control works only *if you use it*.

There is no perfect form of protection. There is no method that works 100 percent of the time—except not having intercourse. The forms of birth control that are the most convenient to use tend to have the most side effects, and those with the fewest side effects are not as convenient to use.

It might seem strange to you that a country as technologically advanced as ours can't produce a safe and perfectly reliable method of birth control. There's really no excuse for this, but one of the reasons it has happened is that sex is such a controversial subject, there's not much money given out to find ways to separate sex from pregnancy. Many people aren't willing to say that it's OK to enjoy sex without wanting to get pregnant, so they don't support programs to find better birth control methods.

The money that is available for birth control research often goes toward finding ways to keep the world population down, especially in underdeveloped nations. That means developing easy-to-use methods, such as the pill or the IUD. The problem is that those methods have by far the greatest health hazards. They work to prevent pregnancy, but many women get seriously hurt in the process.

When enough people say, ''We won't stand for methods that endanger our health'' and ''We want to use birth control that is safe, effective, and easy,'' then maybe researchers will come up with the ''perfect'' method. Until then, we have to choose from what there is.

SPECIAL NOTE ON THE PAGES THAT FOLLOW

Because most of the methods are designed to be used by females, much of the discussion that follows is directed mainly to girl readers. We use ''you'' to refer to the girls who are reading. On the other hand, in the instances where we are speaking about birth control used by boys, we use ''you'' to refer to the boys who are reading.

We believe that birth control is the responsibility of both sexual partners, and we believe their relationship is enhanced when both respect each other enough to talk about and use birth control. The more a boy knows about the methods, the more understanding and helpful he can be to his partner, if she is the one using the method.

Condoms and Foam. A condom is a birth control device for boys to use; foam is for girls. We'll talk about them together because when they are used together they are much more effective than when either is used alone.

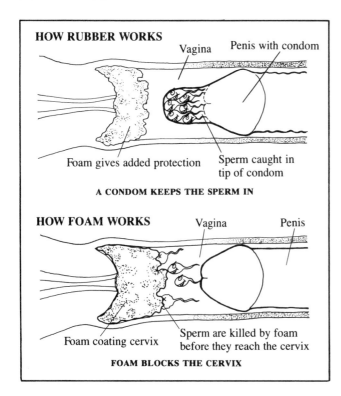

HOW RUBBER WORKS

Vagina Penis with condom

Foam gives added protection Sperm caught in tip of condom

A CONDOM KEEPS THE SPERM IN

HOW FOAM WORKS

Vagina Penis

Foam coating cervix Sperm are killed by foam before they reach the cervix

FOAM BLOCKS THE CERVIX

What are condoms? Condoms are one of the oldest methods of birth control available. They are the *only* effective temporary form of birth control that men and boys can use.

Condoms (also called rubbers, safes, Trojans, prophy-

lactics, sheaths, bags, protection) are thin latex rubber or animal membrane sheaths that fit over a boy's *erect* penis to catch the sperm and fluid that come out during ejaculation. If used alone, condoms are about 90 percent effective, but *when a boy uses a condom and his partner uses foam at the same time, the effectiveness rate climbs to 98 percent*. That is as good as the IUD or the diaphragm.

Foam is a fluffy white cream that looks a lot like shaving cream. It contains a special sperm-killing chemical. Using an inserter, the girl applies some foam to the inside of her vagina, coating the opening to her cervix. If sperm try to get in the cervix, they are killed by the foam. Foam is about 80 percent effective when used alone.

Together condoms and foam work by blocking the sperm from approaching the cervix and killing any sperm that break through the blockade. *They are excellent protection against pregnancy and also against sexually transmitted diseases.*

Types of condoms. There are many different brands of condoms. Some are made of very thin latex rubber. Some are skin condoms, made of the linings of sheep's intestines. Most people buy the rubber variety, although some claim the skin condoms allow greater sensation during intercourse. That is a matter of personal taste. The skin condoms are more expensive, and they are more porous (since skin is more porous than rubber), so they should always be used with foam.

Condoms can come prelubricated (coated with a wetting substance) or not. Prelubricated condoms are very popular, but be careful because they are more likely to slip off during intercourse. Also, no one has studied whether the lubricating substance might be irritating to the vagina or cervix. If the girl you are having intercourse with keeps getting vaginal infections, try changing to a nonlubricated condom to see if that helps. Some condoms come with a special tip to hold the semen after ejaculation.

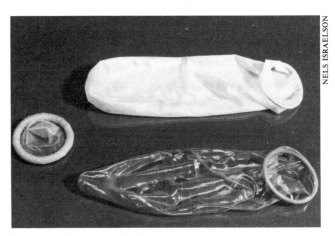

NELS ISRAELSON

(left) rolled condom, before use
(upper right) unlubricated, regular-end condom
(lower right) lubricated, receptacle-end condom

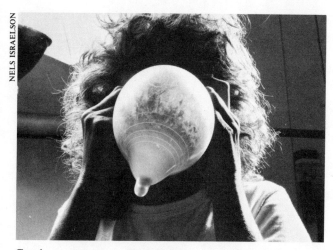

Condoms are strong. They don't burst easily.

Try different brands to see which you like best for yourself.*

How to get condoms. Condoms are sold in drugstores. They are also available in clinics that provide birth control. In some places they can be bought from wall dispensers in men's rooms.

In stores condoms are sometimes kept in the open aisles with the other forms of birth control and personal-hygiene products. If not, ask the druggist for them. Some boys told us that can be embarrassing. Steve, a seventeen-year-old from Michigan, said:

> Getting protection is harder than using it. I usually spend about ten minutes outside the store psyching myself up to go in. The first time was the worst. I was sure everybody was watching me, so when I went in I tried to act real casual. The druggist was actually pretty cool about it. But he asked me what brand I wanted and I didn't know shit about brands, so I said "Trojans" because I'd heard guys talk about Trojans. I said it as if I'd done it a million times, but when he gave them to me and I paid the cashier, I just about tripped over myself getting out of there.

A lot of people think getting birth control is the hardest part, but try to remember that almost everybody does it, and they've all had a first time. If stores or men's rooms in your area have vending machines for condoms, it may be easier for you to buy them that way, but if the supply in the machine hasn't been changed in a long time, you may be buying old condoms. These days most packages of condoms have the date of manufacture written on the outside of the package. Try to avoid using condoms that are more than two years old.

*There is an excellent report on condoms in *Consumer Reports,* October 1979, pp. 583–89. Your library should have a copy. It names and rates the different brands. Sheik #54 and Sheik #28 unlubricated had the fewest problems. Horizon Stimula "had highest resistance to breakage" of any model tested.

In many areas the local Board of Health runs clinics that give away condoms or sell them at very low cost. Also, hospital clinics may offer condoms as part of their outpatient services.

You don't have to be "fitted" for condoms the way girls have to be fitted for diaphragms because condoms come in only one size, which adjusts to the size and shape of your penis.

Condoms come in boxes of three or twelve. A box of three costs between $1.00 and $1.50. In most states there is no age requirement for buying condoms. Anyone—man or woman, boy or girl—can buy them.

How to use condoms. Condoms come individually wrapped in small tinfoil packets. You tear open the packet and take out the condom, which is rolled up. Unroll the condom onto the *erect* penis. This has to be done *before* intercourse—in fact, before your penis gets near your partner's vagina. The pictures below show a man putting on a condom.

Leave about one half inch free at the tip of the condom to catch the sperm when it comes out. Some condoms come with a special tip for that purpose; others don't. If you pull the condom on without leaving room at the tip, the semen may come oozing out the other end and get into the girl's vagina that way. Condoms rarely burst.

After the condom is on, it is safe to enter the girl's vagina. If your condom is not prelubricated, you might want to coat it with a little K-Y jelly (which can be bought at the drugstore) or some other lubricant. Even saliva will work. That may make entry easier.

> After intercourse when you pull out of the vagina, BE SURE TO HOLD ON TO THE OPEN END OF YOUR CONDOM so it won't unroll or slip off as you are pulling out (see picture). The object is to keep the semen inside the condom. Remember, your penis will not be as hard after you ejaculate, so the condom may easily slip off if you don't hold on to it and pull out right away.

When you pull out after intercourse, remove the condom and throw it away. Make sure you are away from your partner's vagina when you remove the condom because your penis will be wet with semen. Sperm will die shortly after being exposed to air. Make sure you are dry before you go near your partner's vagina again. *If you have intercourse another time, be sure to use another condom.*

Storing condoms. Condoms should be kept away from heat, because heat can dry out the rubber and make it crack. Prelubricated condoms last longer than unlubricated ones do. Generally, an unopened package of condoms can be kept for as long as two years if it has been kept away from heat.

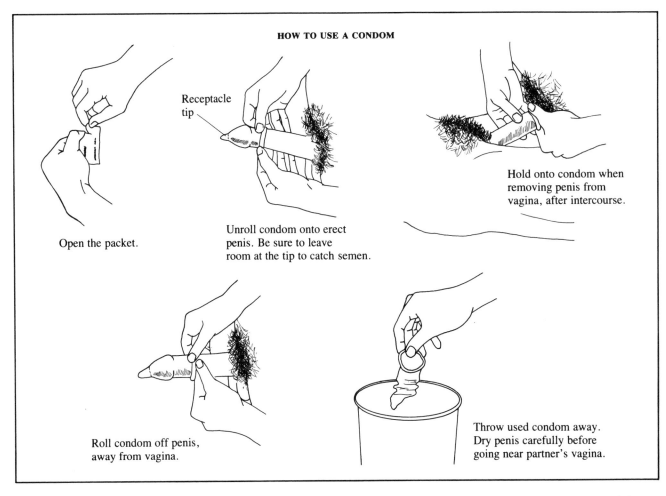

HOW TO USE A CONDOM

Open the packet.

Receptacle tip

Unroll condom onto erect penis. Be sure to leave room at the tip to catch semen.

Hold onto condom when removing penis from vagina, after intercourse.

Roll condom off penis, away from vagina.

Throw used condom away. Dry penis carefully before going near partner's vagina.

Some boys keep condoms in their wallets, but that's not a great place to store them for more than a few weeks, especially if you keep your wallet in your pants pocket. Your body heat may cause the rubber to deteriorate.

Also, before getting a condom from a dispenser in a washroom, make sure the dispenser is not located close to the heater. If it is, the condom may be dried out by the time you buy it.

Good points about condoms. Condoms are safe, effective and cheap. They can be bought in any drugstore. They have no side effects or health hazards. In the rare cases when they leak or burst, even that won't be a disaster if the girl is using foam.

Aside from not having intercourse, condoms are the best way for a boy to share in protecting against pregnancy. When LeRoy, a high school senior from Newark, went to the clinic to pick up more condoms he told the counselor:

My girl and me don't do it that often, just once in a while, so that's why I use rubbers. When we do it, I'm ready and she doesn't have to be on the pill for all that other time.

LeRoy didn't want his girlfriend to have to be on the pill unnecessarily. That's one of the best reasons for using condoms. It gives the boy a chance to take some of the responsibility for birth control off his partner's shoulders. It gives him a chance to protect her from having to take the pill or use the IUD, which both pose serious health risks.

Condoms are small and portable. It's easy to have one with you, just in case you should need it. Many girls carry condoms in their purses. Sally, a tenth-grader from Denver, said:

We used a rubber the first time I had intercourse. It was easy—I bought some and had them in my room. Then when my boyfriend came over one day and we got into it, we didn't have to stop to go get some at the drugstore. I had them right in my drawer.

Another important reason for using condoms is they are excellent protection against catching sexually transmitted diseases (STD). (See p. 166 for a complete discussion about condoms and VD prevention.)

Condoms, used together with foam, are the best way to be ready for intercourse. You can buy them beforehand and keep them until you need them. You don't need a doctor's prescription to get them.

Bad points about condoms. One seventeen-year-old boy who lives in Chicago said that he uses condoms all the time now, because last year he got his girlfriend pregnant. She wanted to have the baby and keep her, so now he's paying child support. He doesn't want that to happen again. But, he said:

I don't really like the way those rubbers feel. I just don't get full satisfaction when I use them. It's not the same as being bare.

One of the most common complaints about the condom is that it interferes with the man's sensations during intercourse. Some boys say it's like "wearing a raincoat." People who feel this way might try "skin" (animal membrane) condoms that are supposed to feel as if you are not wearing anything. And people who use lubricated skin condoms say that there is nearly no difference between them and bare skin.

Another problem with the condom is that some people think it interferes with the spontaneity of sex. Unlike the diaphragm, the condom *cannot* be put on beforehand. It has to be put on during lovemaking, after you have an erection but before you enter the vagina. Some couples who have learned to include that as part of their sex play find it exciting. And since almost every girl appreciates the fact that the boy cares enough about her to use a condom, no boy has to feel embarrassed to put a condom on in front of his partner.

The biggest and most serious problem with the condom is that it is only 90 percent effective. Here are some reasons why a condom may not work:

— sometimes sperm leak out of the open end of the condom and find their way into the vagina;
— if a boy enters the vagina first, then pulls out to put on a condom before ejaculation, sperm may have already gotten into the vagina (often some sperm comes out of the penis before ejaculation, and it only takes *one* sperm to start a pregnancy if the girl is fertile at the time of intercourse);
— on rare occasions condoms burst.

How to use foam. Foam is inserted into a woman's vagina. It must be inserted *no more than fifteen minutes before intercourse*.

Foam comes in a metal container. Shake it very well before use. The more bubbles you shake into the foam, the better it works. The first time you buy a package of foam be sure to buy the package that comes with a plastic applicator. You need the applicator to insert the foam into your vagina.

Put the plastic applicator over the top of the can and bend or press down on the top, according to the instructions on the package. The foam will squirt out, filling the applicator. When the applicator is full, remove it from the can and push it gently into your vagina. Then push the plunger all the way to the top of the applicator; this releases all the foam (see pictures below). Since you want

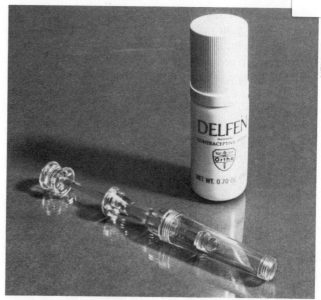

Foam with applicator.

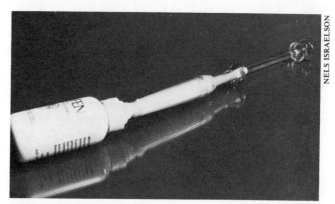

Filling the applicator.

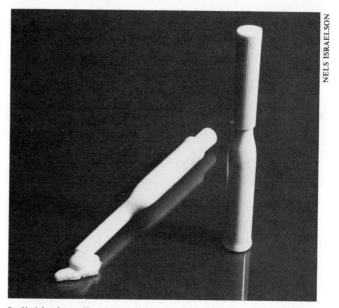

Individual applications of foam.

the foam to coat your cervix, try to aim the applicator at a slant up to your cervix. Most women like to lie down while they are inserting foam.

To be safe, *use two applicators full of foam*. If your partner is using a condom, one application is enough.

> Be sure to use another applicatorful of foam *each time* you have intercourse, even if the second time is within a few minutes of the first. Don't swim, douche or bathe for at least six hours after your last intercourse. Give the foam the time it needs to kill all the sperm that may be inside you.
>
> *Keep an extra can of foam around just in case you run out at the wrong moment*. The way foam is packaged now, there is no way to tell when you are getting close to empty.

Types of foam. There are four main brands of foam: Delfen, Emko, Dalkon and Conceptrol. The first three come in metal containers that hold about twenty applications. You can buy them with or without the plastic applicator tube. Conceptrol comes individually packaged with disposable applicators. It's used the same way a tampon is used and it can be easily carried in a purse. Six individual packages come together in a box.

How you get foam. Foam is sold in drugstores and some supermarkets. Anyone can buy it. Sometimes you have to ask the druggist for it, sometimes it is found in the open aisles. *Be sure the package says contraception or contra-ceptive*. That means the product is a method of birth control.

A medium-sized can costs about $3, and a box of six individually wrapped applications costs about $3. The can is much cheaper, since it gives over three times as many applications for the same price. But some people find the individual applications more convenient.

You can also get foam at birth control clinics and health-care centers. It may be free there or sold at a discount. In most states there is no age requirement for buying foam. You can call a local clinic to be sure.

Storing foam. A container of foam is effective up to a year and a half after manufacture. Keep it away from heat.

Good points about foam. Foam is very easy to use; it is readily available; and when used together with a condom it is *very* effective against pregnancy *and* some types of sexually transmitted diseases.

Many of the teenage girls we interviewed liked foam. This is what fifteen-year-old Chris, a sophomore from Chicago, said about it:

> I feel like I'm too young to take the pill or get an IUD. I haven't even had a pelvic yet, so I don't want to be messing around with doctor's appointments. So my sister told me about foam and I went to the drugstore and got some. I got the kind that looks like Tampax, and you put it in the same way.

Gloria, a senior from Los Angeles, said:

> Foam and rubbers are just about the only kind of birth control you can use when you need it and forget when

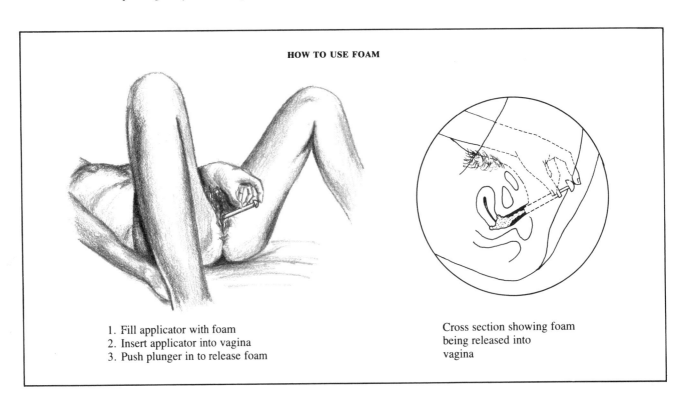

HOW TO USE FOAM

1. Fill applicator with foam
2. Insert applicator into vagina
3. Push plunger in to release foam

Cross section showing foam being released into vagina

you don't need it. I carry those little tubes of foam in my purse when I go out with my boyfriend and it's just like carrying Tampax, which everybody does.

If you have sex irregularly and don't want to use a daily method of birth control like the pill or the IUD, foam may be a good method for you—especially if the boy you're with uses condoms too.

Bad points about foam. Several girls we interviewed said they think foam is messy. If you have intercourse more than once at a time, you might end up with two or three applicators full inside your vagina. After sex, some women who use foam put a tampon in to keep the foam from leaking out.

Another problem with foam is that some brands can be irritating to some people. Carol, a college freshman who goes to school in Boston, told us:

> I went out with this guy and we used foam. Well, he didn't use a rubber and after he pulled out he felt sore, and when he went to pee, it burned him. He thought I gave him the clap, but I knew I didn't. It turned out he was allergic to the foam.

If the boy you are with seems to have a reaction to one type of foam, try using another brand. Usually the symptoms don't last very long, but they can be uncomfortable and even painful to some people. That's another good reason to use a condom and foam both. The condom will protect the boy's penis from irritation.

Less frequently, foam is irritating to the vagina. If that happens to you, change brands and see if that helps.

A third problem with foam when used alone is that it has a high failure rate. Shirley, a seventeen-year-old mother from Dayton, told us:

> See this baby? She's a foam baby. Loreen was born nine months after I used foam, so I guess I did something wrong.

When used alone, without a condom, foam fails about one out of every five times. Sometimes it fails because the person didn't put it in properly. You have to make sure it's covering your cervix. Sometimes it fails because it's put in too far in advance of intercourse. Put it in *no more than* fifteen minutes before you need it. Sometimes it fails because not enough was put in. If the boy doesn't use a condom, be sure to use *two* applicatorfuls of foam each time. Sometimes it fails because the girl is too active after she puts it in and some leaks out before intercourse. Don't go dancing or do acrobatics after you use foam until you're pretty sure it's had a chance to work. It takes about six hours for all the sperm to be killed.

If you use both foam and a condom you have double protection: if either method fails, the other one is there to back it up.

The Diaphragm.   *What is it?* The diaphragm (*dye-uh-fram*) is a small rubber cup. It is soft and flexible and comes in different sizes to fit different women and girls. The purpose of the diaphragm is to hold contraceptive cream or jelly in place around the cervix. Before intercourse a girl coats the inside of the diaphragm with a sperm-killing jelly and then pushes the diaphragm into her vagina so that it covers the cervix. Then she is protected.

If it is used properly *every* time you have intercourse, the diaphragm is 97 to 98 percent effective against pregnancy. It has been a popular form of birth control for over one hundred years. It has *no* dangerous side effects.

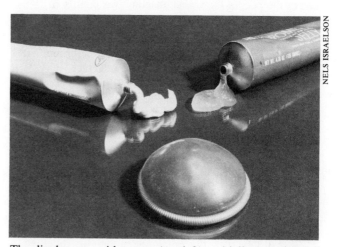

The diaphragm, with cream (top left) and jelly (top right).

How the diaphragm works. The diaphragm works in two ways. By itself it helps to block some sperm from getting into the cervical opening. But because sperm are tiny, many get around the rim of the diaphragm. That's why the diaphragm is always used together with sperm-killing jelly or cream. The sperm that get past the diaphragm itself will be caught in the jelly and killed.

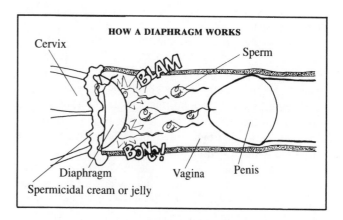

Contraceptive jellies. There are many different brands of contraceptive jelly or cream to use with your diaphragm. Each of them is effective. Sometimes, however, you or your partner may be allergic to one particular brand, or you may find that one brand smells worse than another. If that happens, switch to another brand.

Contraceptive jelly and cream are also good for protection against sexually transmitted diseases (STD, VD; see p. 216). Girls who use a diaphragm with cream or jelly are giving themselves protection against both pregnancy and VD. Some girls like the fact that the jelly or cream used with the diaphragm helps to lubricate their vagina. If you have a tight vaginal opening, that extra lubrication will help.

A seventeen-year-old birth control counselor told us that one of the people she was counseling was confused:

> I was telling this girl about how to use her diaphragm and I thought she understood what I was saying. But then the next day she called me up at the clinic and said, "Do you think strawberry or grape jelly is best?" I said, "What do you mean?" and she said, "With my diaphragm. I don't know which jelly to use."

The counselor quickly told her that contraceptive jelly is entirely different from fruit jelly!

You can buy contraceptive jelly or cream in any drugstore and in some supermarkets, usually in the same section that the store keeps sanitary napkins and tampons. In most states there is no age requirement for buying these products. They are also available at birth control clinics.

A small tube of jelly, containing enough for about ten or twelve uses, costs between $2 and $3. A large tube with about twenty applications costs about $5. Your local birth control clinic may give the tubes free. Be sure to keep an extra tube on hand, just in case you run out at the wrong moment.

NOTE: K-Y jelly is *not* contraceptive jelly. It is for lubrication, and it does not kill sperm.

How to get a diaphragm. Diaphragms come in different sizes because people come in different sizes. To get the right size for you, you must be fitted at a doctor's office or a birth control clinic.

The procedure is very simple. First someone in the office will ask you about your medical history. Then you will be shown into an examining room. If the doctor is planning to give you a thorough examination, you will undress totally and slip on a hospital gown. You should have a complete exam if you haven't had one in a year or more. If you are just going to be fitted for a diaphragm, you will only need to undress from the waist down.

When the doctor comes in to check you, he or she will ask you to lie on the examining table with your knees bent and spread apart. The doctor will put one hand inside your vagina to feel around your cervix. Then he or she will take a sample diaphragm and insert it. If it fits comfortably and covers your cervix, it is the proper size. If it doesn't fit, the doctor will take that one out and try another size.

Tell the doctor how the diaphragm feels to you. If it is uncomfortable, that probably means it doesn't fit well. Sometimes it feels funny just because you may not be used to having something inside your vagina.

The doctor will remove the sample diaphragm, and then it will be your turn to try to put it in. Someone will show you how to do it. If you have any questions, be sure to ask. If it feels as if it is going to fall out any minute, you probably haven't pushed it in far enough. Try again. Keep trying until you are sure you know how to do it. Remember, you're going to have to do it yourself at the time you need it most.

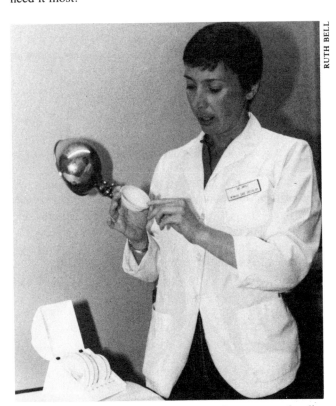

RUTH BELL

A health care specialist will show you how to use the diaphragm.

If the doctor forgets to ask you to put the diaphragm in yourself, remind him or her. Don't leave the office or the clinic without practicing. That way, if you have trouble putting it in or taking it out, someone will be there to help you. Also, ask if you can come back within the next week or two if you continue to have problems or questions. Once you learn how to use the diaphragm it will be easy, but ask as many questions as you want to while you're learning.

Cost. At a birth control clinic you may receive your diaphragm and jelly free of charge or at a very small cost. If you go to a private doctor, he or she will charge you for the visit ($35 to $75 in most areas) and write you a prescription for a diaphragm. You will go to a drugstore to have the prescription filled. Just hand the prescription to the druggest and he or she will give you your diaphragm. It may cost you about $5. Usually your first diaphragm will come in a package together with some contraceptive jelly or cream, an applicator for the jelly and a plastic case for the diaphragm. If the diaphragm doesn't come with jelly or applicator, be sure to buy them too while you're in the store.

Learning to put in the diaphragm. As you can see in these pictures, first you put about a tablespoon of jelly or cream on the inside of the diaphragm. Spread the jelly around with your finger to coat the inside and the rim of the diaphragm.

After it is coated with jelly, the diaphragm is ready to be put into the vagina. Some women like to lie down while they put it in; others stand with one leg up on a chair or the toilet seat; others insert it while sitting on the toilet. Experiment with different positions to see which is the most comfortable for you. The object is to fold the diaphragm and slide it up into your vagina. You have to push it all the

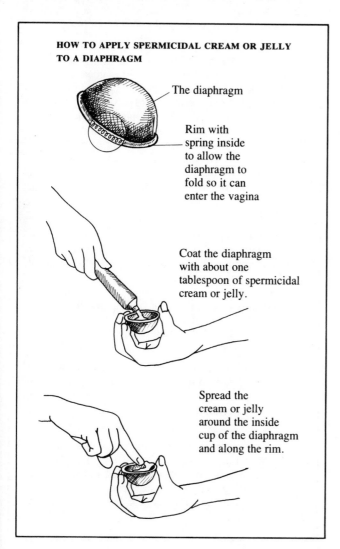

HOW TO APPLY SPERMICIDAL CREAM OR JELLY TO A DIAPHRAGM

The diaphragm

Rim with spring inside to allow the diaphragm to fold so it can enter the vagina

Coat the diaphragm with about one tablespoon of spermicidal cream or jelly.

Spread the cream or jelly around the inside cup of the diaphragm and along the rim.

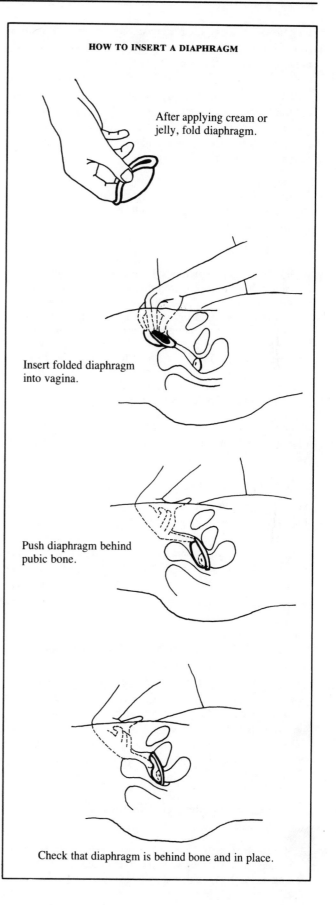

HOW TO INSERT A DIAPHRAGM

After applying cream or jelly, fold diaphragm.

Insert folded diaphragm into vagina.

Push diaphragm behind pubic bone.

Check that diaphragm is behind bone and in place.

way in so the back rim goes past your cervix and the front rim fits inside the pubic bone. You'll be able to feel the pubic bone at the top front of your vagina.

Your vagina *does not* open into the rest of your body except for the tiny opening in the cervix, so there's no way for the diaphragm to get lost inside. It stays in your vagina, just as a tampon does.

Here's how sixteen-year-old Elizabeth described her first attempt at putting in a diaphragm:

> Well, the first time I tried to use it it totally slipped out of my hand and flew across the room. Really. But after that it worked pretty well, except it felt a little funny until I got used to it.

Larra told us:

> The first couple of times I tried to put it in I spent about a half-hour in the bathroom with that thing slipping and sliding all over the place. The jelly was all over my hands and my legs and I couldn't get a grip on the diaphragm enough to push it up far enough so it would stay in there, so it kind of hung halfway out. It was a mess. Finally a friend told me not to use so much jelly. I was using so much because I wanted to make sure I wouldn't get pregnant, but when I cut down on the jelly it was much easier to put in.

A tablespoon of jelly is enough. If you use too much the diaphragm might slip out of place as Larra described. Give yourself some time to practice before you have to use it the first time.

You may want to take time first to look at and touch your vagina. Bring a hand mirror with you into the bathroom. Close the door and undress from the waist down. You can hold the mirror between your legs and look at your vulva. If you spread apart the lips of your vagina you'll be able to see inside. Try putting one or two fingers into your vagina. Do it gently and slowly. See how it feels to you; see how far up you can put your fingers. Some people feel a little funny about touching their genitals. Take your time.

While you're in the doctor's office or if you have a women's clinic near your home, you can ask them to teach you how to see your cervix. You insert into your vagina a speculum (see p. 157), which holds the lips apart for you, then when you hold a hand mirror between your legs with one hand and shine a flashlight on the mirror with the other, you'll be able to see your cervix, the tip of your uterus. You'll see the tiny opening, and you'll understand that the diaphragm has to cover that opening to block sperm from getting in.

Sixteen-year-old Rebecca, a high school junior from Los Angeles, said:

> I used to think I'd never be able to use a diaphragm because it was creepy for me to even think about putting it in. I thought that whole area down there was

---

HOW TO USE A DIAPHRAGM

Here are some rules for using the diaphragm correctly:

1. Contraceptive creams and jellies lose their strength after several hours. Some people say you should put your diaphragm and jelly in *no more* than two hours before you have intercourse. Other people think four hours is OK. If you're going to have a lot of activity like running or dancing or even just standing up a lot before you have intercourse, the jelly may leak out and leave you unprotected. *The closer you insert your diaphragm and jelly to the actual time of intercourse, the safer you will be.*

2. After you have intercourse you must leave your diaphragm in place for at least *eight* hours. By then all the sperm that was left inside your vagina will have leaked out or been killed by the cream or jelly.

3. Do not douche, take a bath or swim during those eight hours. Water that gets into your vagina may wash away some of the jelly and allow any remaining sperm to get through into your cervix.

4. If you have intercourse again, or several times again, during the eight-hour period, insert more jelly or cream each time *before* the penis goes into your vagina. Don't remove your diaphragm for eight hours after the *last* application of jelly.

   To insert extra jelly: Most diaphragm kits come with a plastic inserter for extra applications of jelly. Squeeze jelly into the inserter, or applicator, all the way to the top. Put the inserter filled with jelly into your vagina and push the plunger to release the jelly into your vagina, as in the pictures below. It will coat the outside of the diaphragm, which remains in your vagina.

5. When you are ready to remove your diaphragm, wash your hands first. Then put your index finger into your vagina. Reach up until you feel the rim of the diaphragm. Carefully pull it out. It should slide out easily, but if it doesn't, try again. You'll get it. Sometimes squatting down or putting one leg up will help you feel the diaphragm. The first few times may take a while; after that you'll become better at removing it.

6. To clean your diaphragm, wash it with mild soap and warm water. Make sure it is clean. Dry it with a towel. Never boil it, because that will cause the rubber to deteriorate. *Clean your diaphragm after each use.*

7. To store your diaphragm, dust it with some corn starch or potato flour. Don't use talc because that may contain asbestos particles. Then put it back in its container and store it until you need it again. Don't store your diaphragm near heat; heat can dry out the rubber.

sort of disgusting. But one day one of our teachers took the girls in our class to the women's clinic near our school and they did this demonstration for us, where they showed us their cervix and everything and some of the girls in the class even did it. Right there. Nobody forced you or anything—only if you wanted to do it. But everybody wanted to look. It was really amazing. Everybody's cervix looked a little different. Some were big, some were little, some holes were open pretty big and some were pretty tight. Then they showed us how the diaphragm goes in and covers up that hole. It made it seem logical.*

Once you understand how the diaphragm works, and why it works, it will probably be easier to use. When you get it in, it should feel comfortable. Try walking around. If that feels all right, you've put the diaphragm in right.

After the diaphragm's in place, you may want to wash your hands and the outside of your vagina if they are covered with jelly or cream.

Checking your diaphragm. If you take care of it, your diaphragm should last at least two years. After that time, get it replaced because the rubber will begin to weaken and might rip apart unexpectedly.

Before each use, check the diaphragm to make sure it has no holes or worn places. If there is a hole, sperm might be able to swim through, though if you use enough jelly, that is likely to kill any sperm that get through.

There are a couple of different ways to make sure there are no holes in your diaphragm. One is to hold the diaphragm up to the light and look through it. You should be able to see any tears or pin holes if there are any. Another is to fill the cup of the diaphragm with water. If the water leaks out, then there is a hole.

You may need a different-size diaphragm if you gain or lose more than ten pounds, if you've been pregnant and had a baby or an abortion, or if you've grown a lot taller or broader since your original fitting.

Have your size checked whenever you have a gynecological exam. Bring your diaphragm into the clinic or doctor's office if you think you might need a new one.

Good points about the diaphragm. The diaphragm is safe, cheap and effective. It's easy to put in, once you get used to it. Many girls and women like using the diaphragm because *it doesn't have any harmful side effects or complications.* A seventeen-year-old girl who had been on the pill for a year switched to the diaphragm:

I couldn't use the birth control pill. I went back to the clinic and told the doctor that I didn't want to use the

*Thanks to Carole Downer and Ginny Cassidy of the Feminist Women's Health Center in Los Angeles.

pill anymore because I was getting really bad headaches and they were making me have strange periods and I was scared of what they might be doing to me. So I stopped taking them. We went through everything else and it seemed like the diaphragm was my best bet, so I got one and I've been using it for about six months now. And I haven't gotten pregnant yet, so I guess it works.

If you use the diaphragm according to the instructions, and if you remember to *put it in before intercourse every time*, then it will keep you from getting pregnant. Irene, a seventeen-year-old from Los Angeles, told us:

My boyfriend and I are really close and he helps me put in my diaphragm. Like he'll put the jelly on for me and he'll hold me while I put it in. That relaxes me and makes it easier for me to put it in. He's really into using birth control because once he got a girl pregnant and he nearly freaked out over it. He had to raise the money for her abortion, and it was a big scene. So he's as careful as I am.

Some people prefer putting their diaphragm on alone. You can do it in the bathroom before you start making love, or even before you go out on your date. Remember: if you put it in longer than two hours before you have intercourse, be sure to check that it is in place and use an extra application of jelly.

One of the best points about the diaphragm is that it is a *temporary* form of birth control. There's no need to use it except when you're going to have intercourse. The pill and the IUD have to be used continually, whether or not you are having sex regularly. Several girls with whom we spoke gave that as their reason for using the diaphragm. Sixteen-year-old Jennifer from Des Moines said:

Since me and my boyfriend don't have sex that often, mostly because we don't have that many places we can go to be alone, we pretty much know when we're going to do it, and that gives me plenty of time to put in my diaphragm before we go out.

And Lucy, a junior from Denver, explained:

Peter is away at school, so I don't have sex that often. It doesn't make any sense to me to have something in me all the time, since I know I'll only get to see Peter on holidays.

Another good point about the diaphragm is that it reduces your chances of catching sexually transmitted diseases (see p. 216).

Finally, the diaphragm helps you get used to touching your body. It gives you a chance to learn about yourself and feel comfortable with your genitals. And it gives your partner a chance to participate in birth control if you and he want him to.

Bad points about the diaphragm. The major problem with the diaphragm is that you have to use it every time you have intercourse. *Every time*. Sometimes people forget to use it. Sometimes people don't want to stop the action to go put in their diaphragm. Sometimes people don't have it with them when they need it. Evie, a seventeen-year-old from Los Angeles, hasn't had sexual intercourse yet, but she was talking about which form of birth control she might use if she did want to have intercourse:

> If I were having sex just for the sake of having sex, not with someone I loved, I don't think I'd want to use the diaphragm. I think I would feel uncomfortable about putting it in with someone I didn't know too well. I could see using the diaphragm if you're really into the guy you're with. Like if you've been going out together for a long time or something. I'm scared of the pill and the IUD, but I just think I might be embarrassed to use a diaphragm.

A number of girls we talked with said the same thing: they would feel funny putting in their diaphragm around someone they didn't know well. Sixteen-year-old Dolores, who lives near Chicago, said:

> Those diaphragms are messy. You got to go into the bathroom and say, "Oh, excuse me, I have to go to the bathroom now" and the men know all about it.

And Susanne, a high school junior from Seattle, said:

> I wouldn't want to put in my diaphragm with the guy around. I mean, could you be in front of your date and say, "Oh, excuse me, honey, I'm going to go put in my diaphragm now"? I couldn't do that.

One good way around that embarrassment is to put your diaphragm in before you go out on your date. If you don't have the opportunity to put it in beforehand and you are embarrassed to use it, you may decide to forget it when the time comes. And then you are taking a very big risk: *pregnancy*.

If you think embarrassment will keep you from using the diaphragm every time you need it, it's probably better to get another form of birth control, such as the pill or the IUD, that doesn't have to be applied at the time of intercourse, or to use foam and condoms, which you and the boy use together. But first, give yourself a chance to think about what might cause you to be embarrassed in the first place.

Part of the embarrassment may come from the way many girls are taught to avoid their genitals. They're taught it's private or dirty or smelly or some other negative thing "down there." So they feel funny touching themselves or even thinking about that part of their body.

Part of the embarrassment comes directly from the sexist way we've learned to approach relations between males and females. If our attitude is that girls aren't "supposed" to want to have sex or that girls are "supposed" to be seduced into sex by boys, then it follows that girls aren't

supposed to be prepared for sex. They're supposed to be taken by surprise. So they don't come prepared with protection and then they are in a weak position, totally dependent on the boy to use rubbers or to pull out, if he chooses to.

Bringing along a diaphragm is a sure giveaway that you weren't exactly taken by surprise. It is a statement against sexist attitudes because it shows that girls think about sex too. It is a way of saying that you want to protect yourself and not leave yourself completely dependent on your partner. After all, he doesn't get pregnant; you do.

Also, by using a diaphragm a girl is saying, "I want to use a form of birth control that is *safe* as well as effective." The pill and the IUD may be more spontaneous and they may be less involving for the boy, but they are far more dangerous to a girl's health.

Another drawback to the diaphragm is that some people say it's too mechanical. Unless you put it in prior to going out, you have to stop at some point before intercourse to put it in.

It really only takes a minute to insert the diaphragm, once you're used to it, and some people don't think of it as an interruption. In Massachusetts we met Susan and David at a birth control clinic. David said:

> Me and Susan talked a lot about birth control because we really don't want to sweat a pregnancy. We tried using rubbers at first, but they weren't so great. We decided the pill and the IUD were just too risky, so we thought we'd give the diaphragm a try. I actually like watching Susan put it in. It turns me on.

The Cervical Cap. *What is it?* The cervical cap is a rubber cup like the diaphragm, but it is smaller and fits snugly around the cervix. It can stay in place and remain effective for longer periods of time than the diaphragm.

It is not yet widely available in the United States, although it is being distributed in several European countries. Some women's health centers and clinics in this country are offering the cervical cap now, and when it has been tested more fully and becomes better known, it will probably be offered by most other birth control clinics too.

How the cap works. You apply a small amount of contraceptive jelly to the inside of the cap. Then you insert the cap into the vagina and push it up to cover the cervical opening. It should fit the cervix snugly so that suction is produced. The theory is that suction will hold the cap in place, and while it is in place it blocks sperm from entering the uterus. Like the diaphragm, it must not be removed for eight hours after intercourse, but unlike the diaphragm, it can remain in the vagina for days (maybe even weeks, according to some accounts) and still be effective without applying more jelly.

Several women's health clinics advise people to remove the cap after three or four days to wash it out. New jelly can be applied then, and it can be inserted again. The cer-

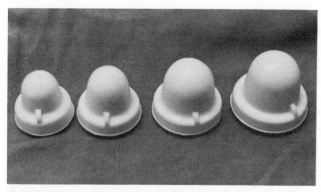

SOME CERVICAL CAPS IN DIFFERENT SIZES

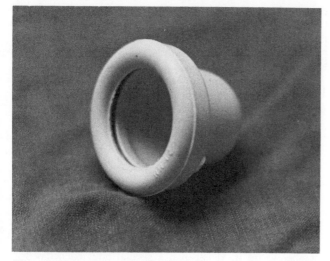

The cervical cap fits over the cervix.

vical cap allows for more spontaneous sex, since it can be inserted hours or even days before intercourse.

Girls remove the cap during their periods to let the menstrual flow escape.

Where do you get a cervical cap? At present cervical caps are not widely available, though some clinics and doctors may have them. Call your local clinic or doctor to see if they are carrying the cap yet.

The cap has to be fitted to your cervix, so an examination is needed. That will be very much like the examination to fit a diaphragm (see p. 172).

How much does it cost? Women's clinics charge around $12 for the cap. Some of these clinics have a sliding scale according to your income. There may be an extra charge for the examination. When you call for an appointment, be sure to ask about cost.

Contraceptive jelly has to be used with the cap, but much less is used over a period of time than with the diaphragm. In the long run the cap is probably cheaper.

Problems with the cervical cap. Although there are many sizes, the cervical cap is not a perfect fit for all girls or women. When it doesn't fit exactly, the cap has been known to slip away from the cervix, leaving the cervical opening unprotected. In the near future it is possible that individually molded caps will be available. That would mean a perfect fit for as long as your cervix stayed the same size. Pregnancy, childbirth, abortion, physical growth and weight gain or loss can change the size of a cervix.

Some people say the cap is harder to insert and remove than the diaphragm. A few women we talked to said that the suction holding on the cap becomes quite strong and it can be difficult to pry the cap away from the cervix. Of course everyone we met was able to remove their cap in a little while—it just took more of an effort for some than with their diaphragms.

Women and girls are advised not to use the cervical cap when they have cervical or vaginal infections. The cap may prolong the healing process because it keeps the cervix covered. If you tend to have heavy secretions from your cervix, you may not want to leave the cap in for more than a day or two at a time.

Positive reaction to the cervical cap. Many girls and women are enthusiastic about the cervical cap, because if it can be perfected it will be the first birth control device that is effective and free from dangerous side effects *that doesn't have to be applied each time before intercourse.* Ask if the cap is available in your area. The more people ask for it, the better chance there is for it to receive wider distribution.

The Birth Control Pill.   *What is it?* The birth control pill is a small round tablet made of synthetic (human-made) hormones. It has been on the market for twenty years, and it is used by millions of women and girls. As of now, there is no birth control pill for men. The pill is easy to use and very effective—99 percent effective—against pregnancy if used properly. But it has dangerous side effects for some women, and since it's only been around for a little over twenty years, no one really knows what its long-range effects will be.

How the pill works. The pill stops ovulation, which means girls don't release ripe eggs during the time they're on the pill. If you, as a girl on the pill, have sexual intercourse, sperm won't find any egg waiting in the fallopian tubes, so no pregnancy can start.

When a woman becomes pregnant, her female hormones (estrogen and progesterone) stay at a pretty high level throughout the pregnancy. That tells the ovaries not to produce any more ripe eggs. The pill copies the effect of pregnancy by keeping the hormone levels high all through the month. It doesn't make the woman pregnant, of course, but it makes her ovaries stop producing eggs, just as if she were pregnant. That's why during their first few months on the pill many girls and women experience the symptoms of early pregnancy: tender breasts, nausea, tiredness and water retention. Seventeen-year-old Beth-

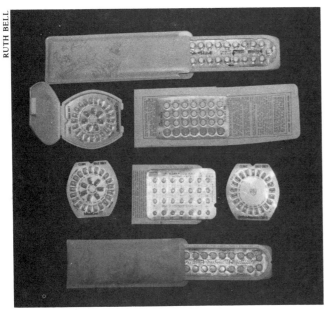

There are many different brands of the birth control pill.

Ellen came to the clinic to complain to the counselor about the pill:

> I started the pill about three weeks ago and I've been feeling shitty lately—I've been gaining weight. A lot of weight. I mean I'm hungry all the time. You can't believe how I've been porking out. And plus I feel sick all the time. I'm nauseous and I have diarrhea, and I feel like if this keeps up I'm just going to have to go off the pill altogether.

The pregnancy-like symptoms usually go away after three months, but there are other annoying side effects and some very dangerous side effects connected with the pill. We'll discuss those more on p. 181, under the heading "Bad Points about the Pill."

A girl doesn't get her period while she is pregnant, but a girl on the pill does get something like a period. She stops taking the hormones for one week each month, and that drop in the hormone level brings on bleeding. (See Types of Pills, p. 179.)

How to use the pill. Carole, a senior in high school in Virginia, explained:

> Until I was in the eleventh grade I used to think that taking the pill meant that you would just take one before you had sex each time. I thought it was like taking aspirin for a headache—you took a pill when you had sex.

Carole didn't understand how the pill works. You don't take just one pill each time you have sex. For the pill to work, you take a pill every day for three or four weeks each month. The instructions will be on your particular package of pills, and the doctor or nurse will tell you how to take them. The point is to keep your hormone level high

enough to stop ovulation, and that means taking the pill all the time, not just before having sex. When you want to go off the pill, you stop taking them altogether.

Each pill contains about twenty-four hours' worth of chemical hormones. If you go longer than twenty-four hours before taking the next pill, or if you forget to take a pill one day, the hormone level in your body begins to drop. That might cause your ovaries to release eggs again.

> If you want the pill to work properly, you should take one pill every day at about the same time each day. That way you are distributing the hormones evenly. Just as one pill's effect is wearing off, you take the next one to keep the hormone level up. If you have a special hour each day for taking your pill, you have a better chance of remembering to take it.

If you don't take your pill at the same time each day, it's pretty easy to forget it. That's what happened to Janet:

> I've only been on the pill one month and I've already forgotten to take my pill twice. I haven't gone a whole day forgetting yet, but I have let about six hours go before I remembered to take it. Now I'm having this discharge, almost like a period, and so I'm beginning to wonder if the pill is working now.

Janet said it's not that she's usually forgetful, it's just that when you aren't used to doing something, it's hard to remember to do it. If she had a special hour each day for taking her pill—for example, just before dinner, or just before school, or at lunch—she probably would be less likely to forget it.

> DURING YOUR FIRST MONTH ON THE PILL, USE AN-OTHER FORM OF BIRTH CONTROL DURING SEX. IT TAKES THE PILL A MONTH TO BE EFFECTIVE AND IT TAKES YOUR BODY A MONTH AT LEAST TO GET USED TO THE PILL. BE SAFE. USE FOAM AND CONDOMS OR A DIAPHRAGM AND CONTRACEPTIVE JELLY WHEN-EVER YOU HAVE INTERCOURSE DURING THE FIRST MONTH.

Evie, one of the girls we met in Boston, told us:

> I wasn't taking my pill every day. I couldn't stand to swallow them. I never was good at swallowing pills, so I'd sort of let myself forget to take them. That's how I got pregnant. I missed too many and they just didn't work for me, I guess.

Forgetting a pill. If you forget to take one pill, take it as soon as you remember it; then take the others at their regular time. If you forget to take your pill during one whole twenty-four-hour period, then take *two* the next day. You probably will still be safe. But if you forget to take two pills in a row, take two each for the next two days and *don't count on the pill alone that month*. Use foam and a condom or a diaphragm and contraceptive jelly whenever you have sex that month. You may start spotting (discharging some blood) from having missed two pills, because your hormone level will have dropped. Call a birth control clinic or your doctor right away and ask them exactly what to do. *Remember, use another form of birth control until you start your next packet of pills.*

> If you keep forgetting to take your pills, then you probably should find another method of birth control. The pills won't work if you don't take them.

Important note. The pill may not work as well if you have severe diarrhea, or if you vomit a lot during one or more days during the month, because your body may not absorb all the hormones on those days when you're ill. If you're sick for more than two days with vomiting and/or diarrhea, use another form of birth control for the rest of that month—until you start your next packet of pills.

Also, some drugs can alter the pill's ability to protect you. These drugs will keep the birth control pill from being effective: barbiturates (such as sleeping pills); meprobamate (brand names—Miltown and Equanil); Dilantin (used in treatment of epilepsy); rifampin (used in treatment of tuberculosis); ampicillin (an antibiotic). All these drugs change the way your body metabolizes estrogen, which means they may decrease the pill's effectiveness. *Before you take any medication, be sure you check with a doctor and tell him or her that you are on the birth control pill.*

As far as we know at this point, marijuana and alcohol don't affect your body's ability to use the pill, although, according to *The Birth Control Handbook* by Howard I. Shapiro, M.D., women on the pill are more likely to be affected by alcohol and for a longer period of time than women who are not on the pill. It's always best *not* to mix drugs and/or alcohol. Just as important is that marijuana and alcohol may make you forget to take your pill.

Types of pills. There are a wide variety of birth control pills available—over forty different types. The doctor who prescribes the pill for you should know the difference between the various brands in order to decide which will be the best for you. The types of pills vary according to the amount and type of synthetic hormones used. Most brands are called combination pills because they contain a combination of the hormones estrogen and progestin. A few brands are progestin-only pills, called mini-pills.

The combination pills are 99.3 percent effective against pregnancy. They come in two different forms. Some are in packets of twenty-one pills each. You take a pill every day for twenty-one days. Then you *stop taking them for approximately seven days*. Periodlike bleeding should come two to four days after the twenty-first pill. Counting the

first day of your period as Day 1, you begin taking a new packet of pills on the fifth day of your period.

The reason your period comes during those days off the pill is that once you stop taking the synthetic hormones, your level of estrogen drops enough to start the bleeding. You can't get pregnant even then, because during the rest of the month the high level of estrogen has kept you from producing a ripe egg.

Some brands of combination pills come in packets of twenty-eight pills. Twenty-one of these are synthetic hormones; seven contain no hormones and are a different color from the others. Usually the seven pills contain iron, which is good for your body during a period. Your period will come two to four days after starting the nonhormone pills. Many girls prefer the twenty-eight-pill packet because that means remembering to take a pill every single day with no interruptions. Discuss this with your doctor or counselor when you go to get the pill.

The birth control pill called the mini-pill does not contain estrogen, so it does not stop ovulation. It depends on increased cervical mucus and faulty development of the uterine lining to keep you from pregnancy. It is less effective than the combination pill, 97 to 98 percent effective, but since it does not contain estrogen, it is safer for some girls. The mini-pill is newer than the combination pill, which means that less is known about its complications or long-term effects.

One important point about the mini-pill is that *you must not miss even one day of taking the pill*. They are to be taken according to instructions every day, and if you miss even one day you run a very high risk of pregnancy. If you do forget one, use another form of birth control for the rest of the month.

Missing a period. Some people do not get their periods during their first month on the pill. Your body has to get used to the sudden increase in hormones.

> Since your body needs time to adjust, you must *not* rely on the pill alone for birth control during the first month. Use foam and condoms or a diaphragm if you have intercourse during that first twenty-eight-day period.

If your period doesn't come, most clinics will recommend starting the next package on time anyway. To be safe, call your clinic for advice. If you miss two periods in a row, have a pregnancy test right away and be sure to check with a doctor. The pill can have dangerous effects on the fetus, so you may want to consider having an abortion.

While you are on the pill your period may be lighter and shorter than it was before. You may also have less cramping.

If you have some bleeding during the middle of your cycle (when your period isn't due), that may mean the pill you are taking isn't a strong enough dose of estrogen for you. Check with the doctor.

How you get the pill. The birth control pill has to be prescribed by a doctor. You can go to a private doctor or a clinic.

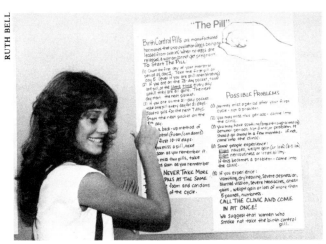

A teen counselor explaining how to use the birth control pill.

During your appointment, the doctor or an assistant will ask you questions about your medical history. They want to know what sicknesses you've had, what medication you take, if you have any special medical problems, what illnesses run in your family.

> Many women have severe complications from taking the pill. Your medical history will help the doctor determine if the pill will be relatively safe for you, or if it might be a health hazard. It's very important for your own safety to be completely honest with the doctor. Remember, it's your body, and you will be the one to suffer any consequences.

The doctor will want to know if you have a family history of diabetes, obesity, heart disease, high blood pressure, varicose veins, cancer, strokes, blood-clotting disorders or epilepsy. Also be sure to tell the doctor if you are a heavy smoker. Any of those conditions can make the pill dangerous for you to take.

After the doctor or counselor talks to you about your medical history, you will go into the examining room for a complete physical checkup, including an internal exam (see p. 156 for a description and discussion). Eighteen-year-old Leah went to Planned Parenthood to get the pill. She said:

Anytime I have to have an examination I always freak out. But they were so nice to me it wasn't so bad.

They were so neat about it—they tried to cool me out and make me relax. And then when it was over, they gave me the pills and told me how to use them. They were super nice people.

When your examination is over, you will get dressed and talk to the doctor about whether you and he or she both feel that taking the pill is a good idea for you. Only take the pill if it is safe for you to do so.

Don't ever start taking the birth control pill without having a thorough checkup. For example, *never* borrow a package of pills from a friend. Each person is different and the dosage of hormones in the many kinds of pills is different. The doctor will prescribe a dosage that is suitable for you, considering your size, your age and your medical history.

If you think the doctor has not given you a thorough examination, do not accept his or her prescription for pills. In that case you can protest your poor treatment and refuse to pay the bill. Explain that no doctor should give a girl birth control pills without following the procedures we described above.

Cost. A package—which is one month's supply of pills—can cost between $2 and $4, depending on the drugstore. Many doctors and clinics, especially teenage clinics, give pills and other forms of birth control free. Before you make an appointment to see the doctor, ask whether they give pills free or whether you have to purchase them.

Good points about the pill.

You've got to use a spontaneous kind of birth control. I mean what if you're driving home from the movies and you go parking and it's twelve o'clock at night. What are you going to do then? Drive around all night looking for a place that sells rubbers?

Sarah, who was just quoted, has been using the pill for a year now. She is eighteen, and she and her mother talked about birth control when she was sixteen, before she had sexual intercourse. They both decided that the pill would be the best form of birth control for her.

Other girls said:

You don't have to plan on the pill. It's real convenient. And I feel safer with it.

I was using foam before and that was messy, so I wouldn't always use it. The pill doesn't get in the way at all.

I got my pills at a family planning clinic when I was only fourteen and nobody gave me any hassle. I had been having sex with my boyfriend for a couple of months and we weren't using anything and I started getting really worried that we were taking too many chances. I feel so much safer now.

The best thing about the birth control pill is that it works: if you take it every day according to instructions, you're almost 100 percent sure not to get pregnant. It is now the most effective form of birth control on the market when it is used exactly according to instructions.

The birth control pill regulates the menstrual cycle—at least for most girls. It brings your period on at a predictable time each month, and it usually reduces the cramps and premenstrual tension that you might have felt before you started taking the pill. Fifteen-year-old Francie, a ninth-grader from California, said:

I used to get real bad cramps with my period, so bad that I couldn't do anything but stay in bed for the first day or two. Now that I'm on the pill my cramps aren't as bad. That's a great extra bonus that I wasn't expecting.

Also, the pill might help clear up your skin, as it did for Geri:

I never had any problems with the pill. In fact, it cleared up my pimples, and after a couple of months I even lost weight. I've never had any headaches or anything with it.

Everyone is different, though, and some girls have reported getting skin problems after going off the pill when they didn't have them before.

Bad points about the pill. Seventeen-year-old Mary-Jo said:

I can't stand the idea of poisoning my body with all these chemicals day after day, year after year. It's like committing suicide.

There are many dangerous side effects and serious health hazards associated with the pill. Not all of the problems are even known yet, since the birth control pill is a fairly new product. A lot of teenage girls wonder what will happen to them in the future if they start taking the pill at a young age. One of the girls helping us with the research for this book said:

You think about it—girls fourteen, fifteen, sixteen using the pill maybe until they're in their thirties. What's going to happen when they're thirty-five or forty? That's a long time to be taking a drug every day.

The pill interferes with the normal functioning of a girl's body. It keeps you from ovulating for as long as you take it. That's why most doctors agree that the pill is *not* recommended for girls who have not had regular periods for at least one year. It takes your body a while to adjust to the cycle of ovulation and menstruation. The pill may interfere with that adjustment process, so you might have problems returning to normal later, when you decide to go off the pill:

As far as we know now, the pill alone does not seem to cause cancer. But there have been studies showing that

---

WHO SHOULD NOT TAKE
THE BIRTH CONTROL PILL

Over the years doctors and researchers have found that the pill is especially dangerous to the health of women who have:

> Blood clotting disorders
> Cancer
> Diabetes
> Epilepsy
> Heart trouble
> High blood pressure
> Liver trouble
> Migraine headaches
> Sickle cell anemia
> Varicose veins

Women who have these disorders or who have a family history of these disorders should not take the pill.

Also, you should not take the pill if you smoke, if you are seriously overweight, or if you are pregnant or nursing a baby.

Be careful—your health is at stake.

---

women over thirty-five who both smoke and take the pill have a much higher chance of getting cancer of the cervix and heart attacks. So if you are a heavy smoker you should *not* take the pill.

Another side effect to consider is that the pill does not protect you against getting sexually transmitted diseases the way the diaphragm and jelly or foam and the condom do. Barrier methods help block the germs. The pill leaves you completely open to germs.

The pill also seems to weaken your body's natural immunity against infections, especially virus infections for which there are no cures yet. Sandy, a sixteen-year-old junior from Rhode Island, came to the clinic to find out about other methods of birth control because, she said,

I had really bad side effects from the pill—bleeding and this vaginal infection that just wouldn't go away. I mean *really* wouldn't go away. I've had it for months now. Finally I decided to go off the pill because my doctor said he thought that might be causing it.

Two other serious side effects are headaches and depression. One girl we interviewed said:

Ever since I started taking the pill I've been getting these terrible headaches before my period. They knock me out.

And another girl said:

There have been times during the last six months that I've been on the pill that I've felt so depressed I couldn't even do anything. I just wanted to stay in bed with the covers over my head. I thought it was just me, but then my friend told me that maybe the pill was causing it. If that's what it is, I'm going off the pill right away.

THE PILL AND GOOD NUTRITION

Studies have shown that the synthetic estrogen in most birth control pills will interfere with your body's ability to absorb some vitamins and minerals. The particular vitamins mentioned are vitamin B6, vitamin B12, vitamin C, riboflavin, thiamin and folic acid. The mineral most affected by the pill is zinc.

Check with a doctor or nutritionist to see which vitamin supplements you should take if you are on the pill. Without adequate supplies of the B vitamins, your body may be more susceptible to anemia and depression. Vitamin C is important in fighting off infections. Zinc deficiency can lead to skin and hair problems.

Food sources for these vitamins and minerals are:

Vitamin B6: whole grains, liver, wheat germ, meats, fish, soybeans, peanuts, corn, bananas, organ meats.

Vitamin B12: milk, eggs, meat, cheese. Strict vegetarians are advised to take B12 supplements.

Riboflavin (Vitamin B2): brewer's yeast, milk, organ meats, whole grains, seeds, leafy green vegetables.

Thiamin (Vitamin B1): whole grains, bran, rice (especially brown rice), pork.

Folic Acid: leafy green vegetables (uncooked or lightly cooked), fresh fruit, dried beans and peas, whole grain breads.

Vitamin C: citrus fruits, leafy green vegetables, fresh strawberries and other fruits, tomatoes, potatoes, cabbage, bean sprouts, green pepper, squash.

Zinc: oysters, yeast breads, wheat germ, dark muscle meats.

Some of the common side effects of the pill may be caused by the vitamin and mineral deficiencies created by the pill. For example, depression may be connected to insufficient vitamin B, especially B6. Anemia is related to lack of B12 and folic acid. Loss of sex drive can be caused by a zinc deficiency. Headaches, color blindness, skin and hair problems, and nervous tension may all be related to the way the birth control pill keeps your body from adequately absorbing these vitamins and minerals.*

A small group of women develop even more serious complications from taking the pill, some of which can lead to death. They are: blood clots, which can move to the

*We recommend the book *Diet and Nutrition, a Holistic Approach,* by Rudolph Ballentine, M.D., published by the Himalayan International Institute, Honesdale, PA 1978. ($7.95.)

lungs or brain; epilepsy; heart attack; sterility; liver problems; and gall bladder disease. These illnesses rarely affect teenage girls, but longtime use of the pill increases a person's chances of developing these or other complications.

Before you decide to take the pill as your form of birth control, be sure to understand what risks are involved. It is your responsibility to yourself not to take chances with your health.

The IUD (Intra-Uterine Device). *What is it?* IUD are the initials for intra-uterine device, meaning inside the uterus. The IUD is a very small plastic device that a doctor puts inside a girl's uterus. It comes in a variety of sizes and shapes.

There is now an IUD containing copper, which is often recommended for teenage girls because it seems to stay in the uterus better than the others and to be more effective.

How the IUD works. The IUD is a good method of birth control—about 97 to 98 percent effective against pregnancy, but, strangely, no one is exactly sure how the IUD works. There are three different theories.

One theory says that the IUD causes the egg to move so fast down the fallopian tube that it doesn't allow time for fertilization by a sperm. Another possibility is that the IUD

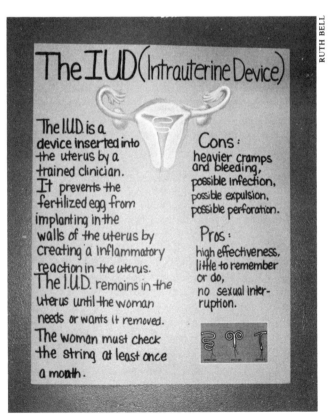

Sign in a teen clinic about the IUD.

causes an exceptionally high number of white blood cells to develop in the uterus, and these destroy the sperm before they can reach the egg. IUD's with copper are supposed to cause the highest rate of white blood cells to be produced.

The third theory is the most widely accepted. According to this, the IUD constantly irritates the inside lining of the uterus and causes a low-grade infection which keeps the lining from developing properly each month. If this is correct, the IUD doesn't necessarily prevent the sperm and egg from meeting, it just doesn't give them a place in the uterus to develop into a baby.

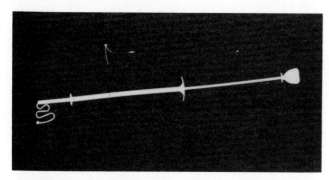

An IUD in an applicator

Important Note. Since the IUD may work by causing an infection in the uterus, it may not be effective while you are taking drugs, such as antibiotics, which destroy infections. An article by Katherine Roberts in *Women and Health* (July/August, 1977) suggests that antibiotics may clear up the infection in your uterus and, under certain circumstances, allow a pregnancy to implant. *Always* use another form of birth control along with your IUD when you take antibiotics. Foam and condoms or diaphragm with contraceptive jelly are good alternative methods.

The staff of the Women's Community Health Center in Cambridge, Massachusetts, also advises using alternative birth control methods while taking aspirin or other anti-inflammatory drugs. Anything that decreases the irritation of the uterus caused by the IUD may lower the IUD's effectiveness.

How you use the IUD. The IUD seems like the simplest method of birth control to use: once it has been placed in the uterus the girl doesn't have to do anything else. But since IUD's have been known to come out, if you have an IUD inserted, the doctor or counselor will advise you to check the string attached to the device. The string will dangle through the opening to your cervix. To check it, place a clean finger into your vagina and feel around your cervix. If you feel a silky thread, your IUD is in place.

Who can use the IUD. The IUD should fit inside a girl's uterus without puncturing its walls, so if you want an IUD, your uterus has to be big enough to hold an IUD. Development is individual, so while some fifteen-year-olds may

be full-grown, other girls don't mature until they are older. Some doctors and clinics refuse to give IUD's to girls under seventeen. Other places make individual judgments depending on the particular person.

There are some people who should *not* use an IUD no matter what age they are. Girls who have an unusually shaped uterus or a severely tipped uterus should probably not use IUD's because the chance of perforation (tearing the walls of the uterus) is too great. Also, girls who have pelvic inflammatory disease, or PID (see p. 39), or any other serious infections of the female sexual organs must not use an IUD until their infection is completely cured, and probably should *never* use an IUD because it increases your chances of future PID.

Girls with cancer of the cervix, cancer of the uterus, or fibroid tumors in their uterus should *not* use an IUD. Also, people who have very heavy periods with lots of bleeding and cramping are advised not to use the IUD because it usually increases menstrual bleeding and sometimes increases cramping.

How to get an IUD. The IUD has to be inserted by an experienced and skilled doctor. It is a very simple procedure, but it takes care to insert it without puncturing the uterus. Go to a doctor who is experienced in putting in IUD's.

Private medical offices, hospital clinics, women's clinics and birth control clinics all have doctors trained in fitting IUD's. Call you local Planned Parenthood or the women's health clinic nearest you for names of recommended physicians. Tell them you are a teenager.

As you can see in the picture, the IUD is inserted into your uterus through the opening in your cervix, called the os. It is best to have the IUD inserted on a day you are having your period because your os is more open then. That makes the procedure more comfortable for you, since opening the cervix can produce some cramping.

Call the doctor or clinic to make an appointment for the time when you are expecting your period. If there's no way for you to judge when your next period will come, tell the nurse or the counselor that you will call them as soon as you get your next period.

When you get to the clinic or doctor's office you should be asked about your medical history. The doctor will want to know about your periods, whether they come regularly and how long they last. He or she will want to make sure you are not pregnant, so you may be asked to take a pregnancy test. IUD's aren't inserted in pregnant women because the device can harm the fetus. The doctor will also want to know if you've ever been pregnant or had a miscarriage or an abortion. That helps him or her decide what kind of IUD is best for you, because a woman who's never been pregnant has more of a chance of expelling her IUD. IUD's with copper seem to be most effective for people who have never been pregnant.

INSERTING THE IUD INTO THE UTERUS

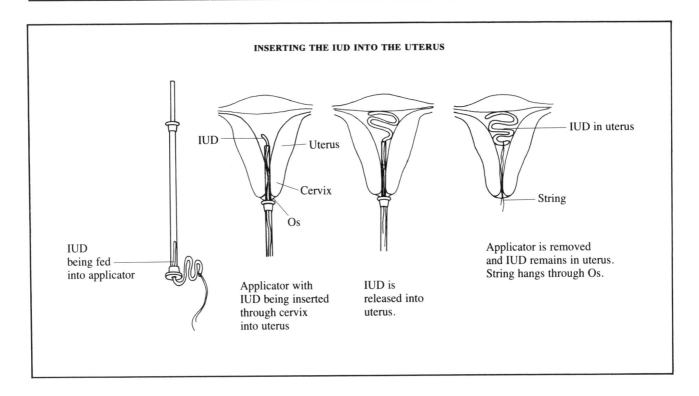

IUD being fed into applicator

IUD — Uterus
— Cervix
Os

Applicator with IUD being inserted through cervix into uterus

IUD is released into uterus.

— IUD in uterus
— String

Applicator is removed and IUD remains in uterus. String hangs through Os.

THE IUD IN PLACE

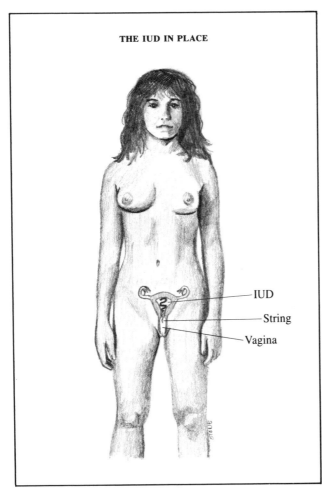

— IUD
— String
— Vagina

In the examining room you will receive a thorough checkup. The doctor will probably place a special instrument into your uterus to find out what size it is. The instrument is called a uterine sound. A clean sound is inserted into your uterus and it comes out wet up to a certain point. That measures the depth of your uterus.

Inserting the IUD. After the sounding, the doctor will put your IUD into an applicator that looks like a long drinking straw. The IUD is squeezed inside, and when the applicator is inserted into your uterus, the doctor pushes out the IUD and it returns to its original shape.

As the doctor inserts the IUD you may feel cramps.

When the doctor pulls out the applicator, the IUD will be in place inside your uterus. The string that is attached to the end of the IUD will be hanging through the os. Feel the string yourself before leaving the examining room to be sure you know how long it is and what it feels like. It may be a little stiff right after insertion, but it will soften up within a week or two. If the person you're having intercourse with feels the string with his penis, that may be because it is still stiff. It may also mean the IUD is coming out. Have it checked to be sure.

After the examination. When the exam is over and the IUD is in place, some girls have painful cramps. Sometimes a pain-killer is given before the insertion, but even so, you may feel cramps when the drug wears off. It's hard to tell beforehand how your body is going to react to the IUD, so it's a good idea to bring a friend along to your appointment, just in case you need a hand to hold or someone to take you home.

Be sure not to leave the doctor's office until you're feeling strong enough to walk. If you feel faint or nauseated, tell the nurse or counselor and lie down. They will help you.

During the next few days your body will be adjusting to the IUD. You may have cramps and you may experience heavier bleeding than is usual with your period. Take care of yourself by resting. (See p. 34 for advice on how to handle menstrual discomfort.) *Be sure not to have intercourse for the next twenty-four hours at least.* Most girls prefer to wait longer than that. You may not want to masturbate to orgasm either, since that might cause cramping of the uterus.

Checking your IUD. As we said before, in some girls the IUD slides out of the uterus. This usually happens, if it's going to, during the first month or two after insertion. After that, if the IUD comes out, it is likely to come out with a period, when the os is slightly open and the blood and tissue in your uterus flow through. That's why it is very important to check for the string each month *after* you finish menstruating.

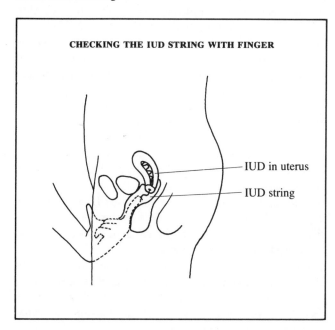

CHECKING THE IUD STRING WITH FINGER

— IUD in uterus

— IUD string

During your period you can wear tampons or napkins, but be sure to look the used ones over before you throw them away. The IUD may have come out and attached itself to the cotton.

If you find your IUD on a tampon or napkin, or if you see it in the toilet after you go to the bathroom, *don't try to put it back in yourself.* It is full of germs now and can cause a very serious infection in your uterus. Save it and bring it with you to the clinic when you go for another insertion. They'll want to know what kind it was. If you can't find it, just tell them at the clinic that your IUD came out and you want another one put in.

If you know how to use a plastic speculum, mirror and flashlight to see your cervix (see p. 27), you can see whether the string is there. You can also feel it by reaching a clean finger up into your vagina and feeling around your cervix.

If you don't feel the string, or if it feels a lot shorter than it did the last time you checked, call your doctor or clinic right away. That may mean you've lost your IUD or that it's moved deeper into your uterus and possibly torn through.

Cost. The most expensive thing about the IUD is the cost of the doctor's bill. If you go to a private gynecologist you can expect to pay a pretty large fee, from between $35 to $75. You will pay much less, and possibly nothing, at a birth control clinic. Most of the time the charge at a clinic is according to how much you can afford to pay. Call first for price information. The IUD itself costs only a few dollars.

Once the IUD is in, there is no further cost except doctor's checkups twice a year and the fee for removing it when you decide to have the IUD taken out. Again, clinics generally charge much less than private doctors.

Having the IUD removed. When you decide you want to become pregnant or when you want to switch to another form of birth control, go back to the clinic and have your IUD taken out. The doctor simply pulls the string very carefully and the IUD squeezes out.

Never try to pull out your own IUD because you could tear your cervix or your uterus in the process.

For most women removal is much easier and less painful than insertion.

Having the IUD changed. If you have a plastic IUD with no copper or the hormone progesterone in it, and if it is giving you no trouble, then you can probably keep it for three or more years without having it changed. You should have checkups every six months to make sure it is still in place and that you don't have an infection.

If you have an IUD with copper in it, you *must* have it changed at least every two or three years because the copper loses its effectiveness after that. The IUD's that contain progesterone must be changed *every year.* When you have your IUD inserted, the doctor or counselor will tell you what type of IUD you have and how often you should have it changed. If they don't tell you, be sure to ask. They may give you a card with that information on it to keep in your wallet.

Good points about the IUD. The best thing about the IUD is that it is the most convenient form of birth control, since once you have it in you don't have to do anything but check the string. A seventeen-year-old college freshman said:

I never could use birth control. I tried the pill for a while but I kept forgetting to take it. And I always figured I wouldn't feel comfortable using a diaphragm because I'd always have to carry it with me. But with the IUD, it's just in there and I don't have to do anything about it. I feel much safer with the IUD than I ever did before.

And Susie, a sixteen-year-old from Los Angeles, said:

I was on the pill for a couple of years, but I started having this bleeding in the middle of the month and the doctor told me I better get off it. So I was really worried because I didn't know what I'd use for birth control. I'd already been pregnant, so I didn't want that to happen again for sure. I didn't want to get an IUD because a friend of mine had terrible cramps from it for a long time. But after I thought about it I knew I had to use something and I didn't want to chance rubbers. So I got an IUD after all. It didn't hurt me half as much as I expected.

Bad points about the IUD. Rachel said:

The IUD worked for me for about a year, but after that I started having these real long periods. They would last more than a week, and then my next period would start early. It kept getting worse and worse and then I started bleeding a little in the middle of the month too, so by the end of about three months I was bleeding just about every day—not much, but enough to have to wear a tampon. It was a real drag. So I went and had my IUD out and almost right away the bleeding stopped.

Rachel's problem is one that several girls we interviewed had—the IUD made them bleed so much during the month that they felt they always had to wear a tampon. Some people said that it became so bothersome that they had to have their IUD removed. Excessive bleeding can lead to anemia, so be sure you are taking iron supplements if you're on the IUD, and include foods rich in iron in your diet; lean meats, liver, oysters, beans, molasses, raisins and leafy green vegetables are high in iron. If you are bleeding a lot, call your doctor or clinic and report it.

Other problems with the IUD are even more serious. The following are some to watch out for.

Sexually transmitted diseases. IUD users are *more* susceptible to gonorrhea germs than are girls who use foam or a diaphragm. The IUD gives *no* protection against the germs and it increases the chances of germs getting into the uterus and tubes. The string attached to the IUD that goes through your cervix is a perfect ladder for germs to climb.

Other infections. The IUD is a foreign object in your sterile uterus. It increases your chances of introducing infectious bacteria into your system. If you get an infection in your uterus or other internal organs, *you must seek medical treatment immediately.* The longer you wait, the more serious your illness will become. It will not go away by itself. Such diseases can lead to sterility by blocking your fallopian tubes; they can also lead to other problems.

> Warning signs of infection are: high fever, chills, severe pain in the pelvic area, unusual bleeding, nausea, generally sick feeling. If you have severe, sharp pains in your lower stomach or if you feel faint, *go immediately to an emergency treatment center.*

Women of any age who use the IUD are definitely at a higher risk of getting pelvic inflammatory disease (PID). PID is one of the most common causes of sterility in this country.

Perforation and embedding. The IUD may puncture a hole in the uterus. This is called perforation. The IUD may also attach itself to the inside of the uterus. This is called embedding. Both of these conditions can happen during insertion if the doctor is not extremely careful. They can also occur by themselves if the IUD moves up in the uterus during cramps or strong contractions of the uterus. That's why it is so important to feel for the IUD string at least once a month, usually just after your period, to make sure the IUD hasn't moved. If the string seems shorter, or if you can't feel it at all, there's a chance that your IUD has moved. Call the doctor or clinic right away if either of these things happens, and in the meantime, use another form of birth control.

Sometimes the only way to remove a misplaced IUD is by performing surgery to locate it and take it out.

Pregnancy. The IUD doesn't work for a small number of girls, and they may become pregnant even with their IUD in place. If you become pregnant, there is a 25 percent or more chance that removing the IUD will create a miscarriage. It is a good idea to have the IUD removed in any case, though, because it increases the chance of infection, which can lead to miscarriage and, in rare instances, to the death of mother and/or fetus.

Most of the time girls become pregnant because their IUD has come out accidentally without their knowing it. *Some people choose to use foam or a diaphragm during their fertile days to take extra precaution against pregnancy even with an IUD in place.*

Ectopic pregnancy. An ectopic pregnancy is one which implants in someplace *other* than the uterus, usually in the fallopian tube. Since the IUD may not stop the sperm from meeting the egg, it may not protect women from ectopic pregnancies as other forms of birth control would.

Ectopic pregnancies can be dangerous. The fallopian tube can burst due to the increased size and weight of the growing fetus. Before it bursts you will experience a sharp pain in the stomach or shoulder and you may have shock symptoms—nausea, dizziness, chills, fainting. *Go immediately to an emergency treatment center and tell them you may have an ectopic pregnancy.*

Girls with IUD's should watch very carefully for all signs of pregnancy: enlarged and tender breasts, tiredness, increased urination, in some cases nausea and vomiting—especially in the morning and early evening—and *missed periods*. If you think you might be pregnant, go for a pregnancy test (see p. 192). Then if you are pregnant, watch for signs of an ectopic pregnancy.

Lovemaking Without Intercourse. One of the most widely used methods of birth control is to make love without having sexual intercourse. Heterosexual couples throughout history have developed techniques for giving each other sexual pleasure without putting a penis into a vagina. When you don't want to or can't risk pregnancy, the *most* effective way to avoid it is by not having intercourse.

Every part of a person's body can be a source of pleasurable sensations, and often by focusing on intercourse, people overlook the pleasure the rest of the body holds. Teenagers from all across the country told us they prefer to have sex without intercourse because they don't want to have to worry about pregnancy. They experience intimacy, passion, tenderness and orgasm in other ways, which they say are just as satisfying, if not more so.

We discuss this more thoroughly in Chapter IV on p. 93.

Natural Birth Control. *What is it?* Natural birth control means having sexual intercourse only when you're sure the girl or woman can't get pregnant. A girl can get pregnant only around the time of ovulation, so you can have unprotected intercourse the rest of the time without having to worry about pregnancy.

That may sound great to you. It sounds great to most people. The problem is that it is very hard to tell exactly *when* a girl is going to ovulate, and it is more difficult to know exactly when she is fertile and when she is not fertile. If you make any mistake in your calculations, you can end up pregnant.

How does it work? There are three different ways to try to figure out when ovulation is about to occur. The first is the calendar method, the second the mucus method, and the third the temperature method. Each is fairly complicated to use, and *none is as effective used alone as it is when used in combination with the other two.*

The methods are *not* recommended to most teenage girls because in order for them to work: (1) you have to have regularly spaced periods; (2) you have to be willing to avoid intercourse during ten to twelve days each month; and (3) you have to be very conscientious about keeping daily records—without records, the methods are likely to fail completely.

Natural birth control takes much more time and cooperation than do the other methods we've described, but it involves no chemicals, no foreign bodies, no devices and no permanent changes.

The calendar method (also known as the rhythm method). Let's imagine that Joanne has a perfectly regular menstrual cycle. Her period comes every 28 days without fail. She's never late and she's never early. We're imagining this because it doesn't happen very much in real life. No one is that regular all the time. Even if your period has come right on schedule so far, it's probably going to be early or late one time or another.

But Joanne is our made-up example, so her period comes every 28 days and it always will. That's why she's able to use the calendar method very easily. She knows that ovulation occurs 12 to 14 days before menstruation. She also knows that she has a 28-day cycle. So she subtracts 14 from 28—and she gets 14. That means she can expect to ovulate on the fourteenth, fifteenth or sixteenth day of her cycle—counting the first day of her period as Day 1. (For more information about ovulation and menstruation see pp. 29–31.)

Joanne also knows that sperm can stay alive inside her body for up to 6 days. This means that to be safe, she can't have intercourse for 6 days before she ovulates. Otherwise there might be some live sperm waiting for her to release the egg. To account for those 6 days she subtracts 6 from 14 (the first possible day of ovulation) and that leaves 8. So starting on Day 8 of her cycle, Joanne is not safe. She can't have unprotected intercourse starting on the eighth day after her period begins.

Once she ovulates, Joanne stays fertile for about 2 days, but to be safe, most experts say you should wait 4 days. Joanne adds 4 to 16 (the last possible day of ovulation) and gets 20. She can start having intercourse again on the twentieth day after her period began. And she can continue to have unprotected intercourse until 8 days after her next period starts.

If Joanne's period came every 31 days, she would subtract 14 from 31 to find out when she might start to ovulate. Seventeen is the answer, so Joanne of the 31-day cycle could ovulate on the seventeenth day after the first day of her period. She subtracts 6 from 17 to get 11. That means she must not have unprotected intercourse starting on Day 11 of her cycle. Adding 4 to 19 (the last possible day of ovulation), she gets 23, which means she can resume unprotected intercourse on Day 23.

Remember: *this only works if you have an absolutely regular menstrual cycle (which almost no one has).* You can work out an approximate schedule by checking your menstrual cycle on a calendar for six months or more. See if a pattern develops.

To find out how to use the calendar method with a less than regular cycle, call Planned Parenthood or your local birth control clinic. Their counselor will give you the information you need, but he or she will probably advise you not to rely on the calendar method. There are *lots* of calendar-method babies born every year.

Problems with the calendar method. The biggest problem with this method is that no one can count on their period coming exactly when it's supposed to. Sickness, travel, weight gain or loss, anxiety, tension—all these things can cause a woman's period to come early or late. Some people never have a regular cycle; they never know when to expect their period. Other people are regular for a while and then suddenly, for no apparent reason, go off schedule. That's why it's not a good idea to trust the calendar method alone.

The mucus method. This method is based on noticing the different types of mucus coming from a girl's cervix during the month. When a girl is not fertile, there is either little mucus around the cervix, or else there may be some thick white mucus present. As a girl becomes fertile—just before ovulation—she begins producing clear mucus that gets stringy, like raw egg white, immediately prior to ovulation. This slippery, clear mucus is perfect for helping sperm swim up to the fallopian tubes where they meet the egg. Without this mucus, most sperm can't survive the journey. After ovulation the mucus disappears until the next time ovulation occurs.

A girl should *not* have unprotected intercourse during the entire time she finds clear mucus in her vagina. And she must wait four days after the mucus disappears before she can have unprotected intercourse again.

Usually the mucus appears between four and six days before ovulation and you must wait until four days after ovulation. That means no unprotected intercourse for eight to ten days. Some people who have taken classes in this form of birth control say that they don't usually have to abstain that long. They feel that they become very familiar with their own signs and know when they can have unprotected intercourse and when they mustn't. However, to be safe, you should not have unprotected intercourse for those eight to ten days.

To check your own mucus put a clean finger into your vagina and rub it gently around your cervix. When you pull out your finger it may be fairly dry, with no mucus, or there may be some kind of mucus. If the mucus is clear, assume you are fertile. On fertile days you will also probably feel a wetness in your vagina.

Problems with the mucus method. Any girl who feels strange about touching her genitals won't be able to use the mucus method, since she'd have to put her finger into her vagina once or twice *every day* to check the mucus. If you forget a day, you may miss an important sign.

Another problem is that sperm look and feel like mucus, so if you've had intercourse and some sperm are still in your vagina, you may confuse sperm with mucus. But

people who have learned how to use the mucus method say they can distinguish mucus from sperm.

Our brief description of the mucus method has not given you enough information to use it effectively. It takes supervision and lots of training to use well. If you're interested, call your hospital or local clinic to see if they will instruct you on how to use this method properly. There are several good books about the mucus method.* But even the books suggest that you take a class before using the method. Don't try to use it without supervision from a trained instructor.

The temperature method. There are slight changes in your body temperature around the time of ovulation. If you take your temperature every day, *using a special thermometer,* you can record the changes. Just before ovulation your temperature will dip a little, then just after ovulation it will rise several tenths of a degree.

Problems with the temperature method. Using this method carefully should let you know the day or two before you are going to ovulate, and it will tell you that you have ovulated. But since you can get pregnant by having intercourse three, four, five or six days before ovulation, the thermometer won't help you with that. If you use the calendar and mucus methods, along with the temperature method, you will have a better chance of avoiding pregnancy.

The temperature method is really more effective in helping people who *want* to get pregnant. It tells them exactly when ovulation is occurring so they can have unprotected intercourse then.

Withdrawal. *What is it?* Withdrawal is a form of birth control that boys can use, *but it is not effective.* We recommend condoms for boys who want to be responsible about birth control.

Withdrawal is taking your penis out of the girl's vagina before ejaculation (coming). When a boy says, "Don't worry, I'll pull out in time," he is talking about using withdrawal as his method of birth control.

How does it work? If sperm doesn't get into the vagina, a girl can't get pregnant. So if you pull your penis out of the vagina *before* any sperm are released, no pregnancy will start. But! Even if you are able to pull out before ejaculating, very often drops of sperm escape from the penis during intercourse. You may be leaving some sperm in the vagina before ejaculation, without even knowing it. It takes only *one* sperm to start a pregnancy when the girl is fertile.

Also, sometimes a boy pulls out just as he is beginning to come, and some sperm land on the outer lips of the vagina or on the girl's thighs. This can lead to pregnancy,

---

*Here are two books we recommend: *Avoid or Achieve Pregnancy* (Emergency Publications, 185 Beacon Hill, Ashland, OR 97520); Christine Garfink and Hank Pizer, *The New Birth Control Program* (New York: Bolder Books, 1977).

since sperm have been known to find their way back into the vagina and from there they don't need a map to find the fallopian tube.

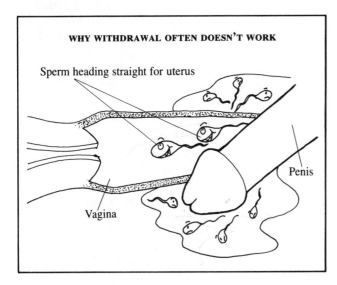

Good points about withdrawal. The only good point about withdrawal is that it's better than using no form of birth control at all. It doesn't cost anything, and you don't have to go to the store or the clinic to get it. But it is the *least* effective of all the methods available. *You can't count on it to work.*

Bad points about withdrawal. The withdrawal method *causes* pregnancy in 30 percent of the couples who use it for birth control. It is the riskiest method.

You may get so excited you forget to pull out, or you don't realize you are about to ejaculate until it's all over, so you don't pull out in time. Withdrawal puts a tremendous burden on you if you are conscientious about using it properly. You have to keep part of your mind on it at all times so that you will remember to pull out *before* ejaculation starts.

With all the responsibility on the boy, that puts the girl in a totally dependent position. If you don't pull out, *she* can get pregnant.

Since there is so much chance for error, both of you may feel tense and worried that something might go wrong. You may not be able to enjoy the lovemaking because of that. You don't have to put yourself in that situation. Choose one of the other, more effective methods of birth control.

Vaginal Suppositories and Tablets. *What are they?* Vaginal suppositories and vaginal tablets contain sperm-killing chemicals. A tablet or suppository is placed into the girl's vagina between fifteen minutes and one hour before intercourse. The sperm-killing chemicals dissolve and spread when they are inside, and they are supposed to cover the cervix, the way foam does. They come in small packets, in boxes of ten to twelve to a box. You can buy

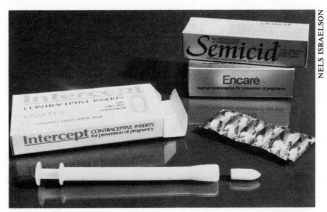

Some vaginal suppositories used for birth control. With an applicator.

these suppositories in drugstores and in some supermarkets.

Be sure to buy only those marked *contraception* or *contraceptive*. Some vaginal tablets or suppositories are not meant for birth control purposes.

Problems with suppositories and tablets. The major problem with these preparations is that they are not very effective. The chemicals do not always spread evenly, so the opening to the cervix is often left unprotected. Also, they can be irritating to a boy's penis.

We do not recommend them, because foam and condoms are much more effective. But like withdrawal, contraceptive suppositories are better than no method at all.

Injectable Contraception. *What is it?* There is a new form of contraception being used in many countries in the world. It is a drug that is injected into a woman every three months to stop ovulation. The most familiar brand is Depo-Provera.

We do not recommend this form of birth control under any circumstances.

Problems with Depo-Provera. Although this drug is being used as birth control in many underdeveloped countries, our own Food and Drug Administration has not approved it for use in this country. That is because there is evidence that Depo-Provera may increase the risk of breast cancer, birth defects and bleeding problems. Once the chemical is in your system, there is no way to get it out until it runs its course.

We recommend the educational comic book *Protect Yourself from Becoming an Unwanted Parent,* by Sol Gordon and Roger Conant (Ed-U Press, 760 Ostrom Avenue, Syracuse, NY 13210; 40¢ each).

So You Think You Might Be Pregnant

Girls can get pregnant. Boys can't. That certainly doesn't come as a surprise to any of you, but we wanted to say it at the beginning because it will help you to understand why we've written this section the way we have. You'll see that a lot of this section is directed to the girls who read it. We say "you" many times when we really mean "those of you who are girls." At the times when it is clear we are talking to the male readers, we say "you" to mean "those of you who are boys." We think the distinction will be easy to see.

We decided to direct much of the discussion to the girl readers because unmarried teenage girls often have to figure out what to do about their pregnancies by themselves—without the support of the boys who helped them get pregnant. In the end it is the girl who makes the decision about what she wants to do, and we believe that is her right, since it's her body and since it's usually she who has to raise the child.

We hope that if you are a boy involved in a pregnancy, you'll want to participate in the decision-making as well as in the parenthood if you decide to have the baby. Many fathers are choosing to be active parents to their children these days, and all of us benefit from that. If you are a boy facing unplanned parenthood, we offer this section as an invitation to join your girlfriend in one of the most important decisions either of you will ever have to make.

How Can You Tell You Might Be Pregnant?

To get pregnant, a girl has to have had intercourse or have been with a boy who ejaculated very near the opening of her vagina. *If you have been having sex you could be pregnant,* even if you're very young, even if you've had sex only once, even if you had sex only during your period, and even if you were using some method of birth control.

Here are some of the signs of pregnancy:

—YOU MISS YOUR PERIOD
—your breasts are tender and seem to be bigger
—you have to urinate a lot
—you feel sick to your stomach in the morning or late afternoon or all the time
—you're more tired than usual, and you feel sleepy during the day, or you get dizzy
—your clothes feel tighter

Not everyone who is pregnant has these symptoms and not everyone who has these symptoms is pregnant.

But if you have had sex with a boy and you have some of these symptoms, plan to have a pregnancy test done as soon as possible.

Missing Your Period. A missed menstrual period is usually the first sign of pregnancy. Some women have a period that is shorter than usual and with less bleeding even though they are pregnant. It's not a normal period. If you miss a period or have a period that doesn't seem quite right, *you may be pregnant.* If you miss a period and have even a few of the other signs of pregnancy, that's a pretty sure indication that you *are* pregnant—but it's not 100 percent sure. The only way to tell for sure is to have a pregnancy test (see p. 192).

A pregnancy won't go away just because you ignore it, and it won't go away because you wish or pray for it to go away.

Once you find out for sure whether you are pregnant or not, then you have a choice. If you are pregnant, you can decide to have the baby or you can decide to have an abortion. If you don't get a pregnancy test right away, then you won't have any choice at all, because by the time your body starts looking pregnant it will be too late to have a simple abortion.

Feelings about a Possible Pregnancy

If you think you might be pregnant, you may have lots of feelings, thoughts and fantasies about it. There are no right or wrong feelings. You don't have to be ashamed of having negative feelings. Lots of people feel angry, upset, scared, shocked and very sad when they find out they are pregnant. You may also feel happy, glad, excited and joyful, and you may have these positive feelings even if you know you don't want to have a baby right now. Lots of people do.

Many people are confused, with negative feelings and positive feelings all mixed up. Here's how fifteen-year-old Carol felt:

We were having sex on the safe days and I wasn't very sure about it but I wasn't getting pregnant, so after a while I started thinking, Well, maybe I can't get pregnant. Then one month I didn't get my period. I didn't want to face it—I kept putting off telling my boyfriend. It was funny because I was sort of glad to find out I could get pregnant but I was miserable about being pregnant.

Sixteen-year-old Bev, a sophomore from San Francisco, told us:

Last semester I got pregnant and I would sit in bed at night, every night, and say, "I don't believe this, this can't be happening to me. Go away. Leave me alone. I can't handle this." I mean, I know that sounds ridiculous, but I didn't know anything and I was so frightened I just thought I'd force my body not to be pregnant.

It's important to remember that many girls and women have been through this same situation. You may feel very alone, but you're not. To get clear about how you're feeling, try to put your feelings into words. You can write out your thoughts in a private diary or journal. You can talk about your feelings with someone you trust, someone who can help you sort out your confusion. Don't let your confusion or fear or anger prevent you from acting, as Roberta, a fourteen-year-old from New Jersey, did:

I thought I was pregnant because I missed my period, but I tried not to think about it. I didn't want to talk to anybody because I was too scared. My mother would have never let me forget it, so I didn't want to tell her, and I didn't want to tell any of my friends because I was afraid word would get around school. But finally I told my boyfriend. He found out where I could get a test done, but I was scared. I'd make an appointment at the clinic and then I wouldn't go. Weeks were going by and finally I talked to my counselor at school who I really like. She was great. She explained everything to me. I went and got the test and it wasn't so bad. But what came out was that I was already five months pregnant, so now I have to have the baby. I can't have an abortion because I'm too far along.

Some people, like Roberta, think they might be pregnant but don't go for a pregnancy test right away because they think it will be a hassle or they worry it will hurt them or they think they'll feel embarrassed. Some people worry that an adult will give them a lecture or they won't have enough money or they won't be able to get to the doctor's office or clinic. Many people don't go for the test because they don't want to face knowing for sure that they are pregnant.

If these kinds of worries are on your mind, remember, it's natural to feel worried. But if you want to have a *choice* you have to have a test done soon. And if you already know you want to have the baby, you need good medical care starting right now—you should eat right, take special vitamins, and stop taking drugs, smoking or drinking alcohol. A healthy baby needs good prenatal care.

If you are pregnant and want to have the baby, we recommend reading the chapters about pregnancy, childbirth and postpartum (after the baby is born) in our book *Our*

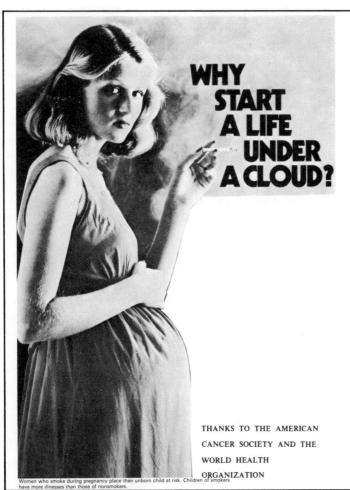

WHY START A LIFE UNDER A CLOUD?

THANKS TO THE AMERICAN CANCER SOCIETY AND THE WORLD HEALTH ORGANIZATION

Women who smoke during pregnancy place their unborn child at risk. Children of smokers have more illnesses than those of nonsmokers.

DANGER!

Studies by doctors and research institutions have proven that *taking drugs, smoking, using caffeine* and *drinking alcohol* can each cause serious complications for the unborn fetus.

Drugs are especially dangerous. All drugs, even aspirin and cold remedies, cross the placenta and reach the fetus. Hard drugs can cause physical deformity and addiction in the baby. Check with your doctor before you take *any* drug, even a prescribed drug, while you are pregnant.

Heavy smokers tend to have low-birthweight babies who are more susceptible to infant death and brain damage.

Caffeine, in cola drinks, coffee, tea and "stay awake" drugs, such as No-Doz, can cause deformities in the fetus.

Alcohol can stunt fetal development both physically and mentally.

You may not find out about the pregnancy until you are one or two months into it. All the drugs and alcohol you might have had during those first months can affect your baby too. That's why if you are having sexual intercourse without using effective birth control, *you should be very careful about what you take into your system. You could be pregnant without knowing it.*

Bodies, Ourselves (pp. 248–316). There are other good books about pregnancy and childbirth available in bookstores and libraries.

The Pregnancy Test

To be sure you are or are not pregnant you need two procedures: (1) a urine or a blood test (the urine test is more common); (2) a pelvic exam—the doctor can see by looking at your cervix and feeling your uterus whether you are pregnant and about how pregnant you are. (See p. 156 for a complete description of a pelvic exam.)

Where to Get the Test Done.   The urine test is available at doctor's offices, clinics or special pregnancy labs. Some of these places offer the blood test too. Some will also do a pelvic exam.

To find a place near you where you can get a pregnancy test:
—Look in the Yellow Pages under Birth Control, Health Agencies, Pregnancy Lab, Abortion, or Family Planning. There should be places listed with phone numbers.
—Call the Planned Parenthood office nearest you. There is probably a Planned Parenthood in some of the major cities in your state.
—Call a women's group or women's health clinic or a local chapter of the National Organization of Women. Ask for a referral. Tell them you think you might be pregnant.
—Call a hospital, public health clinic, free clinic, teen clinic or abortion clinic. Getting the test in an abortion clinic does *not* mean you have to choose to have an abortion if you are pregnant.

When you find a place, call them for an appointment. Your call can be anonymous, which means you don't have to give your name if you just want information. If you like the way they sound, ask if they do pregnancy tests on teens and, if this is important to you, whether they will do it without contacting your parents. Most places do tests for teens and don't contact parents. Some of you will care about this, others won't.

If you make an appointment, get directions about how to get to the place. *Ask about costs.* If money is a problem for you, ask if you can pay in installments. Some places have reduced fees for people who can't afford to pay.

At a lab or health facility a urine test usually costs about $5. The blood test costs more than that, depending on where you go. Some places do free pregnancy testing.

The fee for a pelvic exam and a urine test both can range from a few dollars to more than $60, depending on whether you go to a clinic or a private doctor's office.

Hospitals that accept federal money *must* perform a certain amount of free care.

The Urine Test.   *What is a urine test?* If you are pregnant a special hormone called HCG is released into your urine. A urine test can tell whether HCG is there. A chemical is mixed with your urine, and if the urine reacts one way it means you are pregnant; if it reacts another way it means either you are not pregnant at all or you are not pregnant enough to have enough HCG in your urine yet.

There are several kinds of urine tests available. The one most used can be accurate about forty-two days after your last normal period or about two weeks after your missed period was due. This test is the simplest; it takes about two minutes to complete.

Another kind of urine test can be done sooner, around the time of your missed period. It takes about ninety minutes to complete.

For these tests you must bring a sample of your urine. When you get up in the morning, instead of urinating in the toilet bowl, you hold a *clean, dry* jar under you and urinate in that. Try to get at least a half cup of urine in the jar, then cover the jar. If you aren't going to bring the urine sample into the lab right away, store it in the refrigerator, or if you can't do that, put it in some other cool place (away from the heat) until you can bring it in. The first urine of the morning is usually the strongest and will produce the most accurate test.

You can do a urine pregnancy test for yourself at home if you buy a kit at a drugstore for about $10 to $15. It is very important to follow the instructions *exactly* and to remember that these tests are sometimes not accurate. If the test shows you are pregnant, you should see a doctor for a pelvic exam to make sure. If the test shows you are not pregnant *but you still do not get your period,* have another test done at a lab.

Urine tests done at home or at a lab may not always be accurate. Sometimes the results are wrong because:

—You didn't use your first urine of the morning.
—The sample got too warm by the time it was tested.
—You are too early in your pregnancy for the HCG to show.
—You are too late in the pregnancy for the HCG to be recognized.
—The jar wasn't clean. (If it had chemicals or perfume in it before, that might affect the test. Be sure to wash the jar thoroughly with hot water and make sure it is dry before you use it.)
—You are taking drugs or medicine, such as aspirin in large doses, marijuana, Thorazine, Mellaril, heroin, methadone. Drugs may affect the test.

If the urine test says you are pregnant, believe it. You are probably pregnant, especially if you have other symptoms. To be absolutely sure, have a pelvic exam.

The Blood Test.   *What is a blood test?* HCG is also released into your blood when you get pregnant. A sample of your blood is taken and then a special lab test is run to see if HCG appears.

The blood test for pregnancy is like other blood tests. You go the doctor's office or clinic and a nurse or doctor takes a sample of blood from your body. Usually they draw the sample from a vein in your arm. It may hurt for a second as the needle sticks you. Some nurses and doctors are so good at taking blood that they can do it almost without your noticing.

The blood test can tell if you are pregnant ten days after you miss your period.

Unless you have to find out about the pregnancy immediately, you can wait another week and have a urine test done, which is less expensive and not at all painful.

The Pelvic Exam.   On p. 156 there is a description of what a pelvic examination is like. Read about it so you'll know what's going to happen. Millions of women have pelvic exams every year, because that's the way to get a PAP smear and to check for infections inside your vagina or in your reproductive organs. If you are having sex, you should have a pelvic exam done at least once a year even if you know you're not pregnant.

Lots of women and girls feel uneasy about pelvic exams. That's natural. It takes practice to get used to a doctor examining your insides. But *don't let your nervousness keep you from getting this important exam*, especially if you think you might be pregnant.

If you are pregnant, the examiner will be able to tell because your cervix, which is usually pink or red, will look bluish (because of the enlarged veins filled with blood), and also because your uterus will feel bigger and softer than normal.

Fifteen-year-old Gretchen went to a clinic in Los Angeles for her pelvic exam. She told us:

> When my period was late I knew I could be pregnant and I had to find out for sure because I knew I wanted to have an abortion if I was pregnant. I was so nervous about it because I had never been to the clinic before and I was afraid the people there would be critical of me for being pregnant. I had this dream that this nurse called me to come into the room by shouting so everybody could hear: "*Miss* Blake, how old are you?!!" I woke up scared. But when I finally went everybody was so nice to me. The nurses were all real understanding. I took my best friend with me to the appointment and she was great too.

In Texas, seventeen-year-old Dorrie had this experience:

> When I missed my period I told my sister and her girlfriend, and they were great. They took me to a birth control clinic to get the test done. The clinic was real busy, and I felt like they were rushing me. Everything seemed real impersonal, like they didn't care about you very much. I asked if my sister could come

into the examining room with me when I went in, and at first they said no. But I just about cried and I promised them I would do better with my sister in there with me. Finally someone talked to the nurse and she said OK. This nurse was wonderful. Really. She told me all about what she was doing and the exam was fine. Even my sister learned a lot of stuff she didn't know.

It can be very helpful and comforting to go with someone you trust when you have your tests done. Some places let you bring a friend (even your boyfriend) into the examining room. Other places don't. Some girls prefer to go alone. Decide what will make you most comfortable. Suzanne, a high school senior from Utah, said:

> I went alone for the test because I didn't really have anyone to go with me. The guy I got pregnant by went back to his old girlfriend and I was too embarrassed to tell anybody else about it. I felt pretty funny walking into the clinic, but the people there were so nice I relaxed right away.

Most places that do pregnancy tests for teenagers are set up to make you feel comfortable. Everyone understands that you may be nervous and worried and upset. Lots of times there will be counselors there to talk with you and explain the procedures. They may go over with you all the choices you have if you are pregnant. In most places your visit and your conversations are confidential. Check to be sure.

Finding Out You ARE Pregnant

After the test you will know whether or not you are pregnant. If you are, you may feel relieved to know for sure at last. But you may also be depressed and a little panicky. It's important to try to sort through your feelings to find out what you really want to do now. It's possible that even though you think you might want to end the pregnancy, you still feel glad or proud that you are pregnant. That's very normal. Thirteen-year-old Patty felt that way:

> I knew I couldn't have the baby. I mean I thought, I can't have a baby, I'm just a kid myself. But I had been so worried and so miserable and so sick that I was really glad to find out for sure that I was just pregnant and not dying or something. I mean I felt terrible that I was pregnant, but at least I knew I could do something about that.

When you find out for sure that you are pregnant, you may feel like crying. Lots of girls do. People will understand. You may feel angry and want to scream at the guy who helped you get pregnant. Luisa said that's how she felt:

> I'm so angry I can't stand it. I told Noah I wasn't using birth control, but he said, "Oh, don't worry, I

know what to do.'' How could I have let him talk me into doing it. I was stupid, but he kept saying, ''Don't you love me?''

Barbara, a sixteen-year-old from Denver, said she felt it just wasn't fair:

Why me? I know lots of girls who are doing it, and they aren't pregnant.

What Barbara probably didn't know before is that if you are having sexual intercourse, it's *not* an accident when you get pregnant. It's not a mistake. Unprotected sexual intercourse leads to pregnancy. It may not happen right away, or it may happen the very first time, but it does happen to four out of every five girls eventually.

Some girls who find out they're pregnant feel as if they're being punished for having had sex. Fifteen-year-old Monique said:

We got stoned, and he wanted to have sex and I didn't, but after a while we did it. And the next day I thought to myself, I'm going to be punished for that. And I was right, because I just found out I'm pregnant.

Monique wasn't being punished for having sex. It's perfectly natural to get pregnant after having unprotected intercourse. It's not that the fates or God or some spirit is against you, trying to punish you. *It's just that, in most instances, intercourse without birth control leads to pregnancy.* That's how our bodies are made. It's not a punishment, it's a fact of life.

If You Are Pregnant, These Are Your Choices. When you know for sure you are pregnant, you must choose to continue the pregnancy and have a baby or to end the pregnancy by having an abortion. It will probably help you to make your choice if you answer this basic question for yourself honestly: *Do I want to raise a child?*

On p. 206 there are stories from teenagers who decided yes, they did want to become mothers and raise children. When you read them you'll have a better sense of what being a mother is like.

If you don't think you are ready to be a mother, you have two choices. You can have an abortion, which will end your pregnancy. (Abortion is discussed in detail on p. 201.) Or you can have the baby and give it up for adoption. (That choice is discussed on p. 214.)

For some teenagers it is easy to decide what to do about pregnancy. For others the decision is confusing, painful and difficult. If you have strong, deep feelings about pregnancy, babies, adoption and/or abortion, those feelings will influence your decision. Try to understand where your feelings are coming from before you decide what to do. Here are some of the reactions and experiences other teens have had when faced with the same decision:

Sixteen-year-old Brenda: I love little kids, so I can't

The decision about your pregnancy is one of the most serious you will ever have to make. Help yourself in these ways:

—Read through the rest of this section so you can be clear about your options, your rights and your values. Even if you think you know what you want to do, read on to find out how other people handled the same problem.

—Talk with someone you trust, someone who is realistic and supportive. Weigh the advantages and disadvantages of each choice. Discuss your needs. Talk about your feelings. Figure out how you are going to manage the choice you make. If you don't have anyone to talk with, call your nearest Planned Parenthood or birth control/family planning clinic. These places have understanding counselors on their staff who will be able to help you make a decision that's right for you.

—Share your feelings with the guy with whom you got pregnant. Many boys want to take seriously their responsibility about pregnancy. If the boy you were with is willing, talk to him about his feelings. Find out what he has to say. Let him know what you're thinking. He may be able to help you sort through your choices and he may be able to help you pay the costs of whichever choice you make.

There is no one right choice to make. The decision is yours and you will have to live with the consequences of the decision you make. Make your decision carefully, and make it early, so that if you decide you want to end the pregnancy, you will still have that choice available to you.

wait to have my own. Welfare will help me out. I'm glad I'm pregnant.

Brenda decided to have the baby and keep it. But after a few months she realized she couldn't take care of it and had to give her baby temporarily to a foster care home.

Seventeen-year-old Jo-Ellen: My boyfriend wants me to have the baby. We were going to get married anyway, so now we'll just get married sooner. I can go to college at night.

Jo-Ellen decided to have her baby, but when Jo was nearly six months pregnant, her boyfriend Bill decided he wasn't ready to settle down. They didn't get married. Bill sees the baby once in a while and helps out a little with expenses. Jo-Ellen's living at home with her baby but she's uncomfortable there. When the baby gets a little older she'll put her in day care and try to get a job. Then she hopes to find a place of her own to live.

Fifteen-year-old Denise: Both my sisters got pregnant when they weren't married and they had the babies, and I think they've had it really tough. I want to have a better life than that. It's tough raising a child on your own, especially when you're as young as I am. I'm having an abortion.

Denise had the abortion, and she said she felt bad for a while, but now she can't imagine what her life would have been like if she'd had the baby.

Sixteen-year-old Lisa: I don't believe in abortion. I think it's killing. I'm going to have this baby, and then I'll decide what to do.

Lisa had her baby and decided to keep him. Her mother helps her out by watching the baby while she finishes high school.

What's the Boy's Role in All This?

If you as a boy helped to create a pregnancy, then you may have strong feelings at this time too. It's natural to want to be part of the decision; it's natural, also, to feel very confused. You may in fact be feeling very left out because all the attention is on the girl. She's the one who gets pregnant, she's the one who has to go for the test, and she's the one who has to have the abortion or go through the childbirth. You may feel that there's no role for you in this process, but that's not true. If you care, if you want to be a part of it, you can participate. You also have a responsibility to the girl to help her in any way you can. Sixteen-year-old Stanley told us:

I know some guys skip town or drop out of sight for a while if they get a girl pregnant, but, man, I figure if you were there for the fun you ought to be there for the hard part too. My girl needs me now. I can't let her down.

Like Stan, a lot of boys are concerned about the girl's feelings and well-being. They wonder, Will she be OK? Have I hurt her? Your girlfriend may act very differently now that she's pregnant. She may be depressed and angry and feel panicky about what decision to make. You may have to be extra patient with her at this time.

You, yourself, may have a lot of different feelings. You may be angry too—angry that you didn't use a rubber, or that you didn't pull out in time, or just angry that something as serious as this could have happened. You probably also are worried about what to do. There's a lot to think about and a lot to decide.

In our society men are taught that it's not so cool to be afraid or sad or to worry. Men are taught that they're always supposed to be in control of the situation. But of course men have those feelings and of course men are panicky and out of control sometimes. Everybody is.

If you're having strong feelings about this pregnancy, it helps to talk with a good, close friend, or a parent or relative, a coach, a minister or a teacher you like a lot. You can call a local Planned Parenthood to find out about talking to one of their counselors. You may be embarrassed or feel bad that you and your girl got into this mess, but with help and understanding you'll be able to get yourselves out of it too.

Try to hang in there. You owe it to yourself, the girl, and the possible child to stay involved. Your decision about what to do will have an effect on at least two people's lives, and maybe three people's lives, if the girl gives birth.

Neither you nor your girl may be sure at first what you want to do about the pregnancy. We hope reading further in this section will help you with your decision. Remember, it is important to talk with each other soon about what to do so she can get an abortion if that's what you choose.

Some boys feel proud that they got a girl pregnant. Sixteen-year-old Peter said, "You know you're a man when there's a kid that's yours." Other boys said things like "I'm a man now. No more kid stuff for me," "My girl isn't having an abortion. That's *my* baby in there."

It's very natural to have feelings like that, to be proud and excited that you started a pregnancy. It can make you forget that being a father is a serious responsibility that will totally change your life. Do you want that responsibility? Are you ready to handle it? It would be a good idea to talk with some other teenage fathers to find out what life is like for them. An eighteen-year-old boy from Wyoming told us:

My brother and his girl had to get married because she was pregnant, but they separated a year after the baby came. It was just too hard a life. They kept fighting with each other, and pretty soon Dave moved out and left Paula with the baby. I didn't think that was fair. Now that my girl's pregnant I really think she should have an abortion.

Steve, a seventeen-year-old from San Antonio, Texas, had a different feeling:

I think it will be nice to have a baby. Everybody in our family loves babies, and they'll all help us out. They're real understanding and are behind us.

You and your girl may discuss getting married and keeping the baby. For some people that will seem like the only decision to make. Others of you will know that that isn't the right decision for you. Before you decide, find out who's going to be there to help you out. How do your families feel about it? Will you be able to finish school if you want to? Where will you live and how will you support yourselves? Who's going to take care of the baby while you work? Many, many teenage marriages don't last because marriage isn't easy for anybody. It takes a real commitment to each other and a willingness to adjust to even the hardest times.

Many times pregnancy causes relationships to break up

before there's any discussion about marriage. In New Jersey fifteen-year-old <u>Dominic</u> said:

> Her parents never liked me. When she got pregnant they just shut me out, and after a while I said to hell with them and I stopped seeing her. I never even knew if she had the baby or not.

And in Florida, seventeen-year-old Jerry said:

> I am embarrassed about the way I treated Linda when she got pregnant. I was afraid she'd start pressuring me into marrying her, so I told her I didn't even think it was my kid. I mean, underneath I knew it had to be, but I said that and it made her feel really bad. I told her she better get an abortion and I gave her the money for it. She wanted to have an abortion anyway, but I didn't know that until after I bad-mouthed her. She broke up with me right away after that.

Some boys act as Jerry did and pretend that the baby isn't theirs, even though they're pretty sure it is. It's natural to feel like running away from the problem, because you're facing a big responsibility if you accept your part in the pregnancy. But if you were there for the conception, you should be there for the pregnancy too.

Sometimes it's true that the girl doesn't know who the father is. Sometimes she'll say she thinks it's you, but you don't think so. If she takes the matter to court and *proves* that it is your baby, you will be held legally responsible and you may be required to pay child support.

Sometimes you know you don't want the responsibility of parenthood, so you try to persuade the girl to have an abortion. Bruce tried to talk Kathy into having an abortion, but she didn't want to:

> Kathy wanted to have the baby, and there wasn't anything I could say. My parents even offered to pay for the abortion, but she didn't want to, so now she's married to some other guy and they have *my* baby. That feels pretty weird.

You can't force your girl to have an abortion. You also can't force her to have the baby. In the long run it's her decision. But if you participate, if you both talk about it together, then you have a better chance of finding a solution that will be best for both of you.

Talking with Your Parents

Most teenagers are afraid to tell their parents that they got pregnant or got their girl pregnant. Here are some of the reasons teens gave:

> They'll be so disappointed.

> I know they think I've never had sex. It will shock them and they'll be so angry.

> My father will force us to get married.

> They'll feel so ashamed in front of their family and friends.

> They'll make me break up with Jimmy.

> They'll force me to have an abortion.

> My mom will never let me forget it.

Parents are people too. They're likely to be shocked that their daughter is pregnant out of marriage or that their son got a girl pregnant out of marriage. Sometimes their first reactions express only how upset they are. They may get very angry, they may cry, they may make you feel terrible, but after they get over the first shock, their reactions may change. Parents are usually more understanding than you give them credit for, and generally they are very concerned about your health and happiness. Most parents can be helpful to you if you let them.

Before you talk to your parents about the pregnancy, try to clear up some of your own confusion. Try to figure out what you think you want to do about the pregnancy. Go through the choices and understand what's involved in each of them. That way you will feel better inside yourself when you talk to them. You'll know what your options are and you can help your parents see the different options too.

One of the pregnancy counselors who worked on this section said:

> Whenever I'm talking to teenagers who are worried about telling their parents, I always advise them to practice what they're going to say. I tell them to go over everything with a friend or with someone they trust. That way it's easier when they finally meet with their parents.

A few parents will just not be able to handle the fact that their child is involved in an out-of-marriage pregnancy. Their own upbringing and their own ideas of what is right and wrong will not allow them to be understanding. You have to decide whether your parents will be able to handle

The Abortion Choice: Deciding to End the Pregnancy

> Abortion is *legal*.
>
> The earlier you are in your pregnancy, the easier, safer and cheaper it is to have an abortion.
>
> For a teenager, having an early abortion is safer than having a baby.
>
> Having an abortion does not, except in rare instances with serious complication, affect your ability to get pregnant again.
>
> *You must use birth control after an abortion if you don't want to get pregnant again.*

the news or not. Of course, if you choose to go through with the pregnancy, at least the girl's parents are *bound* to find out. If you decide to have an abortion, you can do that in most places without your parents' knowledge *if you do it within the first three months of the pregnancy*. After that you will need parental consent for an abortion in most states where late abortions are performed in the hospital.

Only the pregnant girl can sign the consent form legally allowing the abortion to be performed, so no one can force you to have an abortion if you don't want one.

An abortion is a medical procedure that removes the pregnancy from the uterus *before* it develops into a baby that could live outside the mother.

Normally, when a girl gets pregnant, an egg from her body and a sperm from a boy's body unite in the fallopian tube and then the fertilized egg moves down into the uterus and attaches itself to the lining of the uterus to grow. (For more on this, see p. 29.) The fertilized egg is called an embryo and at one month the embryo is the size of a pea. At the end of two months, the embryo, which is now called a fetus, is about one inch long and is beginning to take human shape. At three months the fetus is about three inches long and is beginning to develop recognizable body parts.

Determining How Pregnant You Are

Most doctors can figure out how pregnant a woman is by counting the weeks from her *last menstrual period* (LMP). For example, if you had your last period on January 1 and it is now February 12, you are about six weeks pregnant LMP. That means it's been six weeks since your last period.

The actual fact is that you are probably only four weeks pregnant, since conception usually takes place about two weeks after a woman gets her period. But to make calculations easier, doctors usually go by the date of your last period, and in this section we will use the same method.

It is important to know this distinction because many doctors and clinics will not do an abortion more than twelve weeks after your last period. Susan, a sophomore from New York, was confused about how to count weeks. She counted from the day she had intercourse and this is what happened:

I knew exactly when I got pregnant because my boyfriend came into the city for Thanksgiving and that was the only time we had sex all fall. I thought I had plenty of time to have an abortion, so I made an appointment at the clinic for a time when I knew my parents would be away on vacation. But when I went for my abortion, the people at the clinic said I was thirteen weeks pregnant and that was too late to have the abortion. They said I would have to find another doctor. They only did abortions up to twelve weeks LMP. By my calculations I was only eleven weeks

pregnant, but that's because I was counting from the day we had intercourse.

Susan was tremendously upset to find out she'd have to have a more complicated kind of abortion. Don't wait, as Susan did, until the last minute. If you decide to have an abortion, do it as soon as possible. *Many doctors think that between seven and nine weeks is the best time to have an abortion.*

Deciding Whether to Have an Abortion

Abortion is legal, and as a teenager you have the right to have an abortion if you want one.

Abortion is also controversial, and you will have to decide what you believe is "right" for you. Here are the different reactions some teens had when we asked them if they would choose an abortion:

Abortions are OK for other people, but not for me. I don't believe in it for myself.

I'm worried that I would regret it years later.

I feel so lucky to be able to have the choice. If I got pregnant now, I would never be able to have the baby.

I don't think abortion is killing. After all, the fetus couldn't possibly live on its own when it's only two and a half or three months.

My mother got pregnant for the fourth time when she was over forty. She says her abortion was a blessing.

Abortion is my right as a woman.

I think abortion is a sin. If people don't want to have babies, they shouldn't have intercourse.

feelings

There is a lot to think about when you are trying to decide whether or not to have an abortion. Most important, you have to think about what will happen if you don't have an abortion. Do you want to go through nine months of pregnancy? Do you want to go through childbirth? Are you ready to be a mother? How would you feel about giving your baby up for adoption?

If you don't have an abortion you *will* have a baby. That is the decision you have to make.

Mary Elizabeth is seventeen. She comes from Rhode Island and she got pregnant last year. After giving it a great deal of thought, she decided to get an abortion. Here's her story:

I was raised to think that abortion is killing. I saw some of those films that they show you about babies being left to die in garbage pails after an abortion, and I thought it was like murder. I couldn't imagine how anybody could have an abortion. But then, when I got pregnant I had to think about it a different way. I had to think—What can I do for this child? What kind of a life would this child have? I knew if I had the baby I wouldn't be able to give it up. I just knew that. I knew I couldn't go through nine months of being pregnant and then go through childbirth only to sit up and give my baby away to somebody else. So I decided to go to an abortion clinic to find out what I could do. They explained all about the simple kind of abortion I could have if I did it early. They showed me what it would be like. They told me what to expect. I got to thinking, This sounds OK. I got to thinking, This is better than having a baby who might have a miserable life because I can't provide it with anything. And I also got to thinking that I didn't want to have a baby yet. It would wreck *my* life. I have so many things I want to do before I become a mother.

Lurene, a sixteen-year-old from Washington, D.C., made a different decision. She told us:

At first when I found out I was pregnant I thought I would have an abortion, but when it came down to it I couldn't do it. I was brought up very religiously, and I had a real fear of abortion. So I've decided to keep my baby. I feel like this, I chose my own way to go, so I have to take the responsibility that comes with it. And I know I'm making the right decision for me because I'm in love with my baby and it's not even born yet.

Polls show that most Americans believe each woman has the right to decide about abortion for herself. Some people don't agree with that though. They believe that no one has the right to have an abortion. Some of these people belong to organizations that use scare tactics to try to persuade you not to have an abortion. For example, they may tell you that abortions kill babies, when in fact nearly all abortions are performed before the fetus even becomes a baby. The fetus in most abortions is about the size of a lima bean or a walnut and couldn't possibly live outside the mother.

Wanting to have an abortion does *not* mean that:
—you hate children
—you never want to have children
—you are a bad person
—you do not love your boyfriend or girlfriend
—you like the idea of having an abortion
It means that you have decided not to have a child *now*. Most teenagers who choose to have an abortion do not like the idea of having one, but they feel that it is the best alternative for the situation they are in.

When Rebecca found out she was pregnant, she knew she wanted to have an abortion. She called Planned Parenthood right away to make an appointment. We met her there when she went back for a checkup, and this is what she said:

I had a girlfriend who had her first baby when she was sixteen, and she told me she had really wanted to have that baby. She said she wouldn't think about having an abortion. But after she had the baby she realized what a big responsibility it was. She was up half the night and she never got to go out and she was always changing diapers and always having to be with her baby. So when I got pregnant I knew there was only one choice for me—to have an abortion. I wouldn't want to have a baby until I could take care of that baby myself. I want to have my own job and make my own money before I have a baby. I want to be able to afford baby-sitters and I don't want to have to depend on my parents. I wouldn't even want to depend on my boyfriend because he could leave, and then where would I be?

Other teenagers we interviewed gave these reasons for having an abortion:

Joan (fourteen): I know what it's like to grow up without a father. My father left when I was three and my mother had to raise us alone. She had to go to work, and my brothers and I ran wild. I always felt bad about not having a father, so I don't want to do that to my kid.

Peggy (sixteen): My boyfriend wants me to have the baby. He says he'll support it. But I want someone to give me more than money. I want someone to help me take care of it—be a real father. I just can't see us being together for the next eighteen years!

Mike (fifteen): I feel bad about Suzi having an abortion, but I know I'm not ready to be a father. I'm still a kid myself.

Georgia (sixteen): If I had this baby, I'd have to live at home for the next three or four years. My mother said she'd take care of the baby while I went to school, but then I'd be so dependent on my mother. I think she'd always throw it up in my face that she was taking care of my kid.

Since it is such an important decision, you may want to talk over your feelings about abortion with a close friend, a parent, a favorite relative or a counselor. Find someone whom you trust and feel comfortable with. If they tell you abortion is right or wrong, and they try to persuade you to either have the abortion or not have it, that may not be very helpful for you. The best person to talk to is someone who will listen carefully to what you have to say. Someone who will help you make up *your own* mind, not tell you what they think you should do. If your parents are understanding, they would be the best people to talk to. They may also be able to help you find a place and help you pay for the procedure if you choose to have the abortion.

Your Legal Rights. If you are thinking about having an abortion you may wonder:

—Can my parents make me have an abortion?
—Do I need my parents' consent to have an abortion?
—Will my parents be notified if I have an abortion?

The decision to have an abortion is yours as the pregnant girl. *No one can force you to have one if you don't want to.* No doctor, clinic or hospital can legally do an abortion unless they have *your written consent. Don't sign anything until you read it first, and if you don't understand the language, ask to have it explained to you until you do understand.*

The Supreme Court has ruled that minors (people under eighteen) can get an abortion without parental consent. Some doctors and clinics require parental consent anyway if you are a minor. These places are afraid of lawsuits brought by angry parents. If getting your parents' consent will be a problem for you, ask the people at the clinic when you call for an appointment if they require written parental consent before performing abortions on minors. Many places will perform simple abortions (when you are *under* twelve weeks pregnant) without parental consent.

But most doctors and clinics *do* require the consent of one parent if you are more than twelve weeks pregnant. That is because you are more likely to need hospital care either because of the late abortion or because of complications. Minors must have parental consent for hospital care.

Most clinics will *not* notify your parents if you have an abortion because that would violate your rights to privacy of health care. But just to be sure, ask the doctor or clinic about their policy.

You will have to decide for yourself what is best in your own situation, but many teenagers we talked with said they were glad to have told their parents. Most parents *want* to help their children, especially when their children are in trouble.

> If you have any questions about your rights or if you believe a doctor or clinic has violated your rights, call the National Abortion Federation at 1-800-223-0618. That is a toll-free number, so it will not cost you anything. If you live in New York City, call 688-8516. You may also call your local chapter of the American Civil Liberties Union (ACLU), a local chapter of the National Organization of Women (NOW) or Planned Parenthood.

Where to Get an Abortion

In your community there may be many, few or no places at all that provide abortions. If you live in or near a big city, there is probably at least one abortion clinic there, and there are probably several doctors who do abortions privately. Remember: *abortion is legal.* Just try to find the best person possible to do it.

Some clinics do not offer as good a service as you would want. Some charge more than you should pay. That's why you should check around and choose your doctor or clinic carefully.

To find out about abortion services in your area, call the *National Abortion Federation hot line* at 1-800-223-0618 (a toll-free number). In New York City call 688-8516. This organization has information about clinics all over the United States. You might also call the Planned Parenthood clinic nearest you. This national family planning organization has offices in almost every state. Look in the phone book for their number or call the main office in New York City at 1-212-677-3040.

You can also check the Yellow Pages under Family Planning, Health Agencies, Abortion or Birth Control. If you know of a women's group or clinic in your area, they will probably be able to give you information about where to go for an abortion.

Checking Out Abortion Services.   After you have the names of some clinics and doctors or hospitals that perform abortions, take a little time to check them out. Phone them or drop in for a visit. You'll be able to tell a lot by how friendly they are, how much attention they give you, whether they answer your questions carefully, and whether they make you feel welcome. Does their office seem well run? Is it clean? Some clinics are mostly interested in making money. You can use this checklist to help you make your choice:

—Consider the kind of attention you get over the phone—are all your questions answered with respect?

—Ask if you need your parents' consent and/or if the doctor or person in charge will notify your parents even if you don't want them involved.

—Ask what kinds of anesthesia are offered. After you read about anesthesia on p. 201 you will know whether you want local anesthesia or general anesthesia. Some clinics offer only local anesthesia because that has fewer risks. Not offering a choice of anesthesia isn't necessarily an indication of poor service.

—Ask about emergency backup procedures. What hospital do they use if hospital services become necessary? Are they equipped to provide blood transfusions and/or oxygen at the clinic?

—Ask about the fee. How much will the entire abortion and postabortion checkup cost? If you have Rh negative blood you will need a special shot of Rhogam (see p. 201). Ask if that is included in the price or if it is extra. How much extra? Do they provide birth control services?

—Ask if you will have time to talk with a counselor by yourself, if you would like that. Some clinics only offer group counselor sessions. That can be wonderful, but some people need a private session to really get comfortable.

—Ask if you can bring a friend (your boyfriend, your mother, your sister, anyone you choose), and ask if that person can be allowed into the abortion room with you—if you'd like that. Some people feel much better with a friend holding their hand during the abortion.

—Make sure the person doing the abortion will be a

licensed physician. It is illegal for anyone but a licensed physician to do an abortion.
—Ask if there will be a staff member in the abortion room just for your comfort and support.

Use this list while you're on the phone and go through all these points. You'll be able to tell a lot about the kind of service they give by the way they listen to and answer the questions. If you have a choice, take the clinic that sounds as if it will offer you the best care. If you have some concerns about your choice, call the numbers we listed above for advice. Remember: don't be afraid to ask questions. *You have a right to receive the best care possible.*

Paying for the Abortion

Most health facilities will not do the abortion unless you have the proper amount of money in cash, certified check or money order in hand on the day of the abortion. Many places will *not* take a personal check. When you call the place to make an appointment, find out how they expect to be paid.

For many teenagers abortions are expensive (between $125 and $200) and abortions done after the first twelve weeks are even more expensive (from about $300 up). You will have to be resourceful in getting the money together if you don't have it. Here are some suggestions:

—Talk with your parents about it, if you can, or talk to some other adult you trust. See if they will loan you the money.
—Ask the boy who helped you get pregnant. It's only fair that he pay at least half, especially since you're the one who has to go through the hassle of the actual abortion.
—Ask some of your friends for small loans. Tell them it's for a personal emergency (if you'd rather not tell them it's for an abortion). Remember, if you are afraid to let anyone know you need an abortion, they'll find out for sure if you stay pregnant.
—Call the clinic or doctor and ask about a reduced fee or a partial payment plan (where you pay some money at the time of the abortion and the rest in future payments). *Many clinics have been ripped off by people who asked for a payment plan and then never paid their debt.* That's why not many places offer such a plan anymore. For the sake of other teens, if you are allowed to pay in installments, be sure to continue paying until your debt is cleared.
—See if you are eligible for Medicaid coverage; some states do pay for abortions. The Hyde Amendment has made it impossible for the federal government to pay for abortions, but some states do pay for abortions under Medicaid. Call your local Planned Parenthood or the National Abortion Federation at 1-800-223-0618. We know of no place that offers free abortions. Write to us if you find one. Our address is on p. 232.

—See if your private health insurance will pay for the abortion, although this will probably have to involve your parents.

If none of these ideas works for you, and you can't think of a way to raise the money for your abortion, call one of the phone numbers listed on p. 199 and ask for advice. Or call the local Planned Parenthood and ask to speak to a counselor. Don't be embarrassed. They will be glad to talk with you about your problem.

Remember, the longer you wait to get the money, the more expensive the abortion may be. Abortions within the first twelve weeks are the cheapest.

Risks and Complications Associated with Abortions

For teenagers, abortion is safer than childbirth if the abortion is performed within the first three months. But sometimes there are complications. The most frequent problems are infection, tearing of the lining of the uterus, blood loss—losing more than a pint is serious—and incomplete abortion, which means the doctor missed some of the tissue that was part of the pregnancy.

It is very important to watch your recovery carefully and to follow exactly the aftercare instructions given by the doctor or clinic. (See p. 204 for an example of aftercare procedures.) If you notice any warning signs, such as fever, excess bleeding or extreme pain, *call your doctor, clinic or hospital immediately.*

If you have more than one abortion, every time you have an abortion you run the same physical risks.

There may be emotional complications too. Most women and girls are able to cope with the idea of abortion, and even if they are upset before and after, they are glad to have done it. Other women and girls choose not to have an abortion because they truly consider it wrong and do not want to participate in an act they think of as killing. One teenage mother we met in Michigan had had an abortion two years before her baby was born. She told us that she is sorry she had the abortion:

I wish I had thought more about my decision to have that abortion. At the time I was so desperate I didn't know what else to do. After all, I was only fifteen. But I don't think it's right to say that abortion isn't killing just because the fetus is too small to live outside the mother. That's not the point. If you don't have the abortion, the fetus will grow to be big enough to live. That's the point.

It is important to give your decision about abortion a lot of careful thought. Most people feel relieved and glad they ended an unwanted pregnancy after it's over. But some people feel guilty, sorry and victimized for having had an abortion. You're going to have to consider *beforehand* whether you'd be more upset about an abortion or about having a baby you aren't ready to take care of.

Remember: In the future, the best solution is to use effective birth control whenever you have sex. Birth control is the best protection against having to make this hard decision again.

Anesthesia. Abortions are painful for some women and girls. Early abortions tend to be much easier, with much less cramping than late abortions which usually cause more cramping. Each person is different, and how you experience your abortion will be individual.

To help you cope with the possible discomfort, doctors and clinics provide a variety of pain-killing substances. For very simple, early abortions you may find that a pain-numbing tranquilizer is all you need. Some people prefer to have a shot of local anesthetic. This numbs the area around the cervix. It can be very helpful. Some girls are afraid of the shot, so they choose not to have it. Actually, there are few nerve endings in the cervix, so the shot is generally not very painful at all.

Some clinics and hospitals will give general anesthesia before the abortion, which puts the patient to sleep. This is usually done with an injection of sodium pentothal. General anesthesia will make the abortion painless, since you'll be asleep, but when you wake up you may feel cramping, and some people also feel dizzy, disoriented, or nauseated. General anesthesia affects your entire body, and therefore it has its own risks. *You must not eat or drink anything*—not even water—for twelve hours before having general anesthesia.

Some doctors and clinics give you a choice between local or general or no anesthesia; others provide only one type of anesthesia. If you wish to have a choice, ask about that when you are checking for a place to have the abortion.

Remember, no matter what kind of pain-killer you had, if you had any, after the abortion, you will still probably feel cramping when the medication wears off as your uterus returns to its prepregnant size. This is normal.

Having the Abortion

There are several types of abortions. The type you have depends on how pregnant you are. It also depends on what types are done by the doctors in your area. In this section we will describe in detail three of the most common types of abortion.

Vacuum Suction (Vacuum Aspiration) Abortion. This is the most common abortion. It is used *only* if you are *under* twelve weeks pregnant. It takes about four to seven minutes, and it can be done in a doctor's office, a clinic or a hospital. You do not have to stay overnight, but you should plan to stay for about four to six hours because there will be time needed before the abortion for explanations, pregnancy tests and counseling, and time needed after the abortion for recovery.

If you're having this type of abortion, plan to arrive at the place on time, but since sometimes clinics and doctors run late, you may have to wait. Bring a book and/or a friend to talk with. It's a good idea to bring a friend anyway for support and encouragement.

First you will have lab work done: another urine test to make sure you're pregnant, a blood pressure check and a blood test to see what type of blood you have.

If you have something called Rh-negative blood—about one in ten patients do—you will probably need to have an injection of a medicine called Rhogam within seventy-two hours after the abortion. This will keep you from having certain complications with your next pregnancy.*

After the lab work, some clinics and doctors offer group or individual patient-education sessions. A nurse or coun-

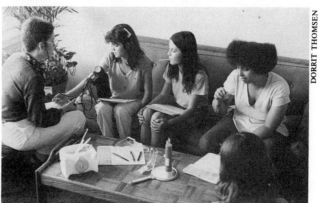

A group counseling session at a women's clinic

selor may tell you about what to expect in the abortion, answer any questions you have, talk to you about your decision to have an abortion. They want to make sure that *you're sure* you want to have one before they do it. These sessions can be very helpful and reassuring. They will probably also discuss methods of birth control and how to use them, so that after the abortion you won't have to get pregnant again until you *choose* to (see p. 159 for a complete discussion of birth control). Here's what Debby, a sixteen-year-old girl from Los Angeles, told us about her preabortion counseling session:

> I went to a women's clinic for my abortion, and they were really great. About five of us were there at the

*Most people have Rh-positive blood. Some people have Rh-negative blood, which means their blood has a slightly different composition. It is perfectly normal, but if an Rh-negative mother is pregnant with an Rh-positive baby, birth or abortion can cause her body to build up antibodies against the Rh-positive blood from the baby or fetus. These antibodies may affect a future pregnancy and harm the next Rh-positive fetus. If Rhogam is given within seventy-two hours after an abortion or childbirth, it will prevent antibodies from forming in the mother's blood. A shot of Rhogam can cost from $50 to $70. If you can't afford it, ask for financial assistance. If you have Rh-negative blood, *it is very important to have Rhogam after every abortion and/or childbirth.*

same time for abortions, and first we all had urine tests and blood tests and stuff like that. I really liked doing the urine test because they let us do our own. First we took turns going into the bathroom to pee in this little cup. Then we came out and mixed a drop of pee with something they gave us and we watched what happened. One girl found out she wasn't really pregnant after all, and we all cheered for her. Then after that we all went into this dressing room where we sat around talking about what the abortion would be like. The head of the group was a counselor who had had two abortions herself, so she told us about what it was like for her. That really made me feel better. I figured if she could do it, so could I. We talked about whether it might hurt. One person said that she'd had an abortion that didn't hurt at all, but someone else said she heard that it did hurt. They recommended we have a shot of local anesthetic. (I decided to have that, and I was glad, because the abortion did hurt me and it would have hurt more if I hadn't had the shot.) We also talked about our feelings about abortions and pregnancy. One person started crying a little, and everyone was real supportive and we told her it would be OK.

In this example Debby was part of a group-counseling session. In many clinics, individual counseling is available. Ask about that when you call places. Some people prefer individual counseling.

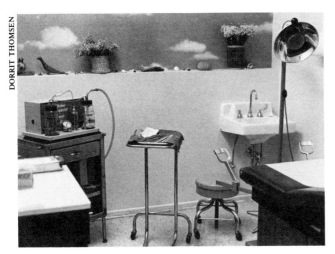

An abortion room

After the preabortion session you will be called when it's your turn for the abortion. You can ask if they will let you bring your friend into the abortion room with you. Some places let you do that. Usually there will be a counselor with you to hold your hand and reassure you. (Ask about that when you call for an appointment.)

The room where the abortion is done usually looks like any doctor's examining room. You'll be asked to undress from the waist down; some places ask you to undress all the way and put on a hospital gown. The doctor will first

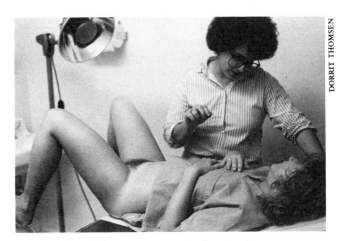

A counselor talking to a woman in the abortion room

give you a pelvic exam, to check to be sure that you are pregnant and that you are under twelve weeks (LMP) pregnant.

If you're having general anesthesia, you will probably get an injection of sodium pentothal in your arm now, fall asleep and wake up after the abortion is over.

If you are having local or no anesthesia, the doctor or nurse will probably offer you some medication to relax you before you even go into the abortion room. It will probably be a tranquilizer, which you should take about a half hour before the abortion. Take the medication *only* under the doctor's supervision. Don't take any drugs at all at home before you come. If you have taken something, be sure to tell the doctor or nurse. (For a complete discussion of the different types of anesthesia, see p. 201.)

After the pelvic exam the doctor will insert a speculum into your vagina so she or he can see your cervix and hold the walls of your vagina open (see p. 157).

If you are having local anesthesia, the doctor will inject a medicine like Novocain (what dentists use to numb your mouth) into your cervix to numb the area. The injection takes a few seconds and may feel a little uncomfortable. Since the cervix is not very sensitive, it may not hurt as much as you might expect. Try to relax during the shot. Breathe deeply and hold someone's hand.

For the abortion, your cervix has to be opened wide enough to allow the suction tube to enter the uterus. The suction tube is about as wide as a piece of chalk. The cervix is the only opening to the uterus, and usually it is almost closed. Opening the cervix often feels uncomfortable. It can cause cramping and pain. Local anesthesia will probably reduce a lot of that discomfort.

For opening your cervix the doctor will use a dilator. Dilators come in different sizes, from the size of a matchstick to the width of a thumb. The doctor will start stretching open the cervix with the smallest dilator and use bigger ones gradually until the opening is wide enough for the abortion. *The later you are in the pregnancy, the wider the opening has to be.*

Dilating takes about two minutes. You may feel sharp cramps at this time or strong pressure. Use breathing exercises to help you relax. Relaxing will ease the pain considerably.

BREATHING EXERCISES

1. Relax as much as you can. Let your legs flop apart and your arms hang loose. Let your mouth drop open too.
2. Keep your toes and fingers relaxed. Try not to let them curl up tight. If there is someone's hand to hold, you may want to do that, but try to keep your toes relaxed.
3. Blow out all the air in your lungs and take a deep breath. Watch your stomach rise as you breathe in. Then breathe out all the air and watch your stomach fall. This deep breathing will help you relax.

If you are feeling too much pain to relax, take a breath that fills your *chest,* then blow it all out slowly. Take another breath and blow it all out. This type of breathing is shallower than deep breathing. Concentrate on blowing all the air out. Make noise if you have to. Keep up the breathing for as long as you want to. The dilation lasts for only a few minutes.

Some abortion facilities use a piece of seaweed, called laminaria, to dilate the cervix. It is the size and shape of a wooden matchstick. It's inserted into your cervix at least six hours prior to the abortion, and some places put it in the day before the abortion and let it work overnight. As the laminaria absorbs fluid, it expands and causes the cervix to open wider. It causes a more gradual opening and may cause less cramping and discomfort.

After the cervix is open, the abortion can begin. A clear plastic hollow tube with a suction tip is inserted into the cervix. It is attached to a suction machine. When the machine is turned on, gentle suction is produced in the tube. The doctor moves the tube around in your uterus and cleans out the embryo or fetus, the tissues surrounding it, and the excess lining of the uterus. (This may hurt, so try to relax and use your breathing techniques. The more you relax, the less it will hurt.) After all that has been removed from your uterus, *you are no longer pregnant.* It takes only a few minutes.

The doctor will check for any remaining particles inside the uterus. With a special utensil she or he will gently scrape along the inside of the uterus to be sure the pregnancy and loose tissue have been completely removed. This may take an extra minute. So the whole abortion itself takes no more than five minutes.

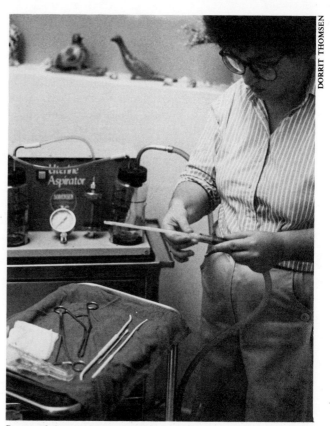

Some of the equipment used to perform an abortion

If you have not had general anesthesia, you will be awake and you may feel mild to heavy cramping. That's because your uterus, which is a muscle, is contracting back to its prepregnancy size.

As soon as you feel ready to get up, usually only several minutes after the abortion, you will put on a sanitary napkin to catch any bleeding and dress yourself. You will then go into the recovery area, where you can relax and have something to eat or drink. Your friend may be allowed to come with you into the recovery area. This is how one fifteen-year-old girl described her feelings right after her abortion:

> What a relief! I mean, *what a relief!* All I can say is thank God abortion was a choice for me because I just could never have made it with a baby.

Give yourself a chance to breathe a sigh of relief if that's how you feel. It's over and you're not pregnant anymore. You may have lots of other feelings too, like sadness, fear, regret, worry, and we'll talk more about those feelings a little later (see p. 205).

Most people feel ready to get up right after the abortion. You may continue to bleed and cramp for a while; most women do. If the cramps stay strong for more than twenty or thirty minutes, ask the nurse for some pain medication. The bleeding may last just a few hours or several days.

Some women stop and then start again. *If you have very heavy bleeding, heavier than your normal menstrual flow, be sure to call the doctor or clinic right away.* That may be a sign of infection or an incomplete abortion.

The doctor or clinic will give you instructions on how to take care of yourself after the abortion. Your body needs a chance to get back to normal. We discuss aftercare instructions on p. 205.

D-and-C Abortion (Dilatation and Curettage). This type of abortion can be done between twelve and fourteen weeks pregnancy (LMP). It takes about seven to ten minutes to perform, and it can be done in a doctor's office or clinic, but it is often done in a hospital. General anesthesia is always used, which means you are put to sleep during the operation. The fee for a D-and-C (or D-and-E, see below) is usually between $250 and $350.

This type of abortion is similar to the suction abortion. Your cervix will be dilated (opened) as in the suction abortion, but since the fetus is larger, the doctor will use a curette—a scraping instrument—to remove the fetal tissue and excess lining from your uterus.

There is slightly more risk with this kind of abortion because your pregnancy is further along and the fetus is larger. Also, scraping is a bit more complicated than the suction technique.

A newer form of abortion, available in some places, combines the D-and-C with the suction method. It is called D-and-E (Dilatation and Evacuation). It can be done between twelve and eighteen weeks of pregnancy (LMP), and it takes about twelve to twenty minutes.

The aftercare for the D-and-C or D-and-E abortions are the same as for the suction abortion.

Induced Abortion. An induced abortion, also called a saline or prostaglandin abortion, is used if a woman is over sixteen weeks pregnant (LMP). This type of abortion is really a medically induced miscarriage. A liquid is injected into your uterus and that causes labor to begin. Your body removes the pregnancy itself. This type of abortion is always done in a hospital and a woman has to stay for two to three days. You can have an induced abortion up to twenty-four weeks (LMP), but with a prostaglandin abortion, after twenty weeks there is a chance that the baby could be born alive.

Your parents will have to give their consent if you are under eighteen and want an induced abortion. It will probably cost between $350 and $500.

In the hospital you will undress and put on a hospital gown. You will lie on a hospital bed. A patch of skin on your belly will be numbed with local anesthetic and then the solution will be injected. The doctor puts a needle through the abdomen, about three to six inches below the bellybutton. This feels like pressure to many women. Some fluid from inside the uterus is withdrawn and it is replaced by a hormone, prostaglandin, or saline, a salt solu-

tion. If saline is used, you may feel bloated and thirsty. It's good to drink a lot.

About five to fifty hours later the uterus will begin to contract and push out the fetus and other matter inside your uterus. This can be painful. There's no way to know in advance how long it will take or how painful it will feel to you.

After the fetus is expelled, the uterus shrinks back to its prepregnancy size. That may cause cramping too.

This type of abortion can be very hard on you not only physically, because it takes a long time and can be painful, but also emotionally, because when the fetus comes out you will see that it looks like a baby. Between sixteen and twenty-four weeks the fetus goes through a lot of growth and development. The earlier you have the abortion, the less like a baby the fetus will be.

Some hospitals offer counseling and some don't. It will be very helpful to you to find someone to talk with before and after the experience. If the hospital allows it, try to bring your boyfriend or an older woman (your mother, your sister, your aunt, a counselor) you like and trust to stay with you during the abortion. If they've been through childbirth, they will be able to reassure you and support you.

Physical Aftercare

Most girls and women have almost no physical aftereffects from the suction-type abortion. They feel fine right away and can leave the clinic within the hour. Later abortions require a little more recovery time.

No matter what type of abortion you had, physical aftercare is very important. Your doctor or clinic will give you instructions on how to take care of yourself. Follow them carefully. The box below contains an example of aftercare instructions.

If after the abortion you continue to have pregnancy symptoms—swollen, tender breasts, increased urination, tiredness, weight gain—you may still be pregnant. In very rare cases the abortion does not remove the fetus. Sometimes the pregnancy is developing someplace other than the uterus. This is called an ectopic pregnancy (see p. 39 for details). Report your symptoms to the doctor or clinic immediately and go in for a checkup.

If you haven't told your parents about your abortion, it may be hard to take care of yourself the way you should, especially if you have a lot of bleeding and/or cramping. You may try to pretend that everything's fine, when really you're not feeling well at all. Sally told us that happened to her:

After my abortion I was really sick for a couple of days. Nothing serious, I just felt awful. But I didn't tell my parents, so I had to pretend I was OK. We had to go on this hike—it was planned and everybody

---

PHYSICAL AFTERCARE

—Watch for fever. Take your temperature in the morning and night for about five days after the abortion. If it goes over 100.5°, call the doctor or clinic.

—Watch your bleeding. It may stop and then start again. It may last a few hours or a few days or even a week. It shouldn't be heavier than your period. If it is heavy and lasts for a long time, call the doctor or clinic.

—Expect your next normal period to come in about four to six weeks.

—Call the doctor if you have severe pain or cramping or an unusual vaginal discharge.

—For *two weeks,* to prevent irritation and infection, don't take a bath, swim, use tampons, have intercourse or douche. In other words, don't put water or anything else into your vagina. You can shower and wash with a washcloth.

—Take it especially easy for a day or two. Don't do anything strenuous. After that you can have normal activity as soon as you feel like it.

—Have a checkup two weeks after your abortion to be sure everything is going well and your body is back to normal.

—*Get birth control so you won't be risking another unplanned pregnancy* (see p. 159).

---

was going, and I was feeling so bad. But I figured, If I don't go, everyone will be asking me what's wrong. I might have been able to tell my mother, but I just couldn't tell my father. He'd be so disappointed if he knew.

Sally never did tell her parents and she did go on that hike, but her bleeding increased, so she had to go back to the doctor to make sure her body was healing properly. The doctor told her she had to get plenty of rest and not even to think about going on another hike until her bleeding stopped. Most girls don't feel sick after the abortion, so they can resume normal activities even before the bleeding has stopped completely.

Most girls and women have almost no aftereffects from the suction-type abortion. They feel fine right away.

Emotional Aftercare

You may have a lot of strong feelings for a while after the abortion. Many people experience that sense of relief we talked about before, but lots of people also feel sad. It's very natural to feel both relieved and sad. It's also normal to feel other things.

For some girls and women it is confusing. They wonder, Why do I feel so sad when I know I really did the right thing?

When you're younger and you think about growing up and having a baby, somehow you never imagine that your first pregnancy might end with an abortion. So even though abortion may be exactly the right choice for you, you still may feel sad about it.

Here are some of the things people feel after they've had an abortion:

Anger. You may be angry with the reaction you got from your boyfriend, parents or friends; or you may be angry with the poor care you got from the doctor or people at the clinic; or you may be angry that you got pregnant in the first place, that your birth control didn't work, that you were careless, that you got ''caught'' when you know other people who haven't gotten ''caught'' yet.

Anger is natural after an abortion. You aren't bad or sick or mixed up to have such feelings. But if you keep your anger inside, it will make you confused and depressed. Talk about your anger with someone you can trust. Fourteen-year-old Susie went to a counseling center in Los Angeles. She said:

After the abortion I was so angry at my boyfriend Billy I couldn't stand him. Everything he did got me mad. The counselor helped me to see that my feelings were pretty normal. After all, *I* had to have the abortion, not Billy. I talked to him about how I was feeling, and, in fact, we had a big fight about it because he said he couldn't help it if boys don't get pregnant. When we made up I was really glad I told him what was on my mind. And now we're both totally committed to using rubbers.

Guilt. You may feel guilty for having an abortion, for not telling your parents, for not telling your boyfriend, for not using birth control, or for having had sex in the first place. Many girls feel guilty for being relieved that they're not pregnant anymore. They feel they should have been punished. Guilt is a way of punishing yourself.

If you had an abortion you probably did it because you weren't ready to be a parent. You were taking care of yourself, and that's very important to remember. You were faced with a very hard decision and you made a choice. If you now think that choice was a mistake, you probably won't have another abortion. But remember, *everyone makes mistakes.* And later in your life you may come to feel that it was a good decision, after all. The important thing is, if you use birth control faithfully from now on, you won't be faced with such a hard decision in the future.

Depression. Some depression after an abortion may be caused by the drop in your body's hormones when the pregnancy is ended, especially if you were pretty far along into the pregnancy. But most postabortion depression is caused by conflicting feelings. You may be feeling angry, guilty, sad, disappointed and vulnerable all at once. Try to figure out where your feelings are coming from. Try not to judge yourself. You did what you thought was the best thing.

Fear. Seventeen-year-old Lynn said:

> I've had two abortions, and I'm worried because I've heard all these things about how too many abortions can keep you from being able to have a baby. I really want to have children when I get older, so hearing those things scares me.

The abortion will not keep you from getting pregnant again, unless you had very serious complications. But each time you have an abortion you run the risk of having complications, so *avoid problems by using birth control.*

Sometimes you may feel scared because you think you ought to be punished for having an abortion. You feel selfish or you feel weak. It might help you to remember that people have abortions because they are not ready to have babies. People have abortions because they don't want to add another unwanted child to the world population. People have abortions because they feel like children themselves and know they can't handle the responsibilities of parenthood. You did what you did because at the time you thought it was the right thing to do. That's not weak, that's strong.

Strength. Many girls feel strong and proud of themselves for coping with such a heavy experience as an unwanted pregnancy. You may feel good that you made the decision you made and carried it through. That was Betsey's experience:

> I felt very grown-up after the abortion. I didn't fall apart. I knew that if I could pull something like this off, I could take care of myself when I had to. It's a good feeling.

Feelings about Sex. After an abortion, many people get reliable birth control for the first time and feel relieved knowing that they can have intercourse without getting pregnant.

But some people feel turned off to sex for a while. It is important to know that this feeling usually changes with time. Some teens say they want to "withdraw and regroup their forces" before they are ready to have sex again.

If this is how you feel, respect it. Don't push yourself. Often, if you had mixed feelings about having had sex in the first place, getting pregnant may seem like a "punishment." You may be afraid it will happen again. Fifteen-year-old Daisy said:

> I was glad when they told me I couldn't have intercourse for two weeks after the abortion. After the two weeks was up, I just never seemed to be in the mood. I kept thinking that I was going to get pregnant again.

Peter, also fifteen, said:

> Neither Nina or I felt like doing it for a long time

after the abortion. I guess we felt badly about the abortion and didn't want to take any more chances until we knew we could handle it.

Barbara, one of the women who helped us with this book, reports:

> As a counselor, many young people have told me after an abortion: "I don't need birth control. I'm never having sex again!" But a lot of these teenagers get pregnant again. Although they feel strongly about not having intercourse for a while, people and situations change. If you are not ready with some form of birth control you are risking another unplanned pregnancy.

Having the Baby: Deciding to Keep the Pregnancy

If you are pregnant and decide not to have an abortion, you are deciding *to have a baby*. Even if you make your decision by just not doing anything—not having a pregnancy test to find out for sure that you are pregnant, not finding out about abortion, trying to pretend that you're not really pregnant—*that* is a decision to have a baby.

But choosing to have a baby is one of the most important decisions a person ever makes. Whether you keep the baby or give it up for adoption, the fact that you had the baby will change your life and your baby's life forever. It's not a decision just to let happen—it deserves a lot of thought and careful planning to make sure you want to do it and are able to handle what will be involved.

In this section we will try to help you figure out if either you really want to be a parent now or you are ready to give a child what he or she needs from a parent.

What Are Your Choices? If you decide to have the baby, you have three basic choices:

1. To keep the baby and try to raise it yourself.
2. To put the baby in foster care until you can care for it.
3. To give the baby up for adoption.

We will discuss these choices in the following pages.

The Choice to Become a Parent

Sixteen-year-old Lucy was attending a meeting at a home for unwed mothers when we met her. She said:

> When I was first pregnant with Heidi I was only fourteen. I could have had an abortion, but there was just this feeling that I wanted to have somebody to depend on me. I wanted to have this little baby who would just love me.

We'll tell you more about Lucy and Heidi in a minute. First we want to talk about Lucy's reason for having Heidi. Many girls we interviewed expressed feelings a lot like Lucy's:

> I like having someone who needs me.

A baby's skin is so soft. They're so sweet and cuddly.

I'm in love with kids. They need you so much.

I'm going to be a great mom. I'll always be there for my baby.

And lots of boys whose girls were pregnant had similar things to say:

I'll be proud to have a kid of my own.

I like having a family to take care of.

I don't want my girl getting an abortion. That's my kid in there and I'm going to take care of it.

The creation of a human life—a baby—is wonderful, and seems magical or like a miracle to many of us. Most of us have very positive and even romantic feelings when we think about having a baby of our very own.

The *idea* of having a baby can be dreamy. We can imagine how good it will feel holding a soft, little, snuggly baby. We can picture what it will be like dressing our baby up and taking him or her out for a walk and having everybody say, "Oh, what a beautiful day."

But having a baby is not just an idea. It will be a reality, and you, as the parent, will have to cope with the reality. Lucy found that it was much harder than she imagined:

After I had Heidi I couldn't believe how my life changed. I couldn't stand just sitting home all the time watching her, so I started going out every night leaving Heidi with my mother, and if my mother wouldn't watch her, I'd drag Heidi along with me. When she was real little she used to get up a lot during the night, and I hated getting woken up. So sometimes I would just let her cry and cry and it would wake everybody in the house up and we'd all be miserable in the morning. Then when she was about nine months old, Heidi got real sick, so sick I had to take her to the hospital. She was in there for almost two weeks. I was so scared that she was going to die because I didn't take care of her the way I should have. That's when I decided I had to grow up and take some responsibility. I decided I'd have to change and not go out partying or running around. I wanted to be a good mother to Heidi, and that meant changing my style completely. I grew up during those two weeks.

Like Lucy, you may be ready to have a beautiful baby who will gurgle and coo and love you. But you may not be ready to deal with a screaming, demanding, fussing baby who wakes you in the middle of the night and who makes you stay home when you want to be out with your friends. Both parts are real, and as Lucy found out, you don't just get the first part when you have a baby.

It doesn't matter at what age you become a parent; if you're not prepared for the hard part you'll be shocked. Many older parents, in their twenties and thirties, say that they weren't at all prepared for the way a baby changed their lives.

In the beginning especially, the baby needs you all the time—to love, feed, change diapers, play with, comfort and watch over when he/she is sick or upset. That means *all the time*. The baby doesn't stop needing you because it's time for you to go to bed, or because you have a party to go to, or because you want some time to be alone. The baby doesn't understand about your needs. That's not because the baby is "bad" or "spoiled." That's just what being a baby is all about. And if you want to give your baby what he or she needs to grow up feeling good about him/herself, then you or some other loving, caring person has to be there *all the time*.

Probably no one is ever completely ready for parenthood, and everybody has some mixed feelings about taking on such a responsibility. But it's easier to be a parent if:

—you are grown-up yourself;
—you like children and enjoy being with them for hours at a time;
—the mother and father are both ready and willing to participate in bringing up their child;
—you have support from people who are willing to help you and listen to you;
—you have enough money for a comfortable place to live, food, clothing, toys, doctor's bills, baby-sitters;
—you are ready to change your life-style to make time for a baby;
—you feel worthwhile as a person and have your own interests.

When you find out about your pregnancy, talk to other teenage parents to see what life is like for them. Some people are making their lives work. Other people are having a very hard time. Of course it would be easy to make the decision if you could gaze into a crystal ball and see how being a parent will work out for you. But since that's not possible, the next best thing is to listen to other teenage parents. Give yourself time to make your decision early enough in your pregnancy so that if you decide not to have the baby, you'll be able to have an abortion if you want to.

Meet Some Teenage Parents. While we were working on this section we talked to many teenagers who had become parents. Here are a few of their stories so you can get an idea of what it's like for them.

Tami is eighteen. Her daughter, Gina, is three and a half now. They live with Tami's mother, brother and two sisters in public housing. The family receives welfare assistance:

I was fourteen when I had Gina. Everyone thinks if you're so young and you got pregnant it was because it was a mistake. But with me I was trying to get pregnant. I was going through a lot of changes—I even left home for a while. I felt lonely and I really wanted something that'd be mine and no one could take away from me.

My mother didn't approve at all. Right off she wanted me to have an abortion, and then when I said no, she wanted me and Tommy to get married. Tommy was twenty and we both wanted the baby, but I didn't feel ready to get married. So my mother was really mad and she said she wouldn't have anything to do with the baby when it was born. That didn't scare me.

The pregnancy was good for me. I didn't have morning sickness like some girls have. I was lucky in that respect, but when it came time to deliver I was very nervous. I didn't know what to expect and I'd heard some pretty gruesome stories. Well, it was very painful and it lasted longer than I thought it would, but, you know, after it's over you don't remember too much.

After I brought the baby home my mother changed about her. She said she'd take care of Gina so I could go back to school, but she got attached to Gina and tried to take her away from me. Like she wanted my baby to call her "Mommy." And my younger sister, she used to tell Gina that I wasn't her mother. I freaked and we had a big thing about it. I got so mad I left the house with Gina and we spent that night riding the subways. I came home the next day and I guess they saw where I was coming from because they stopped doing that stuff. Living at home is OK now, at least better than it was, but I can't wait to move into a place of my own. I don't know when that will be, because I want to get a job first and put Gina into a good day-care place.

When Gina was about a year and a half, I got pregnant again, but I had an abortion. Me and Tommy weren't getting along at all. He was real excited right after Gina was born. He really wanted to have a little girl, so he was all stoked up about it. He would come over every day and sometimes Gina and I would stay at his place for a couple of days. But then he started getting jealous of how much time Gina was taking. He thought I was paying too much attention to her and not enough to him, so I pulled away from him because I thought he was acting like a baby and one baby was enough for me. Gina sees him once in a while now, but she knows we're split.

All in all, I have to say me and Gina are real close. I think having her has done a lot for me. It gave me ambition, you know. Everything got important. Everything I did mattered. I had to start looking to my future—I mean our future.

Tami feels she did the right thing in having Gina. Even though life hasn't been easy for her, she's managing well.

Tom and Becky think that if they had it to do over again, they would have been better off getting an abortion. They got married when they were eighteen and Becky was three months pregnant. Their son, Luke, is five now. Tom told us:

When I look back, I regret the marriage most of all. It's hard to think about abortion now because I can't wish Luke wasn't here, but Becky and I really weren't ready for marriage. We loved each other, sure, but we've had so many problems over these last years—money problems especially. We didn't have anyone to help us out, and I was struggling with a job and night school and Becky was trying to find a job. After a while we would spend all our time together—which wasn't very much anyway—fighting. We hurt each other a lot. We're separated now, and that's real hard on Luke because he lives with Becky but he misses being with me too. I see him as much as I can, but the tension between me and Becky makes that a bad scene.

Sadly, many teenage marriages end in separation or divorce, especially when a child is involved. It's very difficult to take care of yourselves and a baby with no job, no diploma and no help from home.

When you do have help, and when money isn't a problem, life is still hectic but not as desperate. Susan, sixteen, and Neil, seventeen, are in that situation. They live with their one-year-old daughter in an apartment Susan's parents made for them in their house. Both Susan's parents and Neil's parents give them money:

Neil's in his last year of high school and I'm a junior. He goes to school during the day and I go at night, so you can see we don't get much time to be together. Here's what a typical day is like for us:

We get up about seven and Neil gets ready for school and I feed and change Molly. Then I have breakfast and clean the house and take Molly to the supermarket. When we get back, Molly has a nap and I try to fix things up or catch up on chores. Then Neil comes home for lunch and that's when I get a chance to go out by myself. I need that hour because being cooped up with Molly all day isn't easy. I love her very much of course, but I do need a break. When I get back, Neil goes back to school and I finish feeding Molly. Then sometimes she'll take a short nap in the afternoon and that's when I try to study. Neil has a job after school until six, and when he comes home I rush out the door to get to my class on time. Neil takes over with Molly. He plays with her and gives her a bath and puts her to sleep.

When I get back from school about nine, we hang out together for a while. That's really the only time we get to talk to each other. And even then, sometimes we have to use that time to study. We're usually in bed before eleven and we take turns getting up with Molly in the middle of the night.

Susan and Neil both work hard. They both want to go to college. They both want to make a good life for Molly. They are lucky to have parents who help them out.

Carol, who's now twenty-three, didn't have anyone to help her. She had to make it on her own:

I left home at seventeen because my father kicked me out. He called me a slut for having sex with my boyfriend. So I moved in with some friends and then sort of drifted from place to place. It was pretty nice being on my own, but it was also very lonely. I hardly had any friends and I didn't know what I was doing with myself. Now when I look back on it I think I must have been very immature.

My boyfriend and I got along pretty fine. We used birth control some of the time but not always. At seventeen I just didn't think I would get pregnant. Jimmy and I talked about what would happen if I got pregnant and he said, "I'll take care of it." You know how that goes. Anyway, in the beginning everything was cool. When I first found out I was pregnant, Jimmy said we'd get our own apartment and it would be great. Then when I was four months gone, he tells me he can't handle it, so I should get an abortion.

To make a long story short, we split. I just couldn't get myself to have an abortion. I even made four different appointments, but I just never showed up.

I was so scared I tried to forget I was pregnant and I did a lot of drugs and didn't take care of myself. I'll tell you right now I was dumb because Ray was extra small when he was born and he has a hearing problem and I'm sure that was because of the drugs I did.

Finally, when I was six months pregnant, I called a hot line for help and they put me in touch with a maternity shelter. They put me up and gave me food and clothes and a place to stay, but for a while they kept pressuring me to give the baby up for adoption. That was hard for me because no way did I want to give the baby up.

Well, my delivery was pretty easy, but I didn't like being in the hospital at all. I felt sorry for myself because I was in this room with married women who were going home to their husbands and people who cared about them, and I didn't have anyone who cared about me.

When I left the hospital Ray and I lived with another friend of mine until I could get on welfare and get my own place. I thought it would be OK then, but the first few months were like a nightmare. I could only afford this dumpy place and the heat would go off all the time, and Ray was tiny and sick a lot. I had bad dreams because I was afraid to sleep because Ray and I were sleeping in the same bed and I kept being afraid I'd roll over and crush him. I really thought I was going to go crazy. The only nice people I knew were the nurses over at the hospital clinic. They really tried to help me.

Let me tell you. It wasn't easy. I don't think it's ever easy for a single parent who doesn't have any money.

Carol stayed on welfare for a couple of years, but at the time we interviewed her she was working and going to college at night. Ray is five now, and he goes to school dur-ing the day and a baby-sitter takes care of him while Carol goes to school.

Choosing to have their babies hasn't made life very easy for these six people. But they did it, and they are trying their hardest to give their children a good life. Lots of teens don't do as well as these people, because they aren't able to make the adjustment that has to be made when a baby is born.

When you are considering being a parent, remember there will be a real, live, helpless human being totally dependent on you for his or her needs. Babies and children need a lot. Think about yourself. Did you get your need for love and attention and care met when you were a child? If you did, could you provide that for your child? If you didn't, do you know for certain that you could be a better parent to your child than your parents were to you?

Parents need support and love. Children need the same. They also need to know that they will not be abandoned by the grown-ups they become attached to. If you take on the responsibility of a baby, you owe it to that baby to try to love and provide for him or her until he or she grows up.

Helping Yourself. Our society doesn't give parents much help. For some reason we seem to think that once people have babies they can take care of themselves and their babies without too much trouble. All of us who are parents know that that's not true. We need a lot of help.

Try to find other teenage parents or young parents in your area and set up a support group of your own. You can get together with your children to talk and share stories while the kids play together. Sometimes people set up more formal play groups or other baby-sitting arrangements.*

One of the hardest things about being a parent is that it tends to isolate you. You spend most of your time home taking care of your baby. Remember, it's important to make an effort to get out and meet other parents. If there is a maternity home or a home for unwed mothers or some service like that in your area, they may have support groups already established. Don't be embarrassed to call. They'll probably be very helpful and friendly.

Using Foster Care

If you decide to go through with your pregnancy but before or after your baby is born you realize you just can't take on the responsibility of parenthood, you have two choices. You can give your baby up for adoption, which means you permanently give over your rights to the baby. Or you can decide to give your baby to another family

---

*You may want to take a look at a book some of us worked on that is called *Ourselves and Our Children*. It has a lot of suggestions about finding help for yourself as a parent, and it has discussions by other parents about what parents go through. The whole purpose of the book is to support you and make you feel better about yourself as a parent.

temporarily, until you can take care of him or her yourself. This arrangement is called foster care.

> Foster care is help for parents who can't take care of their child now but think they will be able to take care of their child in the *near* future.
>
> Your child will be placed in an approved foster home for a certain amount of time. *You are still the child's mother or father,* so you must be actively involved in your child's life by visiting regularly and helping out financially if you can.
>
> *It is not good for your child to live separately from you for a long time,* so most states do not like to arrange long-term placements. If you don't think you can manage being a parent for your child, it is probably better to allow your child to be adopted by a family who *will be able to* and *will want to* take care of him or her.

There are several different types of foster care available. The first thing to do is call a lawyer or the state Department of Child Welfare or one of the agencies listed on p. 211 to find out your possibilities. In this section we will go through some of the arrangements you can make.

LEGAL RIGHTS

The decision to use foster care is yours unless you can't take care of your child. In that case the court may place the baby in foster care without your consent. Even if you are a minor and your parents have legal responsibility for *you,* they *don't* have legal responsibility for *your child.*

Both parents of the child, whether they are married or not, must consent to the foster care arrangement. When a mother places her child in foster care, she must name the father unless he is unknown or it can be shown that naming him would be harmful to the child. If the father refuses to admit that he is the father, he can be taken to court in a paternity suit.

If one of the parents does not consent to the foster care arrangement, a judge will decide whether to place the child in foster care even without that parent's consent. The judge can also decide that some other arrangement would be better for the child.

Private Foster Care Arrangement. Sometimes foster care is arranged informally, meaning it's not done through the courts and there is no formal, written agreement. If your parent, relative or friend agrees to care for your child until you are able to take care of him or her yourself, you can make a private agreement with that person. It's not done through the courts and no formal legal agreement is written up. The mother, if she is unmarried, still *has the legal right to her child* even though the child is living tem-

porarily with someone else. If the mother and father are married, they both have legal rights to their child.*

Here is an example of a private foster care arrangement. Karen got pregnant when she was fifteen. She was living at home with her mother and six brothers and sisters. Karen's mother told her there would be no room for the baby, and Karen felt she was too young to live on her own. The baby's father had moved out of state and wasn't interested in taking care of the baby. When Derrick was born, Karen looked for someone to care for him temporarily. Her mother's close friend, Mrs. Rowan, loved babies and said she would be able to care for Derrick. Karen brought Derrick to Mrs. Rowan's to live and she visited him three times a week, at least. Sometimes she would take Derrick home for the weekend. When the child was two years old, Karen got married and took Derrick to live with her and her new husband. Karen's arrangement with Mrs. Rowan worked out very well for everyone. Karen kept in close contact with her baby and he grew up knowing that Karen was his real mother.

Even though private foster care isn't arranged through the courts, your legal right to the child can be taken from you if it can be proved in court that you have abandoned or neglected or seriously mistreated your child. That is what happened to Joyce, who was sixteen when Matthew was born. Joyce's boyfriend, Joe, was seventeen. Neither of them was able to take care of Matthew, so a friend of Joyce's aunt, Mrs. Quentin, agreed to take him. Mrs. Quentin had always wanted a son, after raising three daughters of her own. Joyce and Joe said that they would want to take Matthew back in eighteen months, after Joe graduated from high school and could get a decent job. They said they would visit Matthew at least once a week. Mrs. Quentin agreed. Within six months Joe and Joyce broke up. Joe moved out of the state to live with his new girlfriend and Joyce became very depressed. Matthew looked a lot like Joe, so Joyce found it harder and harder to visit him and take care of him. Pretty soon she stopped visiting altogether. Matthew became very attached to Mrs. Quentin and her daughters. He was part of the family and thought of Mrs. Quentin as his mother. After Joyce failed to visit or call for six months, Mrs. Quentin hired a lawyer to try to adopt Matthew legally. Joyce was notified of this action, and she was told that she could have free legal services if she needed them. Joyce decided not to fight the adoption because she knew she couldn't be a good mother to Matthew.

Since a teenager's parents aren't legally or financially responsible for the care of their grandchildren, they may

---

*Note: A recent decision by the Supreme Court gives the baby's father the *same rights* as the baby's mother, even if they are not married. The father must show the court that he wants to have legal rights to his child. The mother has the rights automatically.

be eligible to receive foster care funding if the child lives with them, even if the child's mother or father also lives with them. Other relatives may receive this funding too if the child or the teenage parent and his or her child live with them. If your parents or relatives are willing and able to help you by providing a home for you and your child, or just for your child if that's what you'd prefer, contact a social service agency to see if they can receive financial assistance as foster care parents.

Many teens feel better putting their children in private foster care, since it is usually with someone they know and someone who they know likes children.

If you make a private arrangement for your child, it's up to you to visit the child and help out the foster parent as much as you can. If you neglect your duties as a parent, the person who cares for your child may try to have your legal rights taken away from you. It's important to a child's health and sense of security to know that he or she is loved and appreciated. If you aren't able to give that affection to your child, he or she might be better off with someone who can.

Voluntary Placement for the Child. If you can't or don't want to make a private arrangement for your child, you can place your child legally in a temporary foster home, which is paid by the state for taking your child. This is not an around-the-clock baby-sitting service for your child; it is a place where he or she can be cared for *until you can provide adequate care yourself.* That means you should have good plans to care for your child in the near future—after you graduate from high school, or as soon as you find an apartment, or when you get a job.

There are two kinds of placement: short-term, which is under three months, and long-term, which is over three months. The type of home your child is sent to will depend on whether you say you want short-term or long-term placement. If you arrange short-term placement and then change your mind, your child may have to move from one foster home to another because the people he or she is with aren't prepared to keep him or her for a long time. That is generally not very good for the child. Many children who have been placed in one home after another grow up feeling they don't belong anywhere and aren't wanted.

How to make the arrangement. There are many agencies that help people make foster care arrangements. Here is a list of some that do:

—United Community Services
—State Department of Child Welfare (sometimes called the Bureau of Child Welfare), which operates its own foster care homes and cooperates with other voluntary agencies
—Religious organizations: Catholic Charities, United Federation of Jewish Philanthropies, Federation of Protestant Welfare Agencies, placements made through local churches or temples

---

This poem was written by a fifteen-year-old girl who spent her childhood in six different foster homes.

REALITY

Her eyes were of wonder
As she saw her new home.
She quietly began to ponder
All the places she had been sent to roam.

Alone at night she would cry—
(Her mother's death came as a shock),
Hoping and praying the days would pass by,
Having something to say but not wanting to talk.

Now on the verge of insanity,
No one will listen.
Is this the fault of fate or society?
For now her eyes no longer glisten.

—Groups that are against abortion, such as Birthright or Right-to-Life
—Foster care agencies in your area (call the Bureau of Child Welfare for information about private agencies)
—Maternity homes or shelters, which sometimes can help you arrange foster care

To get in touch with these agencies, look in the phone book to see if they have a number listed. If you live in a very small town, try the phone book of the biggest city near your home. The library should have the city phone books. You might also try calling information to get the numbers.

If you know before your baby is born that you will want to make use of foster care, get in touch with the agency while you are still pregnant. The arrangement will be easier, and you will feel better knowing that you have someone to look after your baby right away.

The agency you contact will assign a social worker or counselor to help you make the arrangements and write up the agreement. He or she will be able to answer your questions and help you think through your plans.

Children in foster care can be placed in a private foster home, licensed and paid by the state and approved by the agency; or they may go to a child care institution run by the agency. Children living in an institution live in a group and are cared for by special child care workers. Children living in a foster home are part of the foster parents' family.

The final decision about where your child is placed is up to the social service agency, but you can request that your child be placed in a family and you can ask that the family be of a particular race or religion. The agency usually will try to do what you ask if they think it's reasonable, or if they have the facilities. Marilyn's experience was like that:

> When Frankie lost his job, he couldn't get another one because he got sick, so I had to go to work. We couldn't afford baby-sitting for our baby and there wasn't any day care near us that would take a one-year-old. So we talked to our baby's doctor, who put us in touch with an agency that arranges foster care. We told them that we had a friend of Frankie's family who was a foster mother to another kid, and they got in touch with Mrs. Polk and said the baby could live with her until we got on our feet again. Mrs. Polk loves kids and needs that extra money she gets from foster care agencies. She kept our baby for a year, but we visited him every weekend and he always knew that we loved him and would take him back as soon as we could. It took us a year to get it together, but then we got Mark back and now we're living together again.

The foster care agreement. Foster care is usually seen as a last resort, because temporary placement is generally not as good for a child as permanent placement. You and the agency you work with may want to explore all the other possibilities, such as welfare, family day care, help from parents and relatives, and adoption, before you decide to use foster care.

If you and the agency agree that foster care is the best thing for your child, they will ask you to sign an agreement that legally transfers the care and custody of your child to an authorized agency. When you sign that agreement, the agency becomes the legal guardian of your child.

Be sure to get and keep a copy of the agreement. If any legal problems come up, you will need it. If you have to contact a lawyer, he or she will want to see the agreement.

The agreement will probably be written in confusing legal terms, so be sure to have the agency explain everything to you in language you understand. Remember your rights and your baby's rights are at stake. You may even wish to speak to a lawyer before signing the agreement. If you don't have much money, you are probably eligible for *free* legal assistance. Ask about it.

It is especially important that you understand what you are being asked to sign. The agreement will say how often you are supposed to visit your child; how long your child will be kept in the foster placement; whether you have to give any money to the foster parents. The agreement will also say that you have to keep in contact with the agency social worker.

Be sure to follow the rules of the agreement completely, because if you don't, you risk losing your rights to your child.

Your child will be released to you at the time and under the conditions stated in your foster care agreement. If the agency feels you have not met the terms of the agreement and that you can't take good care of your child, it can refuse to return the child to you. If you don't agree with this decision, you will have to appeal it in court.

Feelings about foster care placement. A lot of teenagers who put their children into foster care do it because they feel they have no other option. They want the best for their child, and they know *they* can't provide it at the time.

Here is how two teenagers described their situation:

> Mary (fifteen): I could never give my baby up for adoption, but I really couldn't take care of her myself either. My mother and I never got along, and after I got pregnant she made me move out. I've been living here and there since then and that's really not the best situation for a baby. Welfare thinks I'm too young to have my own place. They said I should go into a foster home with my baby, but no thanks! Then you got a curfew and rules and stuff like that, and I've been on my own too much already for that. So foster care for Tammy seemed like the only way. I get to visit Tammy at least once a week, and I'm going to start a waitressing job and save enough to get my own place together. By that time I'll be old enough for welfare to help me out and then I'll get Tammy back. I feel like it's the right way for us.

> Gregory (sixteen): My girlfriend and I are still living at home. We want to live together as soon as I can get a job that pays enough, but right now I'm finishing school. Melinda's mom is very sick and it would just be too much for her to have the baby around, and Melinda's dad travels a lot, so he can't be counted on to help. And my mom, well, she was really mad when she found out about the pregnancy. She never liked Melinda. She thought Melinda was a bad influence on me, and she told me she doesn't ever want to see Melinda or the baby around here. I keep hoping she'll change her mind someday because, I mean, she is my mom and I know she loves me, but right now Mel and I figure the baby will be better off in a foster home.

Many of the teenagers we spoke to said that they feel upset about having to put their child in foster care. Jody, a sixteen-year-old mother from Texas, said:

> I felt so empty after I left the hospital without the baby. There just wasn't anything else I could do, but it's very hard for me to visit her. When I'm with her I don't want to leave. She's a year old now, she clings to me and cries and I just about break down every time myself.

Lois, who's fifteen, told us:

> My daughter's foster family treats her so well. She's always clean and dressed in pretty things and she has so many toys. God, *I* never had so many toys. But it

really hurts me when I hear her call her foster mother ''Mommy'' and I feel like maybe I don't have a right to her anymore.

Brian is a seventeen-year-old father. He and his girlfriend Sarah visit their son every week, but Brian said that's just not like living with him:

> When Sean took his first step, he was with his foster mother and somehow it's beginning to feel like he's going to grow up without me. I'm trying like mad to get something going for us—to find a job that can support us all—but until then I guess me and Sarah are just going to miss out on some of those important moments.

Beverly, a seventeen-year-old from Washington, told us:

> I used to wake up in the middle of the night with the same dream. I'm walking on the beach and I see my daughter with her foster family. I try to catch up with them but I can't. I run as fast as I can, but even when they see me they ignore me, like I'm not really there.

Seeing your child in a foster care situation is bound to bring up lots of feelings like these, and you may also worry that your child isn't getting good care.

Talk all this over with the social worker from the agency, or with some other person you trust. It will make you feel better to share your worries and your sadness and to get out your anger. Your mixed emotions are natural.

It's also natural to have an emotional reaction to getting your child back when the placement is over. It will almost certainly take time for you and the child to feel comfortable living together after having been separated. Give yourself the time it takes to get adjusted. Talk about your feelings, the negative ones and the positive ones, with someone who will understand. You're not bad or mean or wicked to have mixed feelings about being a parent. Most parents have mixed feelings.

Some problems with foster care. Once you sign the foster care agreement, your child is the legal responsibility of the foster care agency. They can make decisions about your child that you may not agree with. For example, they can transfer your child to another home without your consent; they can refuse you the right to take your child for an overnight visit; they can decide that you are not able to care for your child and bring your case to court. You have the right to appeal in court any decision made by the agency.

If you do not follow the instructions in the foster care agreement, the agency may decide you are an unfit parent and may set up court proceedings to release your child for permanent adoption. That is how Janis lost her daughter, Suzi.

Janis, who was seventeen, gave birth to Suzi in April and signed an an agreement to place her daughter in foster care until she was able to find a good place to live, get a job, and arrange good child care. Janis visited Suzi twice a month for the first three months, but after that she didn't see Suzi for almost a year. She told her social worker that she was busy looking for a job and just could never make the visits. She never showed up for appointments with the social worker either. When the social worker called, Janis said she was living with a new boyfriend who didn't like children but she didn't want to give up her rights to Suzi because she was sure she could persuade her boyfriend to let her have Suzi. Janis didn't call her social worker or make any attempt to visit Suzi for six months more and the agency took the case to Juvenile Court.

Though she knew about the hearing Janis didn't show up in court. The judge decided not to leave Suzi in foster care until Janis could make adequate arrangements. He ordered the court to begin proceedings to make Suzi eligible for permanent adoption. At that point Janis tried to fight the ruling, but the court ultimately decided that she had not been and would not be a fit mother. Suzi was adopted within a year.

Some other alternatives. Placing your child in a foster home isn't the only alternative. If you are still a minor, you may be able to find an arrangement by which both of you (or, in rare instances, the three of you—father, mother and baby) are placed together in a foster home. Other possibilities are family day care, where the baby stays during the day at someone else's home while you work; foster care funding going to your parents or relatives for providing a home for your baby; welfare assistance, if you live alone with the baby. These alternatives can be discussed with a social service agency in your area.

Here's Paula's story:

> I'm sixteen now, but I've been in foster care myself since I was four. When I was pregnant with Tasha, I lived at a maternity shelter. Then when she was born, she and I went to live together in a foster home. The shelter helped us find a place. My foster mother is really great. She takes care of Tasha while I'm at school, and she helps me out when I'm home. Like she taught me how to give Tasha a bath, and when Tasha fusses at night, sometimes she'll come and relieve me so I can get some sleep. I'm really lucky; I know a few kids who aren't so lucky.

Fifteen-year-old Carolyn still lives at home, but her mom and dad both work. Since Carolyn wanted to continue her schooling, her agency helped her find a family day care arrangement:

> My social worker told me about this program where they have these families who take care of babies during the day so their parents can go to school or work. You bring the baby in the morning and pick the baby up at night or after school. That seemed like the perfect thing for me until I finish school and Joey and I can get married and have our own place.

For many teenage parents, day care doesn't solve the problem. You still have to take care of the baby when you're tired after school or work; you have to pay for the baby's expenses; you have to provide for the baby when he or she gets sick and can't go to day care. Also, there is usually a waiting list to get into the family day care program.

The Adoption Choice

When you are pregnant, or even after your baby is born, if you decide you are not able to raise the baby, you can choose to put the child up for adoption. In adoption, *you permanently give over your rights as a parent to another person or family.* You will no longer be considered the child's parent in the eyes of the law.

Both biological parents must agree to adoption, even if they are not married. Only when the father or mother is legally declared unfit or cannot be located does he or she lose the right to consent.

If the biological parents disagree about whether to put the baby up for adoption, the court decides what to do. Patrick and Brenda were in that situation. Sixteen-year-old Brenda told us:

> I figured that if he wasn't going to marry me, I wasn't going to be able to raise the baby myself. I didn't even want to raise *his* baby, so I decided to give the baby up for adoption. That way he'd never see it and he'd always know that he made me give his baby away because he wasn't man enough to take care of his responsibility.
>
> But when it came time to sign the adoption papers, Patrick wouldn't sign. He said he wanted the baby and that he would keep the baby with him and his mother. We went to court, and the judge gave custody of the baby to Patrick and his mother. I was so mad I felt like killing Patrick.

Brenda said she felt the decision wasn't fair. She felt they didn't have a right to give her baby to Patrick. But the judge saw that Patrick was the father and that Patrick really wanted to give the baby a good home. Since Patrick's mother agreed that she would be there to raise and care for the baby too, that seemed to the judge to be a better solution than putting the baby in a strange home.

If it is possible, the court will usually decide that it's best for the child to live with one of the biological parents.

Making Adoption Arrangements. *It is best for your child if he or she is put up for adoption as soon after birth as possible.* It is easier for a baby to be adopted when it is newborn, and it is easier for you to give up the baby before you begin to grow attached to him or her.

Most important, it is better for a baby not to be separated from the people who care for him or her. Even very young babies grow attached to the adults who take care of them. So the sooner your baby goes to his or her new

home, the better adjustment he or she will be able to make.

If you can make the adoption arrangements while you are still pregnant, that is best for both you and the baby. Elizabeth, a fourteen-year-old from Los Angeles, did it that way. She told us:

> I don't believe in abortion, but I knew I couldn't take care of a baby. I'm too young to be a mother. So when I got pregnant I knew I'd give the baby up. I got in touch with Catholic Charities and they arranged it for me. I don't know who got my little boy, but I know he'll have a better home than he would have had with me. I think about him sometimes, but I know I did the right thing by him.

Carrie also decided to give her baby up for adoption. We met her at a maternity shelter in Detroit. She was nearly nine months pregnant when she said:

> I know it's not going to be easy to give my baby away, so I just don't think about it. By the time I found out I was pregnant I was already six months gone and it was too late to have an abortion. I came here and they told me about adoption and how that would be the best thing for the baby, since I don't really have anybody to help me out. My mom and dad both work all day and I'm still in junior high. I don't want to quit school. Right now I know it's not real to think that I could be a good mother to a baby. I'm a kid myself. So that's no good. I want to do what's best for this baby, and I think that's to give it to a family who really wants to have a baby. My friend was adopted and she has great parents. I think it will be OK.

No one can make you give up your child for adoption. Even if you are under age, no one can force you to sign an adoption consent, and the baby or child cannot be put up for adoption without your consent. The only way your child can be taken from you legally is a court decision that you are an unfit parent.

The rules of adoption have been made to protect the child. It is better for the child not to be confused about who his or her parents are. It wouldn't be fair to the child if you stayed in the picture. It also wouldn't be fair to the adoptive parents. They want to feel that the child they adopt is their child. They don't want to have to worry that you will come someday and take their child away from them.

In some states there are "grace" periods during which you can change your mind about the adoption. For example, New York State has a thirty-day "grace" period during which you can decide you want your baby back. After that you cannot change the adoption plan.

When they get older, some adopted children try to find their biological parents. In the past all records were kept absolutely secret, so it was very hard to do this. Recently

LEGAL ADOPTIONS

If you want your child to be adopted legally you have to work through a government-authorized adoption agency or arrange a private adoption through a lawyer or state judge. It is always a state judge who gives final permission for an adoption.

Some agencies that can help you are:

—United Community Services
—Catholic Charities; the Federation of Protestant Welfare Agencies; the United Federation of Jewish Philanthropies
—The Department (or Bureau) of Child Welfare in your state
—Adoption agencies
—Maternity homes (shelters), which don't arrange adoptions directly but can put you in touch with an agency that can arrange the adoption

The authorized adoption agency that takes care of your adoption will ask you to sign papers showing that you surrender your child to the agency. Then the agency places your child in a family, if it can find a family to take your child. You will not be told who the adoptive parents are or when the adoption takes place.

You can request that the adoptive family be of a particular race or religion if that is important to you. You can also write special arrangements into the agreement giving instructions as to what to do if your child isn't adopted.

Once your child has been legally adopted, you have no rights to your child. You have no right to visit the child and you have no right to receive any progress reports on your child. You are no longer considered the child's parent.

some agencies have begun to relax their policies, making it easier for biological parents and the children they gave up for adoption to become acquainted years later. You may want to discuss this possibility with your social worker at the time of adoption.

Private Arrangements. It is possible to make private arrangements for adoption. If you happen to know of a family who wishes to adopt your child, you can make the arrangements legally through a lawyer. The agreement must be approved by a state judge.

Be sure to keep a copy of all papers you sign. There may be a time in the future when you will need them or want them.

Illegal adoptions. Since many teenagers who get pregnant are choosing to have an abortion or keep their baby to raise themselves, there are fewer babies available for adoption these days. In some states there are more people who wish to adopt than there are babies available for adoption.

Sometimes pregnant teens are offered money by a doctor or a lawyer or someone else to give their baby up. *This is an illegal act.* The adoptive family is *not* investigated or approved by a state licensed agency.

Usually the person who arranges this illegal adoption makes a lot of money for doing it. The couple who wants to adopt the baby pays a very high price. Their only qualification for adopting your baby is that they are willing and able to pay a lot to buy the baby. Having a lot of money has *nothing* to do with being good parents. This is a very risky way to deal with your life and your baby's.

Feelings about adoption. It's natural to have many powerful feelings about giving your child up for adoption. You may know that adoption is the best choice for you and your baby but still have mixed emotions about it. Fifteen-year-old Patricia told us what it was like for her:

I had no choice, really, and I'm relieved that the whole thing is over now. But whenever I see a baby about my baby's age I feel sad. I wonder how she is and what she looks like. I hope she's happy.

But I try not to dwell on it. It happened, it's over, and I have to get on with my life. I know that I want to do a lot of things for myself before I can be a good mother to anyone. I think that if I had kept the baby it wouldn't have been fair to either of us. It would have ruined both of our lives. At least this way my baby has a chance.

Adoption is a way to give your baby a chance. If you aren't ready to be a parent, if you don't have enough money or support or maturity to provide a baby with the security he or she needs, then adoption is a very positive way for you to love your child.

It will help to talk with someone you trust both before and after the adoption. Keeping your feelings bottled up inside can make you depressed. When you tell someone else about what's troubling you, it almost always relieves some of the pressure. Juliana was seventeen when she gave her baby up. She said:

After I had the baby and gave her up for adoption, I felt very empty inside. I had trouble sleeping because I would keep dreaming about the baby. I had the same nightmare over and over again. I was holding a baby and singing to it. I felt all peaceful inside because the baby was cooing and smiling. But when I went to give it a bottle I realized I was just holding a blanket. The baby had disappeared.

That dream kept haunting me. I'd remember it even while I was awake. Finally I called the adoption agency and they gave me the name of a social worker to call. She was very nice, really, very nice and she didn't mind when I kept crying about the baby. I always felt before that that no one wanted to hear me talk about the baby. My mother kept telling me to try to forget it, and my best friend kept saying I should just not think about it anymore. But of course you

> If you think you may be pregnant or if you think your girl is pregnant, you have some hard decisions to make. There are problems connected with all your choices—abortion, parenthood, foster care, adoption.
>
> Help yourselves by talking over your feelings, fears, doubts and concerns with someone you trust. Try to talk to your parents if they are available. Meet with a pregnancy counselor at a birth control clinic.
>
> Most important, make the decision that *you* feel is right for you, given your situation and your beliefs. And *be sure* to find out about birth control (see p. 159). Stop future unwanted pregnancies *before* they start.

can't just stop thinking about something. I'm sure that I won't always be feeling this way, but for now it's comforting to be able to talk to Mrs. Little. She's very understanding.

Fathers may also have strong feelings about giving their babies up. Seventeen-year-old Ruben was one of the people we interviewed in Iowa. He told us:

It was heavy. I don't talk about it too much. I mean it wasn't like Sharleen was my girlfriend. We just had a good time together. I didn't see her for a while and then the next thing she tells me is that she's pregnant and she's giving the baby up for adoption. I couldn't believe it! First I thought she was kidding. Then I swore up and down that I couldn't be the father, but deep down I think that I probably am. I haven't seen her for a long time now, but I heard she did put the baby up for adoption. Sometimes I think about that a lot. It was a boy, I heard. I keep wondering who adopted him. I wonder if he is mine? I wonder if he looks like me? I wonder how he's doing? I'm sure now that I want to have a kid of my own someday.

Ruben and other fathers we talked to have been deeply affected by the experience of adoption. They think about their babies and wonder about them. It's natural for that to happen.

On the other hand, most parents who give their babies or children up for adoption do it because they feel it is the right thing, the best thing to do under the circumstances. Sad feelings and disappointed feelings and angry feelings may be part of the experience for almost everyone, but there might also be a sense of your own strength for having been able to do what you felt was best for yourself and your baby. An eighteen-year-old boy from New York told us:

My girlfriend and I talk about the baby a lot. He would have been a year old this month. Father's Day just passed and I got very depressed, but I know we did the right thing. Joan and I both know we weren't

ready to be parents. We couldn't have given our baby anything, and now he's probably with parents who really wanted to have a baby badly. I think the whole experience made me and Joan grow up a lot. We're real careful now, we never take chances with birth control or anything like that. We want to plan our lives and enjoy our lives. I think we're a lot closer now.

Sexually Transmitted Diseases (STD's) and How You Can Avoid Them

Most people have prejudices against sexually transmitted diseases. They think you have to be dirty or loose to get them. A fifteen-year-old from Boston said:

Yeah, there's this feeling like, *I* can't get anything like that! You've got these certain kinds of distinctions in your head that say, Wait a minute, he's my friend. He can't have VD.

Actually it's not like that at all. Anyone who is sexually active can get an STD—from a friend, from a stranger, from a relative. And the more sexual partners you have, the higher are your chances of catching a disease.

> NOTE: You've probably heard of venereal (veh-*neer-ee-uhl*) diseases, known as VD. Most people mean gonorrhea (the clap) and syphilis (siff) when they talk about VD.
>
> Actually there are a lot more diseases that are passed through sexual contact—twenty or so diseases, in fact. That's why the name VD has been changed to STD, which stands for sexually transmitted diseases. That covers all of them.
>
> We're going to discuss the most common ones in this section:
>
> | | |
> |---|---|
> | The old standbys: | syphilis and gonorrhea |
> | The new big menace: | herpes (*her*-pees) |
> | Other viruses: | hepatitis and venereal warts |
> | Common infections: | non-gonococcal urethritis (NGU) vaginal infections |
> | Bugs: | pubic lice and scabies |

Everything and everybody alive can get sick, and germs that cause sickness are everywhere. Each time someone with a cold sneezes near you, you run the risk of catching cold. If your body is run-down, you're more vulnerable. Many germs are passed by normal, everyday social contact—people being around other people who are sick. This chapter is about the germs that can be caught specifically when people have sexual contact with each other. Most STD germs love warm, dark, moist places, so most of the sexually transmitted diseases are passed from one body opening to another. For example:

> mouth to mouth
> mouth to penis
> mouth to vagina
> mouth to anus
> penis to vagina
> penis to anus
> vagina to vagina

IF YOU HAVE ANY SEXUAL CONTACT WITH AN-OTHER PERSON, FROM KISSING TO MAKING OUT TO INTERCOURSE, YOU MAY BE EXPOSING YOURSELF TO AN STD IF THAT OTHER PERSON HAS ONE.

A few STD's are tiny parasites that infect a person's body and cause terrible itching and irritation. We talk about these on p. 232. You can catch them from sleeping in the same bed as someone who has them, wearing an infected person's clothes, shaking hands with them, as well as by having closer physical contact.

By now you may be thinking you should avoid all contact with everyone else forever! But that's not the case. Just as there are ways to prevent other illnesses, there are things you can do to keep yourself from catching sexually transmitted diseases too. And that doesn't only mean no sex. There are simple methods everyone can use to prevent the spread of STD's and still enjoy sex with others. Much of this section will describe those preventive measures.

Feelings about STD and Sex

Eighteen-year-old Marsha told us:

> I was brought up to believe that ''nice'' people don't get VD, so how do you think I felt when I got gonorrhea? Shitty. I felt dirty. Like I was crawling with bugs.

And Eric, a sixteen-year-old junior from Milwaukee, said:

> The guy I had sex with knew more about everything than I did. It was my first time. I just let him take care of me and he took care of me good! He gave me the clap.

Anyone can get an STD. Being clean or ''nice'' has nothing to do with it. Being inexperienced won't keep you from them either. Many people don't know about prevention when they first start having sex, so they are even more likely to catch an STD.

One myth is that prostitutes spread STD's, but in fact professional prostitutes have a very low infection rate. Most of them know about preventive methods and use them.

Ginger said she learned about STD in school. This is how she explained it to us:

> Sure, we had that sex ed lecture they give you, but after you hear that, you'd have to be crazy to want to have sex. They make it sound like you'd end up crippled for life or blind or maybe even dead if you do anything. So of course nobody listens to them. I mean, you see plenty of people walking around the street and you figure at least some of them must have had sex without anything happening.

The dangers of sexually transmitted diseases are used to discourage people from having sex in the first place. Many of us were taught that catching an STD was a disgrace, so that was another reason to stay away from sex. Thirteen-year-old Larry said:

> My parents gave me some books on VD and what it can do to you. It's pretty clear that having sex with different people can give you VD if they have it, so I wouldn't do it. If you're going to have sex, you might as well get married.

Many other teenagers we met have decided that sex belongs only in marriage. But Larry's reasons for coming to that decision are partly based on the myth that if you have sex outside marriage you're probably going to get an STD. That isn't true.

What is true is that *if you have sex with more than one partner or if your partner has other partners, then you run a high risk of catching an STD—unless you use preventive measures*. Marriage has nothing to do with it. Married people can catch STD's too.

Another myth is that homosexual couples, gay men and lesbian women, don't have to worry about STD. That is false. Gonorrhea, NGU and hepatitis are epidemic in male homosexual communities. They are less common among lesbian couples, but they exist. Nearly every form of sexually transmitted disease can be passed by homosexual lovemaking as well as by heterosexual lovemaking.

Preventing Sexually Transmitted Diseases

Sex is natural. STD's are simply diseases passed through sexual activity. If you are having sex, learn how to protect yourself. You don't have to start a pregnancy; you can use birth control. You don't have to catch an STD; you can use preventive methods. Here we will name some of the general precautions people can use to help themselves avoid sexually transmitted diseases. Some methods are more effective than others. A condom, for example, is the most effective way to keep gonorrhea germs from spreading through penis-vagina or penis-anus intercourse. Other techniques are helpful when used in combination with each other.

You can catch a sexually transmitted disease only from someone who has one or from someone who is a carrier of one. That's why it's very likely that you won't get an STD if you don't have any sex with a partner at all. A few STD's can start from causes other than sexual contact, so even if you're not having sex, you may get one of them (hepatitis, vaginal infections; see pp. 229 and 230). It's also likely that you won't catch an STD if you're having sex with only one partner, as long as that person has no other partner but you. That is called a monogamous (mah-*nah*-gah-muss) relationship. *If neither of you had an STD when you started the relationship, you are safe until one of you has sex with someone else.* (But there are some infections you can pass back and forth to each other, so keep alert for symptoms. See p. 220.)

If you do need STD protection this chart should help. Luckily, some of the best ways to prevent STD's are also ways to prevent pregnancy.

These preventive measures are safe, effective and cheap. So why doesn't everyone use them?

Lots of people don't feel very comfortable with sex in the first place, so anything extra makes them even more nervous. Others have sex with partners they barely know, which also makes talking about STD prevention difficult.

Still other teens have said they are sometimes drunk or stoned when they have sex, so they aren't exactly thinking about protection or responsibility. It's very hard to take precautions in situations like that.

Many teens and adults say that communication between partners is one of the hardest parts of a sexual relationship. There's a long discussion of that issue in Chapter IV, pp. 105–6. We suggest you read that because it may help you feel more comfortable talking with your partner about sex in general and STD prevention and birth control in particular. Teenagers have told us they think sex is supposed to be like a silent, passionate love scene in the movies. In that kind of atmosphere, how can you stop to ask your partner if he or she has an STD? Or how can you get up the courage to say, "What's that rash on your neck?" Or "Here, wear this rubber or I won't have sex with you"? If you're feeling a little unsure of yourself anyway—and most of us do in new relationships—it's not easy to follow the suggestions on the "Techniques of Prevention and Control" list. It may feel a lot easier just to forget the whole thing.

That's why STD's like non-gonococcal urethritis, gon-

TECHNIQUES OF PREVENTION AND CONTROL*

Condoms are available in drugstores. If used by males during vaginal or anal intercourse, condoms (rubbers, safes) will stop many germs from getting to and from the penis (see p. 12).

Contraceptive creams and jellies can be used by females with a diaphragm or cervical cap to help prevent germs from entering the cervix. But that may not protect the vagina from attack unless a condom is also used in penis–vagina contact (see p. 171). Creams and jellies can be used in the anus by males and females to give some protection. Remember, they only protect the area they actually cover.

Contraceptive foam is more effective because it coats more of the vagina. It can be used in the anus during anal intercourse by both males and females (see p. 166).

Foam and condoms used together are excellent protection against both STD and pregnancy. We recommend them.

Look yourself and your partner over. Examine yourselves carefully. Check for a bad smell, unusual discharge, rashes, sores, bumps, itching or redness. All these can be signs of a possible disease. Don't have sex if you or your lover has one of the signs. If you decide to anyway, *you are taking a chance.* Use foam and condoms. Have yourself checked soon afterward.

Urinating before and after sex *may* wash away some germs, but don't count on that alone. It is only an extra precaution, and it works only for men.

Gargling with hot salt water after oral sex may help to kill STD germs in your throat. It must be done right away. Don't count on gargling alone.

Talk to each other. It can be hard to talk about sex, but it's your responsibility to your health and to your partner's health to discuss STD prevention. If you both use something, that makes it easier. *Protection is the best prevention.*

Have regular checkups. As soon as a person starts having sexual contact with others, he or she should have medical checkups at least once a year and, even better, twice a year. If you are having intercourse or oral sex, make sure the doctor or health workers test you for gonorrhea and syphilis each time you go, and also, but less often, for chlamydia. (See p. 226 for a description of the tests.)

Watch for symptoms. Starting on p. 224, we describe the symptoms of each disease. If you notice any, *go to the doctor or clinic immediately and have yourself checked.*

*Much of the information in this box and in this section was taken from an excellent pamphlet called *Sexually Transmitted Diseases (STD) and How to Avoid Them*, by Peggy Lynch and Esther Rome. It is available through the Boston Women's Health Book Collective, Dept. EP, Box 192, W. Somerville, MA 02144. Send a stamped, self-addressed envelope for one free copy. Inquire about bulk orders.

orrhea and herpes are spreading so rapidly. They are everywhere. In order to stop their spread people have to start taking precautions.

Before women and girls used the pill and the IUD for birth control, fewer people caught STD's because they had to use condoms, foam, diaphragms, and contraceptive creams and jellies to prevent pregnancy. If people would switch back to those methods, STD's wouldn't be passed so easily. One woman we know said:

I think condoms and foam are absolutely the best form of birth control if you have more than one partner. You're not only giving yourself good protection against pregnancy, but you're also protecting yourselves against VD. The pill stinks as far as I'm concerned: it only gives you complications and VD.

How Do You Know If You Have an STD?

Many people find out that they have an STD when they notice some symptoms. Then they can go to the clinic and have themselves tested and treated. They are lucky. A lot of people don't show any apparent symptoms. Or they mistake STD symptoms for those of a more common disease like a cold or the flu. Sometimes the sores or discharge or irritation is hidden deep inside where it can't be seen.

With gonorrhea, for example, 80 percent of the females who get it don't notice any symptoms. Between 10 and 20 percent of the males who get it don't notice any symptoms.

If you don't discover the disease by yourself, there are two other ways to find out that you might have an STD. One is to be told by a sexual partner who finds out that he or she has it. If you had unprotected sexual contact with someone who has the disease, there's a very good chance you've got it too. IT'S VERY IMPORTANT THAT SEXUAL PARTNERS REPORT TO EACH OTHER IF THEY HAVE AN STD. YOU MAY BE SAVING SOMEONE FROM A SERIOUS AND COMPLICATED ILLNESS. The second way is to have *regular* medical checkups. On p. 153 we discuss the checkup in detail, so you will know what to expect. Be sure to tell the doctor or clinic that you want tests for gonorrhea and syphilis as a preventive measure. There will soon be a test for NGU, and you should ask about it. Most clinics like to do those tests routinely anyway, but ask to be sure.

Finding Medical Help for Sexually Transmitted Diseases

Clinics are better for complete STD testing than most private doctors. Because clinics take care of many more people with STD, they are usually better equipped.

When you call for your appointment, ask if the doctor is set up to do all the possible STD tests (see p. 221). As a general rule it is best to have a reliable diagnosis before going ahead with treatment. However, if you know that it's likely you won't be able to come back or if it's very difficult for you to come back to the clinic—you don't have the time or money, you're afraid someone will see you, you're afraid of hospitals or doctors, you can't get up the courage to think about the problem one more time— *then* it's probably better to take an educated guess, based on circumstances and symptoms, and get treatment *right away*. This will make it less likely that you'll endanger yourself by letting the disease get worse or that you'll pass it on before you get around to going back for treatment. Try to remember to call the clinic or the doctor when the test results are expected back to make sure that the right guess was made.

Some people end up being treated and then find out they didn't have an STD in the first place. But most doctors and health professionals prefer treating you with medication while you are at the clinic to letting you go home without treatment, because if you have a disease, you could infect others while you're waiting to hear your results. If you have a disease, it could get worse while you're waiting for the results. Also, some people who go in for the tests don't want to come back another time for treatment. They'd prefer getting it all done in one visit.

If there is a good reason to suspect that you don't have an STD, then it is probably better to wait for the results of your tests before receiving antibiotic treatment.

Tests are usually free, but there may be a clinic charge. If you go to a private doctor you will have to pay his or her fee. Mention it if you do not want the bill sent to your home address. If you pay cash on the spot, there will not be a bill sent. Most places will want you to pay for the services at the time, if there is a charge. Call first. Ask what, if anything, the charges will be, and bring the right amount of cash with you.

Here are some suggestions on how to find medical help:

National VD hot line: From every state but California, call 1-800-227-8922. From California, call 1-800-982-5883. In some areas you don't have to dial (1) first. *This is a free call.* No charge will appear on your bill, or if you call from a phone booth, your money will be returned. The call is confidential—you don't have to give your name.

The hours to call are 8 A.M. to 8 P.M. Pacific Time, Monday through Friday, and 10 A.M. to 6 P.M. on Saturdays and Sundays. We recommend calling this hot line if you want information or if you are having trouble finding a clinic or doctor in your area.

Local VD hot lines: Many locations have their own hot

GENERAL SYMPTOMS OF STD

IN FEMALES

Sores: Painless sores in or near the vagina or anywhere else on your body may be a sign of syphilis. Painful sores and blisters around the genitals may be a sign of herpes.

Discharge: Some vaginal discharge is normal, but an irritating, itching discharge that is yellowish or white should be checked. A discharge from the anus should always be checked.

Burning urination: If urinating hurts or burns, that may be a sign of an STD. If you feel you have to urinate very often (like two or three times in one hour), that should be checked. These signs may mean a bladder infection or an STD.

Sore throat: People get sore throats for lots of reasons, but if you've had oral sex, your sore throat could be a sign of gonorrhea.

IN MALES

Sores: Painless sores around the penis or elsewhere may be a sign of syphilis. Painful sores near the penis or anus may be a sign of herpes.

Discharge: A clear or white "drip" from the penis or anus should be checked. It could be gonorrhea or another kind of infection.

Burning Urination: Same as for females. When this is coupled with a discharge from the penis, it usually means gonorrhea or another kind of infection in the urethra.

Sore throat: Same as for females.

Itching: Itching in the vaginal opening area can be a sign of an infection. Itching anywhere that doesn't go away could be a sign of an STD bug—especially in pubic or body hair.

Rashes: A rash can be a sign of an STD, especially on the soles of the feet or the palms of the hands. Have it checked.

Warts: Warts or other bumps and lumps around the genitals should be checked.

Lower abdominal pain: This may be a symptom of an infection that has traveled from the genitals to the uterus or tubes. *Have it checked right away.* If there is a possibility that you're pregnant, go to an emergency room immediately.

Itching: Itching in the area around the penis opening or anus can be a sign of infection. Itching in pubic, body or face hair can mean STD bugs.

Rashes: Same as for females.

Warts: Same as for females.

Pain in groin: This may be a symptom of gonorrhea or another infection that is spreading. *Have it checked right away.*

Lots of jokes are made about "social" diseases and how they're caught, but getting an STD is no joke. Most can be cured, but if they go unchecked and uncured, they can cause serious infections, painful symptoms and often permanent damage. *Always have your symptoms checked by a medical person as soon as you can.*

---

lines for STD information. Call Information (411) and ask for the number to the VD hot line. Or look in the phone book under VD or STD hot line.

Board of Health: Each state has a Board of Health or a Department of Health that provides *free* STD tests and treatment. Look in the phone book under the name of your city, county or state. There will be a lot of services listed. Find the heading that says Health and look under it for Venereal Disease (VD) Control or Sexually Transmitted Disease (STD) Control. Call the number listed and ask where you can go for tests. Ask if there will be any clinic charge. Ask if you have to make an appointment or whether you can walk in anytime.

Women's clinics: There are women's clinics in many areas. They generally provide treatment for women only, but call to find out what services they offer. Look in the Yellow Pages under Clinics or Health Services. Make an appointment if that is necessary and ask if there will be a charge. Tell them you want to be checked for an STD.

Free clinics; Planned Parenthood clinics; family planning clinics: These places usually provide STD services. Call first to find out and ask if you need an appointment. Planned Parenthood clinics are listed in the phone book. Other clinics can be found in the Yellow Pages (see above). Or call Information (411) if you have the name of a specific clinic. When you call, ask if there is a charge for the service.

Private doctors: If you have a family doctor you trust, or if a friend recommends a doctor, he or she may be a good person to see. Many doctors are glad to treat teenage patients because they want to do what they can to stop the STD epidemic. They are required by law to keep your visit confidential. Mention it if you do not want the bill sent to your home. Some doctors will expect payment at the time of service.

Going to the Clinic or Doctor. Whenever you use a medical facility, you have the right to expect gentle, careful and thorough service. You have a right to be treated with respect by the health workers and doctors. Sometimes teenagers in particular do not get the respect they deserve. If you feel you are not receiving good service, make your complaints known to the clinic manager. If there is some other place to go for treatment, you might choose to do that.

We recommend bringing a friend to the clinic with you. That will make the experience more pleasant, and you will have someone to talk to during the wait before your examination. If you bring your sex partner, you can both be tested and treated. You may, of course, prefer to go alone.

Most people we know say they have felt embarrassed or uncomfortable being in an STD clinic in the first place. They feel ashamed for having caught an STD. Remember: sex is not dirty; it's natural. STD's are not punishments for having sex. STD's are nearly as easy to catch as a cold or the flu. You are taking care of yourself and your future partners by having your STD treated. There's nothing to be ashamed of. In fact, you can be proud that you're acting so responsibly.

Here's how seventeen-year-old Nancy described her experience at a VD clinic in Los Angeles:

Underneath everything I was really embarrassed. I felt like everyone was looking at me, but I played it off like I knew exactly what I was doing. My boyfriend came with me, and we asked the nurse if we could be checked together. She was a little shocked, but she said, "Sure, why not?" So me and Jimmy got to go into the examining room at the same time. Jimmy told the doctor about his symptoms, and I said I didn't have any but I wanted to be checked anyway. They took a Q-tip and touched it to the top of Jimmy's penis, and when it was my turn they had a longer stick with cotton on it for the inside of my vagina. We were really glad to be in there together. He held my hand when I was being examined, and I held his hand when it was his turn.

Many places will allow you to bring a friend with you into the examining room if you'd like to. Other places don't allow it. If you want company, ask if it's OK. The more people ask, the more it will be allowed.

During the checkup the health professional will ask you to describe your symptoms. He or she will check your body for sores, rashes, swelling and infection, and may take your temperature. He or she will order tests for you to find out specifically which germ or bug you have.

The three basic tests are a blood test, a culture and a gram-stain. Depending on what the lab technicians do with each test, they can determine a variety of STD's. Talk to the lab technician or health professional about what they are planning to do. There are other tests as well.

The blood test. A sample of your blood is taken, usually from your arm, and it is sent to a laboratory to be checked. Under the microscope they will be able to see if your body has produced antibodies to syphilis or hepatitis; if it has, this means you have been infected. You may not get the results of your test for two days to a week.

The culture. A sample from the infected area of your body is taken and placed on a culture dish to grow. In girls they should take culture samples from the cervix, anus and throat. In boys they should take culture samples from the penis, anus and throat. The sample is removed with a cotton swab that is gently pressed along the site that may be infected. Some people say this is a little uncomfortable. Others say they can't even feel it.

The culture has to grow for sixteen to twenty-four hours, sometimes longer. At the end of that time it is analyzed by the lab workers to determine if you have gonorrhea.

Culture tests for gonorrhea are only 80 to 90 percent accurate. If the test said you were negative but your symptoms don't go away, go back immediately for another test. If you had no symptoms but you suspect you might have an infection, go back immediately for another test.

There is a new culture test for NGU caused by chlamydia (see p. 226). It is not yet widely available, and it is currently too expensive for use in many places. Some medical professionals are trying to create a more accessible version of the test, so it may be offered in many clinics in the near future.

The gram-stain test. This is a test for gonorrhea that is accurate for males with symptoms, and when done under excellent lab conditions it can be accurate for females too. The gram-stain test is done by taking a sample of discharge and putting it on a slide to be examined under a microscope. The results can be seen immediately.

Treatment for STD's. Different drugs in varying amounts are effective for curing the different diseases. Only the doctor or clinic worker can prescribe the proper medication for you. *Do not try to cure yourself by taking other people's pills. That can make things worse, not better.* We will discuss the specific treatments when we talk about each disease (starting on p. 224).

As we said, it usually takes a few days before the results of your tests are returned. If you were not treated at the time of testing, you *must* return to the clinic as soon as your tests results show that you have an STD. You will need antibiotics if you have gonorrhea, NGU or syphilis. You must start the treatment as soon as you can or else secondary infections may develop. *Do not have sex with anyone until your test comes back negative.*

Seventeen-year-old Jeff told us:

When Lucy and I started having sex, we used foam for birth control. Well, right away I started getting this discharge and it hurt when I peed. I thought she gave me the clap and I was mad because I thought she wasn't being honest with me. She kept saying she couldn't have it because she'd never been with anybody else. I wanted to believe her, but I couldn't figure out what was going on, so we went to the clinic. They gave us each a gonorrhea test, and then they gave us each a big shot of penicillin. Then when I called the clinic two days later to find out the results of the test, they told me it was negative. It turned out I was just having an allergic reaction to the foam Lucy was using. As soon as I started using rubbers and we changed brands of foam, my discharge disappeared. All that penicillin for nothing.

Be sure to take the *whole* treatment prescribed for your illness. Follow the directions exactly. Take the pills according to the instructions each day until they are all used up. That way you will kill all the germs. The symptoms almost always will go away before all the germs are killed.

Some people stop taking the pills as soon as their symptoms start to disappear. That is dangerous because some germs may still be alive inside your body. Without continued treatment those germs will grow, get stronger and keep infecting you.

After you finish all the medication, go back to the clinic for another test. If the results are negative, you have probably been cured. Since the tests are not 100 percent accurate, you need at least two negative tests to be absolutely sure you no longer have the disease.* If you continue to have pain or sores or discharge, *go back to the clinic immediately.*

DO NOT HAVE SEX WITH A PARTNER UNTIL THE DOCTOR SAYS YOU ARE CURED. TELL ALL YOUR PARTNERS THAT THEY SHOULD BE TESTED AND DO NOT HAVE SEX WITH THEM UNTIL THEY HAVE BEEN CHECKED AND TREATED IF NECESSARY.

Telling Your Partners

If you are treated for gonorrhea or syphilis, the doctor or health worker may talk with you about your sexual partners. They want to know who else may have the diseases.

*Three negative tests are recommended by *The VD Handbook*, 1975 ed. (Montreal Health Press, P.O. Box 1000, Station G, Montreal, Canada H2W2N1), p. 26.

They are not being nosy. They are asking because they want to help stop the spread of STD's. Every one of your lovers must be treated and cured for his or her own safety and to make sure that he or she won't give the disease to anybody else. Your name will not be given out. That is a law.

It is hard for many people to talk about their sexual relations. It can be especially hard if you are gay and still in the closet. Seventeen-year-old Allen said he is open about his homosexuality, but he still felt funny talking to the health worker, who assumed he was straight:

When she was talking to me during the exam, she kept saying things that just assumed I was having sex with a girl. It made me really uncomfortable. I wanted to say, What makes you so sure my lover is a girl? But I didn't. Before she gave me the treatment, though, she asked me for the names of my lovers, and when I told her, you should have seen her face!

Part of caring for a person and being a responsible lover is to tell the other person if he or she needs STD testing. Sometimes that's the only way people know they may have it. Marie, a seventeen-year-old girl from Chicago, told us she never would have known about her disease if her date hadn't called her:

I had sex with this guy last week, and a couple of days ago he called me up to tell me he caught the clap from me. I didn't know what he was talking about because I didn't know I had it. But I went to the clinic for a test, and they said I did have it and that it was already starting to infect my tubes. I remembered feeling some pains in my stomach, but I just thought it was a stomachache. Now I think I must have had gonorrhea for about two months at least, because that was the last time I had sex. Anyway, I sure am glad that guy called me. After I found out, I called up my old boyfriend to tell him he better get checked too, and he told me he already got tested last month. He tried to call me but my line was busy, so he just forgot about telling me. I couldn't believe it. I probably could have died and he would say, Oh gee, I meant to call her but her line was busy.

Darrell, a junior from the Midwest, said that telling his date was the hardest part about having gonorrhea:

It's embarrassing. It's just plain embarrassing to call up your date and say, "Oh, Chris, by the way, you better go in for a VD check. I might have given you the clap."

If you are in a relationship with someone and you caught an STD from someone else, telling your boyfriend or girlfriend may bring up issues that you probably should have been dealing with all along. You may be faced with their anger and disappointment that you were with someone else. You may feel humiliated. You may be afraid that they'll want to break up with you. These are serious concerns. But still, *for their safety, you must tell them*. With herpes and syphilis, most people develop symptoms, so they will probably find out themselves, although some symptoms are mistaken for other, less serious diseases. People don't always recognize syphilis symptoms, especially since they go away on their own. Also, women may have a chancre inside the vagina, and gay men may have it inside the anus. Women with NGU often show no symptoms. With gonorrhea, many people don't show any symptoms until the infection starts attacking their insides and causes pain and fever.

Sometimes it's hard to tell your partner because if he or she doesn't have symptoms, you may not be believed. You may find yourself having to persuade him or her to go for a checkup.

If you simply cannot bring yourself to tell your partners, you can report their names to the Department of Health in your county, and a health worker will tell them that they have been exposed to an STD and must be tested and treated. Health workers are forbidden, by law, to give your name. They are *not* the police. They only want to stop the spread of sexually transmitted diseases. If someone at the Department of Health hassles you or treats you harshly, contact the national VD hot line and report it to them.

STD's and Pregnancy

Often people who do not protect themselves against STD also do not use birth control. We have already mentioned how girls can have gonorrhea without knowing it. If one of these girls gets pregnant and gives birth to a baby, the child may develop eye problems or even blindness unless his or her eyes are treated with silver nitrate or antibiotic preparations immediately after birth. Babies can be infected with gonorrhea or chlamydia in the womb or in the birth canal. This can create a serious infection in the baby.

If a girl has syphilis and gets pregnant, the bacteria can attack the unborn child and the baby may be aborted, born dead, deformed or diseased. If the syphilis is cured before the sixteenth week of pregnancy, the fetus is probably not affected. That's why it's so important for every pregnant girl to get tested for syphilis as soon as she finds out she is pregnant. If she catches syphilis after she is already pregnant she must be treated immediately.

Herpes is also very dangerous to newborns. If the mother has herpes, the baby may get the virus and, as a result, may be born with birth defects and brain damage. Even if the virus has not attacked the fetus, if herpes sores are present in the mother's birth canal, the baby may get the disease while passing through the vagina during childbirth. Caesarean delivery is advised in many cases.

Another disease that can cause trouble during pregnancy is non-gonococcal urethritis, or NGU (see p. 226). It has been responsible for spontaneous abortions, stillbirths and newborn death. It can also cause pneumonia in the newborn.

When a woman gets certain varieties of hepatitis late in pregnancy, her infant may be affected. As many as two-thirds of these newborns come down with the disease and may develop persistent infections or become carriers of the disease.

Some forms of birth control also protect against STD. It makes sense to use them.

BIRTH CONTROL AND STD PROTECTION	
Type of Birth Control	*How Does It Protect Against STD?*
Condoms and foam used together	Excellent protection. Two barriers against germs.
Condoms	Good protection for penis and whatever penis touches. More effective as birth control when used with foam.
Diaphragm and jelly or cream or cervical cap and jelly or cream	Good protection. Two barriers around cervix. Use a condom too, to protect vagina and penis.
Creams, jellies, foams used alone	May be protection. More effective when used with a condom or diaphragm.
The pill	No protection.
The IUD	No protection. *Increases* risk of infection spreading to uterus and tubes.
Withdrawal	No protection. Not effective as birth control either.
Natural birth control	No protection.

Facts on Gonorrhea

Common names: Gonorrhea (gah-noh-*ree*-ah) is also known as the clap, dose, drip, morning dew, gleet, hot piss, the whites.

What Is It? Gonorrhea is an infection caused by the gonococcus bacteria. It can only live in dark, warm, moist places inside the body. It dies on contact with air within seconds.

How Is It Passed? The bacteria are passed when mucous membranes (the lining of the body openings) come in contact. The bacteria usually grow in the vagina, the penis, the mouth or throat, and the anus. Eyes can be infected too, if they come in contact with the bacteria. The germs are not spread by doorknobs, toilet seats, towels or clothes.

Gonorrhea has passed the epidemic state and are considered pandemic (widespread epidemic).

What Are the Symptoms? Some symptoms generally show up within one day to two weeks after contact, but many people show *no* symptoms.

Females (80 percent show *no* symptoms)	*Males* (10 to 20 percent show *no* symptoms)
Vaginal discharge with unusual odor; has whitish, greenish or yellowish color	Discharge from penis—sometimes noticed as a drip seen before first urinating in the morning; sometimes a continual discharge
Painful urination	
Lower abdominal pain	
Sore throat or swollen glands	Burning, itching or pain when urinating
Discharge from anus	Sore throat or swollen glands
	Discharge from anus

Tests and Diagnosis. The doctor will look at and listen to your description of symptoms.

For males: if you have a discharge from your penis, the doctor may do a gram-stain test (p. 221), which is reliable; if there is no discharge, a culture (p. 221) is taken from the penis, throat and anus.

For females: the gram-stain test is *not* reliable; a culture is taken from the cervix, anus, throat and urethra.

The culture test is only 80 to 90 percent accurate. If your culture comes back negative, go back to the clinic in a week for another test, especially if you suspect you may have the disease. Two negative cultures usually mean you don't have gonorrhea.

Throat cultures are important if you've had oral sex. Anal cultures are important if you've had anal intercourse. In females, a culture from the urethra (opening for urine) is important since germs can travel from the vagina to the urethra.

Treatment. Penicillin, ampicillin and tetracycline can cure gonorrhea. People allergic to penicillin are given tetracycline, but *pregnant girls should not take tetracycline,* as it is dangerous to the unborn baby's bone and tooth development, and may affect the mother's liver and kidneys. The doctor will give you an alternative drug.

You may be given a shot of an antibiotic or pills or both. Follow the instructions *exactly.* Take the complete dose of medication for as long as you're told to.

Never borrow someone else's medication or give some of yours to anyone else.

Follow-up. NO SEXUAL ACTIVITY UNTIL THE TREATMENT IS COMPLETE AND YOU HAVE HAD TWO NEGATIVE CULTURES.

Some gonorrhea germs are very strong and need two complete treatments before they are all killed. It is very important to return to the clinic for follow-up tests after you complete the first round of antibiotics. If your test comes back negative, go back the following week for a second test. If that comes back negative too, you are cured. Some strains are resistant to penicillin and tetracycline and need different treatment.

If your follow-up test comes back positive, you must continue treatment with a second round of antibiotics. When that is complete, go back for follow-up tests.

Complications. If untreated, gonorrhea bacteria will continue to infect you. *It will not go away by itself, even if the warning symptoms go away.* The germs will spread and cause serious infections in your reproductive organs. It can lead to permanent sterility, which means you will no longer be able to get pregnant or get someone pregnant. It can also cause crippling arthritis in some people. If the germs infect your eyes, you can go blind.

Specific problems in females: PID (pelvic inflammatory disease), which is very serious. It can cause severe pain, damage to the reproductive organs and sterility. If scar tissue forms in the tubes, you may be susceptible to ectopic pregnancies (see p. 39). If a mother has gonorrhea, the baby can develop an infection in his or her eyes during childbirth, which, if untreated, can cause blindness.

Specific problems in males: Chronic urethritis, which is long-term inflammation of the urethra. It may result in problems and pain during urination and ejaculation. Also, epididymitis, which is inflammation of the sperm centers in the testicles. It is very painful and can cause sterility.

Prevention

—Use rubber and chemical barriers (condoms, foam, diaphragm with cream or jelly, cervical cap).
—Check for discharge, strong odor. Do not have sex with a male who has a discharge coming from his penis.
—Gargle with salt water after oral sex.

Extra precaution. If you are sexually active with more than one partner, or if your partner has other partners, have a gonorrhea culture taken at a clinic at least twice a year.

Facts on Herpes

What Is It? Herpes (*her*-pees) is a virus that is highly infectious. It is the newest STD epidemic. *There is no cure for it. Once you catch it, you may have it for life.*

Common-cold sores are one type of herpes. They are

called herpes simplex I. They are the fever blisters and canker sores people get around their mouth.

Genital sores are called herpes simplex II. They are painful sores that appear on and in the penis, vagina, and/or anus. In some cases Type II appears around the mouth also.

The herpes virus invades the body and attacks the cells in that area. It causes the skin to burst out in painful, reddish blisters. When the blisters heal, the virus travels up the nerves to live at the base of the skull, near the spinal column, or in ganglia (collections of nerve cells throughout the body). When a person with herpes is under stress—sick, upset, run-down, tired, or has had too much sun—the virus travels down the nerves again and causes the painful sores to erupt.

How Is It Passed?   The virus is passed by direct contact with sores, or by contact with the area twenty-four hours or less *before* sores erupt. The virus from one person's sores enters the other person's body through cuts, openings in genitals, mouth, eyes, and maybe even through pores in the skin. You can also pass the virus from one part of your body to another when you touch the infected area.

What Are the Symptoms?   Symptoms generally show up two to twenty days after contact, but sometimes they don't show up for several months or even a year.

First symptoms are usually itching or tingling around genitals. Then there is aching in the genital area. There may also be a general achiness, as if you're coming down with the flu. There may be a slight fever, a headache and swollen glands.

Next the sores appear. They are very painful. They may crack and become blistered. Sometimes the sores bleed or ooze fluid.

The sores can last up to two weeks the first time you get them. They may go away and never return. Or they may go away and then return at different times throughout your life, especially when you are run-down. Severity generally lessens with repeated attacks.

Tests and Diagnosis.   The doctor or health worker will listen to your description of the symptoms and will look at the sores. Usually the appearance of the sore tells that it is herpes. Sometimes herpes sores are mistaken for syphilis sores, but herpes is painful. Syphilis sores are not painful.

A sample of fluid may be taken from the sore and tested. You should also have a blood test, to make sure you don't have syphilis, and a culture test for gonorrhea. In girls a Pap smear should be taken (see p. 158). A new tissue culture test is the most reliable way to tell if you have herpes.

Treatment.   At the present time there is no medication to kill the herpes virus. The doctor can only give you things to help soothe the pain of the sores and possibly make them disappear sooner.

The doctor may prescribe pain-relieving drugs, such as aspirin. He or she may also prescribe sulfa creams or viral creams for the sores. Many doctors think the creams only help spread the infection, so they do not recommend them. Home remedies:

—Keep the sores clean and dry.
—Ice relieves the pain by numbing the area. If you feel the attack coming on and apply ice in an ice bag, it may stop the sores from erupting. Keep the area dry.
—Dry thoroughly after baths and showers.
—Eat a balanced diet. Check with a nutritionist for specific supplements.
—Get enough sleep. Try not to let your body get run-down.

Follow-up.   If sores do not go away within ten to fourteen days, go back to the doctor or clinic. Continue going there once a week until the sores disappear. Sometimes a bacterial infection can complicate the healing process. You may need antibiotics to kill the infection.

Avoid all sexual activity until the sores disappear completely. Do not even masturbate, because your hands can pass the disease to other parts of your body.

Girls with herpes should have Pap smears at least every six months.

Keep yourself healthy and rested. You may avoid future attacks that way.

Complications.   For males, herpes is painful and annoying. For females it can be dangerous. It is also dangerous for babies.

In females there is a possible link between the herpes simplex II virus and cervical cancer. That is why girls and women with herpes *must* have Pap smears twice a year. If any abnormal cells appear, the area should be watched more carefully. Girls and women whose partners have herpes should also go for Pap smears twice a year, even if they themselves don't ever experience the sores.

Herpes can complicate pregnancies, causing spontaneous abortions in some people. It can also infect the unborn baby and cause brain damage, birth defects and, in some cases, death. This is especially dangerous during the mother's first case of herpes.

If there are herpes sores in the birth canal, the baby can get the disease as he or she is traveling down the canal to be born. Caesarean deliveries are recommended for pregnant girls and women with active herpes. (See *Our Bodies, Ourselves,* pp. 287–289.)

Herpes can infect eyes and cause blindness.

Prevention.   Most specialists in this field believe that herpes is contagious only during attacks when the sores are present or during the twenty-four hours *before* the sores appear.

—*Never have sexual contact with someone who has genital sores.* Avoid oral contact with someone who has sores around his or her mouth.

—Ask your sexual partner or partners if they have herpes. Ask them if they feel an attack coming on. The symptoms can be like flu symptoms; they may feel run-down. Sometimes there is tingling in the area of the sores.

—If you have herpes, watch for signs of an attack and avoid sexual contact at those times.

There is no method that will prevent the spread of herpes during contact. Some people are naturally less susceptible than others, but the only sure way to avoid herpes is to avoid sexual contact with someone who has it.

Extra precautions

—Use condoms and foam together or other barrier methods during intercourse, although virus germs may be able to pass through these barriers.

—Wash genitals before and after contact.

—Keep yourself healthy. Eat well, get enough sleep, exercise.

—Don't get too much sun. Many people who have had the disease get herpes attacks after exposure. The sun doesn't cause the herpes, but overexposure seems to cause an attack if the virus is already in your system.

IF YOU HAVE HERPES

Watch for common preattack signals:

—Tenderness in genital area or around lips.
—Dry or red spot on skin, crack on lip.
—Fever.
—Flu-like aches and depression.
—Swelling of glands.
—Prickles and tingles on area where sores break out.

If you feel an attack coming on:

—Do not have sex with anyone.
—Get enough rest.
—Put ice on the area. Wrap ice in a plastic bag and hold it on the area for as long as you can stand it. Take it off, then repeat.
—Eat well. Avoid junk foods.

Herpes is spreading fast. A special national organization has been formed to help herpes sufferers get more information about the disease. They share successful home remedies and news about herpes research. Write to them at HELP, P.O. Box 10, Palo Alto, CA 94302. They publish a monthly magazine called *The Helper*. A subscription costs $5 per year.

Facts on Non-gonococcal Urethritis

Common names: This disease is also known as NGU or NSU (non-specific urethritis). Non-gonococcal urethritis is pronounced non-gah-noh-*cah*-kuhl you-reeth-*rye*-tiss.

What Is It? NGU is an inflammation of the urethra (the passageway for urine). It is most often caused by the bacteria named chlamydia trachomatis. It can also be caused by other organisms, such as T-strain mycoplasmas. Along with gonorrhea, NGU is the most commonly caught sexually transmitted disease.

In females, NGU infects the vagina during penis–vagina intercourse. Less frequently it is passed to the urethra.

How Is It Passed? Chlamydia and the other organisms that cause NGU stay alive in dark, warm, moist places and are passed through penis–vagina intercourse. STD specialists think NGU may also be passed through penis–anus intercourse as well as fellatio (penis–throat contact).

It is possible that some people carry the chlamydia organism without showing symptoms and these people may pass it on to their sexual partners.

What Are the Symptoms? The symptoms of NGU are discharge from the penis or cervix; burning sensation during urination; a feeling that you have to urinate more frequently than usual; possible itchiness around the penis or vagina. These symptoms appear gradually within ten to twenty days after contact with an infected partner, but not everyone who has NGU gets symptoms. Most females and some males have *no* symptoms of the disease. The only way a person with no symptoms can tell whether he or she may be infected is being told by a partner to have a checkup. So remember, if you find out you have NGU or some other sexually transmitted disease, tell your partner or partners to go for a checkup. You may be saving them from serious complications.

If the infection goes untreated it may move into the internal organs and cause damage to the organs of reproduction and, in boys, to the urethra also. Most people feel pain in the lower abdominal or groin area if this occurs.

Tests and Diagnosis. Up till now the way the health professionals tested for NGU was to test for gonorrhea and other infections. If those tests were negative, they would assume—by the process of elimination—that your problem was NGU. That is still the procedure in most clinics.

There is a new culture test for chlamydia available in a few labs, which can actually determine if the chlamydia organism is present. This test is expensive and not widely available at present. When you go for your test, ask the lab worker if they are able to run the chlamydia culture test. If they are not, ask if there is a lab in your area that is able to run it.

Treatment. The treatment for NGU is tetracycline, an antibiotic. (Penicillin, which cures gonorrhea, does *not* cure NGU.) You must take the tetracycline tablets for the full period prescribed by the doctor. Avoid dairy products while you are taking tetracycline, because they seem to interfere with the drug's function.

If you are allergic to tetracycline or if you are pregnant,

the doctor will arrange some substitute, probably erythromycin. Pregnant girls and women should not take tetracycline.

If one partner has NGU, the other or others should be treated too. Otherwise they may continue to pass the disease back and forth to each other.

NGU usually occurs when your body is run-down or overstressed. Be sure to eat a well-balanced diet and get plenty of rest while you are recuperating.

Follow-up. After you finish the medication, return to the clinic for another test. Girls should return again a third time one month later.

DO NOT HAVE SEXUAL CONTACT WITH PARTNERS UNTIL YOU ARE SURE THE INFECTION NO LONGER EXISTS IN EITHER OF YOU.

Complications. Some strains of non-gonococcal urethritis are responsible for birth defects, eye damage and pneumonia in newborn infants born to mothers who have the disease. NGU may also cause spontaneous abortions and stillbirths in some cases.

NGU may lead to pelvic inflammatory disease (PID) in girls. PID is an inflammation of the internal organs, especially the fallopian tubes. PID can cause sterility in some girls. It can also cause scar tissue to build up in the tubes, which can result in ectopic pregnancies (see p. 39).

In boys NGU can lead to infections in the testicles, which can possibly result in sterility.

In both boys and girls NGU can leave the urethra scarred, causing problems with urination and in boys with ejaculation.

Prevention

—Do not have sex with a boy who has a milky discharge from the penis, or with a boy or girl who complains of burning urination.
—Use condoms and foam during penis–vagina or penis–anus intercourse.

Facts on Syphilis

Common names: Syphilis (*sih*-fih-liss) is also known as siff, pox, lues, bad blood, Old Joe, haircut.

What Is It? Syphilis is a disease caused by small spiral-shaped bacteria. Once the bacteria infect the body, they enter the bloodstream and attack vital organs. Syphilis is a less common disease than gonorrhea, but it is dangerous and can do serious damage to your body. In the first stages it causes a *painless* sore or blister to appear on the body, usually around the genitals. This is called a *chancre* (pronounced: shanker). Later a rash may appear over the body or particularly on the palms of the hands and soles of the feet. Sometimes the rash appears while the chancre is present.

If syphilis is not treated, the external symptoms will disappear, but the disease will not disappear. It stays alive in the body. If it is never treated it may eventually cause death.

How Is It Passed? The germs are passed when contact is made with the sores or with the rash. The bacteria are commonly passed through sexual contact. The chancres around the genitals or mouth of the infected person pass the bacteria to the genitals or mouth of the other person.

What Are the Symptoms? Symptoms generally appear between ten and ninety days after contact with an infected person.

There are three stages of syphilis, and it is highly contagious during the first two stages.

Stage I:

—Painless sores (chancres) appear at the spot where the germs entered the body. Often just one chancre appears first. In females the sore may not be visible if it is inside the vagina or around the cervix or in the anus if partners had anal sex.
—The chancre(s) will disappear in one to five weeks. The germs are still alive in the body.
—Sometimes a rash appears.

Stage II:

—Months after the chancres disappear some people get secondary symptoms. Other people don't show any secondary symptoms.
—The symptoms are fever, aches, sore throat, mouth sores, patchy hair loss, swollen glands, flu-like ailments.
—A rash may appear all over the body, or it may only be on the palms of the hands and the soles of the feet.
—If not treated, these symptoms will disappear by themselves after a few months, but the germs will still be alive in the body.

Stage III:

—Months or even years later, serious complications may occur.
—The disease may begin to attack internal body organs causing:
  Heart disease
  Blindness
  Muscle incoordination
  Deafness
  Paralysis
  Insanity
  Death

An unborn baby can get syphilis from its infected mother. The germs will attack the baby through the placenta.

Tests and Diagnosis. If you go to the clinic when you notice a chancre, the health worker will take a sample of the fluid from the sore and examine it.

The doctor or health worker will listen to your description of symptoms and check you for fever, swollen glands, unusual discharge, chancres.

You will be given a blood test, called VDRL, which is reliable about one week to ten days after the chancre appears. A VDRL will detect syphilis in Stage I, II or III. If the test comes back negative but you definitely have a painless chancre, go back for another test. There may not have been enough bacteria in your bloodstream to show up the first time.

Every pregnant girl and woman should have a blood test for syphilis when she finds out she is pregnant, and another one during the last three months of pregnancy.

Treatment. The earlier the treatment, the less damage will be done. Long-acting penicillin injections are given to treat syphilis. If you have definite symptoms or if there is good reason to believe you have been exposed to the disease, you will probably be treated when you go in for the test. Otherwise the clinic will call you when they receive the results of your test. If the results were positive, you will be told to come in for treatment.

People who are allergic to penicillin will be given another drug, such as tetracycline. Pregnant girls and women should not take tetracycline. It can cause bone and tooth damage to the unborn baby, as well as liver and kidney trouble in the mother.

Follow treatment instructions *exactly*. If they give you pills, take them according to directions and for as long as the doctor prescribes. Do not stop treatment just because your symptoms have disappeared. There may still be germs alive in your system.

Follow-up. DON'T HAVE SEX UNTIL YOU ARE CURED.

One month after the treatment is completed, go back to the clinic for another blood test. You may begin to have sexual relations when the doctor or health professional gives you the go ahead.

Have blood tests to check for syphilis *every three months for one whole year* to be certain you are free from the disease.

Complications. Untreated syphilis is life-threatening. See discussion under Stage III on p. 227.

Prevention

—Avoid people with sores and rashes. Never have sex with a person who has sores around his or her genitals or mouth, or a rash, particularly on the palms of the hand or soles of the feet.
—Use condoms and foam during intercourse, although theoretically syphilis germs can pass through condoms.
—If you are having sex with more than one partner, or if you partner has other partners, have a blood test to check for syphilis at least twice a year.

Extra precautions

—Urinate before and after sex.
—Wash your genitals before and after sex.
—Gargle with hot salt water after oral sex.
—Don't kiss someone with sores around his or her mouth. Don't let that person put his or her mouth on your body.

NOTE: Not all sores are syphilis chancres, and not all sores are contagious. But unless you are sure that your partner's sores are *not* contagious, don't take chances.

Facts on Venereal Warts

What Are They? Venereal warts are wartlike bumps that usually appear around the inside and outside of the genital organs—the penis and testicles in boys, the vagina in girls. They can also appear around the anus. If they are inside the vagina, intercourse may be painful or itchy.

Venereal warts are caused by a virus, as are other warts. If you do not treat them, they can get larger.

How Are They Passed? They are passed by direct contact between the warts and someone else's skin. They grow in both dry and moist areas of the body. During sex they are passed from the genital area of one person to that of his or her partner.

Not everyone who comes in contact with warts will catch them.

What Are the Symptoms? The warts are hard, wrinkled bumps that appear on the skin or in the genital area within one to three months after contact. They are usually painless, but they can be irritated by rubbing and sometimes they itch. When they are inside the vagina or anus they are usually pink and wet, and they may go unnoticed.

Sometimes these warts are mistaken for syphilis chancres at first, but warts are not filled with fluid as chancres are.

Tests and Diagnosis. The doctor will examine the warts and be able to identify them from their appearance. Tests are rarely done. Sometimes a blood test should be taken to make sure you do not have syphilis.

Treatment. There are three types of treatment to remove the warts. They must be removed or they may get larger and infect a larger area. These treatments should be done by a doctor or health worker at the clinic.

—Chemical treatment. If the warts are small enough they may be removed with an application of an ointment or liquid called podophyllin. This chemical should be washed off after six hours or it can burn your skin. You may need several applications. Pregnant girls and women should not use podophyllin.
—Freezing. Small warts can be frozen off with dry-ice treatment. This is sometimes painful, but only briefly. After treatment the doctor snips off the warts.

—Large warts must be removed surgically. In most cases this is done under a local anesthetic, which numbs the area to reduce pain. In a few cases it may be done under general anesthesia. Pregnant girls and women should avoid surgery.

Follow-up. *Avoid sexual contact until all the warts have been removed.* Have the area checked by a doctor about a week after removal to make sure you are clear.

Do not irritate the area from which the warts were removed for at least one week. That means you must not have sexual contact in that area during that time.

Every time you go for a checkup, have the doctor or clinic check to make sure your warts have not returned.

Complications. The only complication is that if they are not removed, the condition may worsen. The warts can also return even after treatment. If that happens they will have to be removed again. Babies born of mothers with venereal warts may develop problems, particularly growths in or around the larynx.

Prevention

—*Do not have sexual relations with anyone who has genital warts until the warts have been completely removed.*
—Have regular medical checkups if you are sexually active.

Extra precautions

—Use foam and condoms or other barriers during intercourse. These may help to keep the germs from passing from one person to another, although theoretically virus germs can travel through most barriers.

Facts on Hepatitis

What Is It? Viral hepatitis (heh-pah-*tie*-tiss) is a disease caused by several viruses. It mainly infects a person's liver and can cause serious damage to that organ. It makes you very sick because the disease affects the functioning of your whole system. There is no real cure for hepatitis because it is a viral infection. If you get it, you just have to let the disease take its course.

How Is It Passed? There are three different types of hepatitis and they are passed in different ways.

Hepatitis A, which used to be called infectious hepatitis, is caused by feces contamination. It can be passed by direct contact with body wastes, through anal intercourse or mouth-anus or finger-anus sex play. It can be caught through unsanitary living conditions. For example, someone can catch it by sitting on a contaminated toilet seat, or if a person with hepatitis does not wash his or her hands after touching or wiping his or her anus, germs can get on objects he or she touches. Drinking water and certain foods, especially raw or undercooked seafood, can carry the disease.

Hepatitis B used to be called serum hepatitis. It can be found in the body fluids of an infected person. It can be passed through mouth-to-mouth or mouth-to-genital contact or through other sexual contact that brings one body opening in contact with another. Also, Hepatitis B can be passed by puncturing the skin with contaminated instruments, such as the needles used for tattooing, ear piercing, acupuncture, and medical or dental work. The germs can also be passed by using someone else's razor or toothbrush if that person has the disease.

The third type of hepatitis is called Non-A, Non-B hepatitis. Not much is known about this disease, except that it is different from both the other varieties. Its main route of infection seems to be through blood transfusion from an infected donor. It may also be passed through other means, including sexual contact.

What Are the Symptoms? The general symptoms are nausea, muscle achiness, fatigue, fever, loss of appetite, headaches, dizziness. These are similar to flu symptoms, and as a result, hepatitis often goes untreated for a long time because people confuse it with the flu or a bad cold. If they are having sexual relations during this time, they could be passing the disease on to their partners.

In some cases there are only mild symptoms. In other cases there are definite symptoms particular to hepatitis: darkening of urine color, lightening of stool color, yellowing of eyes and skin (jaundice), tenderness in the liver. Contrary to popular belief, though, most people with hepatitis do not turn yellow.

The symptoms may begin to appear within the first month after contact, or they may not appear for up to six months. This usually depends on the type of virus that has infected your system. If you notice symptoms, go to a doctor or clinic right away to be tested.

Tests and Diagnosis. The doctor will listen to your description of the symptoms. He or she will check for fever and look at your eyes to check the color. You may be asked to bring in a stool sample (the fresher it is, the better it will be for testing). You will be asked general questions about your health and living habits. Since hepatitis is a common disease among male homosexuals and among heterosexual couples who practice anal sex, be honest with the doctor about your sex life. It will help him or her make an accurate diagnosis.

A blood test can identify hepatitis after the second week of infection, so a blood sample will be taken for testing.

Treatment. The best treatment is bed rest, lots of fluids and a light, healthy diet. Avoid fatty foods and junk foods. Most doctors advise patients with hepatitis to avoid alcoholic beverages because alcohol can further strain the liver and cause serious injury.

Several people we interviewed said that they were so weak during their bout with hepatitis that they could hardly move. They needed someone to help them take care of themselves and feed them. It will help if you are living with people who care about you and can tend to your needs. They should receive gamma globulin shots for protection.

If you have no one to help you, contact your local Board of Health or call the local Visiting Nurse Association.

Follow-up. Recovery usually occurs within two to three months, and sometimes less. You must take care of yourself and get plenty of rest until the disease is completely gone. Avoid stress. Have frequent medical checkups, according to your doctor's instructions.

You must not have any sexual contact with partners until the disease has passed and a blood test shows that you are cured.

One attack of hepatitis generally gives you immunity from that type of virus and you will not come down with that strain of hepatitis again. *But* some people can carry the virus in their system even after all their symptoms have cleared up and they feel healthy again. They are chronic carriers, and they can continue to infect others even though they themselves seem to be over the disease.

Hepatitis A doesn't lead to a carrier state, but hepatitis B and Non-A, Non-B hepatitis can. Hepatitis B carriers can be determined by a blood test. Non-A, Non-B carriers can't be identified through a blood test yet. The only way they can be identified is by passing the disease on to someone else, usually if they donate blood and a recipient of their blood gets the disease. *Known hepatitis carriers must not donate blood.* Also, carriers should inform their doctor or dentist of their condition. Sexual partners should also be warned because they are at risk of catching the disease.

Complications. Liver problems are the most common complication of hepatitis, since the disease affects the liver. In rare cases hepatitis can cause permanent damage to the liver or even death due to liver failure.

Hepatitis may be the cause of miscarriage during pregnancy. If a girl or woman has hepatitis B during the last months of pregnancy, the newborn may develop the disease and become a chronic carrier. It may be possible to protect the infant with special globulin injections, so any pregnant girl or woman with hepatitis should tell her doctor right away.

Prevention

—Don't have sex with anyone who appears sick or who looks jaundiced.
—Never use someone else's toothbrush, razor, enemas, douche equipment or other equipment that may be contaminated by body fluids, blood or body wastes.
—If you are living with someone who has hepatitis, keep all their food preparation and eating utensils separate, and make sure they have separate towels, bed linen and dishes. If possible, they should use separate toilet facilities. If that isn't possible, careful scrubbing of the toilet after use is essential.
—Do not sit on strange toilet seats. Especially avoid wet or dirty toilet seats.
—Wash your hands thoroughly with soap and water after using the toilet.

Extra precautions

—Wash your genitals, especially your anus and anything that touches it, before and after sexual contact.
—There is a product called Fleet's enema that can be used to clean the anal canal before anal sex.
—Use condoms and foam during anal intercourse.

Facts on Vaginal Infections

We will discuss two vaginal infections: yeast infections (called candida, monilia and fungus) and trichomoniasis.

Normally many bacteria and organisms grow inside the vagina, just as they do in the mouth. Some of them help to keep the chemical balance of the vagina healthy. Under certain conditions, such as after antibiotic treatment, pregnancy or an illness, or during times of stress, harmful bacteria and organisms can multiply and upset the healthy balance. That is when vaginal infections develop.

Infections can also start when girls wear tight pants that cut into their crotch, or when they wear pantyhose or nylon panties that don't allow air to circulate around the vagina. Sometimes infections start because of an allergic reaction to a birth control product, a dye in colored toilet paper, a bath oil or a vaginal deodorant. Douching, too, can cause a bacteria imbalance and create an infection. So can birth control pills.

Yeast Infections. *What are they?* Yeast normally grows in the vagina and also in the anus. If there is an imbalance of organisms, the yeast can multiply and become thick. A cottage-cheese-like discharge will appear. It usually itches a lot and can cause irritation around and inside the vagina. The vagina may become red and dry and painful to touch.

How are they passed? Once you have a yeast infection it can be passed to a sexual partner through genital or oral sex. Even if your partner has no symptoms, he or she can pass the disease to you if he or she has it. Your system may be more susceptible to a yeast imbalance. Careless anal sex practice can cause yeast infections. Always wash your finger and/or penis after anal sex, *before* putting them in the vagina.

What are the symptoms?

—Itchiness around the genitals.
—Cottage-cheese-like discharge.
—Pain or redness around the vagina or the opening of the penis.
—Yeastlike smell in the genital area.

Tests and diagnosis. A sample of the discharge is placed under the microscope. Yeast cells will be easily seen in most cases. You can see them yourself. Ask the doctor to let you look.

Treatment. A drug called Mycostatin or some other form of nystatin is prescribed either in a cream or in vaginal suppositories for girls. The medication can also be taken by mouth by both males and females, according to the doctor's prescription.

The doctor may paint the inside of the vagina, the cervix and the vulva with a substance called gentian violet. It is bright purple, so it may stain your clothes. Wear a sanitary napkin to protect them. Some people have an allergic reaction to gentian violet.

Use these products exactly according to instructions and for the entire time recommended, even if your symptoms seem to go away.

Some girls and women use home remedies to cure yeast infections. One common one is a vinegar-and-water douche.* Use two tablespoons of white vinegar to one quart of warm water. Use this solution as a douche one or two times a day until symptoms disappear, then continue for two days after that. *Always be sure to hold the douche bag below your waist, or squeeze the syringe gently. Pregnant girls and women should never douche.*

After the vinegar-and-water douche, apply plain, unsweetened, unflavored yogurt to the inside of the vagina. That adds healthy bacteria to the area, and will help the vagina achieve a normal balance again. It is also soothing. See *Our Bodies, Ourselves,* p. 138, for other suggestions. If these home remedies don't work, consult a medical person.

Follow-up. Yeast infections can be hard to get rid of. If yours won't go away, try to figure out what may be causing it. Wear cotton underpants. If you wear long skirts, don't wear any underpants at all. The air helps. Don't wear tight pants, at least until your infection clears up. Use only white toilet paper. Don't use anything with perfume around the area. Eliminate bath oils or other bath preparations. *Use no vaginal deodorants.*

Do not have sex with a partner until the infection clears up.

If the symptoms do not go away within three to four weeks after you begin treatment, go back to the clinic.

Sex partners must be treated and cured together or else they will pass the infection back and forth.

Complications. Many girls have recurring yeast infections. A few weeks after one is cured, they develop another one. If that happens to you, follow the advice listed under Prevention below.

---

*Regular douching is not advisable, but during vaginal infections vinegar-and-water douches may help restore the vagina to its healthy state.

A yeast infection can be very hard to cure during pregnancy. Babies can pick it up as they pass through the birth canal. It may cause an infection in the baby's mouth, called thrush.

If you get yeast infections over and over, that could be a sign of diabetes. The yeast infections don't cause diabetes, but they can be a symptom of it. Have yourself checked by a competent medical person.

Prevention

—Keep the genital area very clean. Wash with soap and water at least once a day.
—Don't use perfumed powders or deodorants or bath preparations in the genital area.
—Don't wear pants that are tight in the crotch or thighs.
—Use barrier protection during intercourse.
—Contraceptive jellies may slow down the growth of yeast infections.
—Don't eat too much sugar. High sugar intake can interfere with the normal balance of your body chemistry.
—Use plain, white, unscented toilet paper.
—Make sure your sex partner is clean.

For girls:

—Always wipe from front to back after going to the bathroom.
—Never put anything from your anus into your vagina without washing it first.
—Don't douche.
—Wear cotton underpants.
—If you're on the birth control pill, consider some other form of contraception. The pill increases a girl's susceptibility to yeast infections.

Trichomoniasis. Common name: trichomoniasis (trih-coh-moh-*nye*-ah-siss), or trichomonas vaginalis, is also known simply as trich (pronounced: trick).

What is it? It is an infection, usually found in the vagina, caused by a tiny, one-celled parasite. Many girls normally have trich organisms living in their vaginas that do not cause symptoms.

How is it passed? The trich parasite can be passed through sexual activity between partners. Finger–genital touching can pass it. If you touch your partner's vagina and then touch your own penis or vagina, you can pass the organism to yourself. The parasite can stay alive outside the body for up to seven hours. Penis–vagina or vagina–vagina contact will also pass the bug if one partner has it.

Males can develop trich in their prostate gland and the organism can be part of the semen that comes out during ejaculation.

Trich can also be passed by using someone else's washcloth or towel, or by wearing someone else's bathing suit or unclean underpants. You can even catch it by sitting on an infected toilet seat.

What are the symptoms? In girls: intense itching in the vagina; pain during urination; red, tender labia. There may be a thin yellow-green or gray foamy discharge from the vagina, which will have a foul odor. If you have another infection along with the trich, the discharge may be thicker and whiter. In boys: discharge from the penis; slight tickling in the penis.

Tests and diagnosis. Secretions from the vagina or penis are put under a microscope. The trich organism can be seen swimming around. Ask the doctor if you can see them too. You should have a culture taken, to rule out gonorrhea.

Treatment. A drug named Flagyl is the only medication currently available that kills the trich organisms effectively. Sexual partners must take the treatment together, or they will continue to pass the trich back and forth.

Unfortunately, Flagyl is a very dangerous drug, especially when taken in the high doses recommended to kill trich. Some tests have shown that the drug used to make Flagyl can cause gene mutations. It has caused birth defects in animals and cancer in rats and mice. It produces side effects such as dizziness, nausea and headache in some people.

This is a case in which we are in a no-win situation, since Flagyl is the most effective way to get rid of trich but has dangerous side effects. Most clinics and doctors recommend its use anyway. Talk this question over with your doctor. Call a local women's health center for more information, or write to the Boston Women's Health Book Collective.*

Pregnant girls and women must never take Flagyl or any product containing metronidazole. If you took Flagyl before you knew you were pregnant, you may want to consider having an abortion. Talk to a counselor.

Other people who should not take Flagyl are those with blood disease, peptic ulcers or central nervous system diseases.

There are some vaginal suppositories available that do not contain Flagyl but can be fairly effective in destroying trich. Ask at the clinic. Boys will not be able to use the suppositories, since the opening in the penis is not large enough.

Because of the dangers of Flagyl, the best treatment for trich is to prevent it in the first place. Use foam and condoms.

Follow-up. Trich grows best in an alkaline environment, so vinegar-water douches may keep girls from getting it. These douches may be especially effective during menstruation, since the blood from the menstrual fluid is very hospitable to the organism. This is one time when douching may actually be recommended.

Keep yourself clean. Girls should avoid tampons, vagi-

*P.O. Box 192, W. Somerville, MA 02144.

nal sprays and deodorants, or any perfumed powder. Both boys and girls should wear clean underwear every day. If you can walk around naked from the waist down at home, do it as much as you can. Air will help get rid of the infection.

Girls should have a sample taken from the vagina ten days after treatment began to make sure the disease has been cured.

If you take Flagyl, do *not* drink any alcohol during treatment. Also, avoid vinegar (except in douches) and mayonnaise.

No sexual contact with a partner until disease is cured.

Complications. For girls: inflamed cervix and urethra; abnormal Pap smears. For boys: infected prostate gland, bladder infections, infected testicles.

Prevention. For girls: vinegar-water douches, especially during menstruation, if you seem to be particularly susceptible to trich.

See Prevention advice on p. 230, under Yeast Infections.

Facts on Pubic Lice (Crabs)

Common name: Pubic lice are commonly referred to as crabs, because they look like tiny crabs.

What Are They? They are little animals the size of a pinhead, yellowish-gray in color. They feed on human blood and like to live in moist, hairy spots—for example, in pubic hair, eyelashes, underarm hair and chest hair.

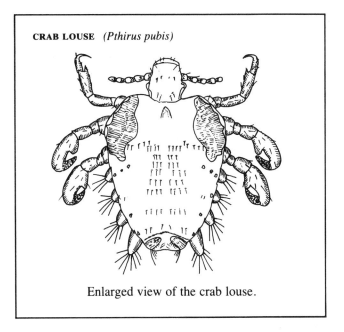

CRAB LOUSE *(Pthirus pubis)*

Enlarged view of the crab louse.

How Are They Passed? Crabs are passed through close contact with a person who has them. They can also be passed by clothes, bedding and upholstered furniture. The crabs from the infected person hop onto another person, pet or warm spot and try to make themselves comfortable in the new host. Since they need blood to survive, they cannot live for more than twenty-four hours without a host. Their eggs can live about a week without human contact.

When two people have close contact, the crabs can move from one host to another. If you borrow the clothes of someone who has crabs, you can become infested. If you sleep in his or her bed, even alone at the time, you can become infested. Sometimes crabs are even caught from sitting in the same chair or couch as someone who has them.

They are *highly* contagious.

What Are the Symptoms? The first symptom of crabs is usually intense itching in the site where the crabs have established themselves. They are generally found in pubic hair initially, but they can move to other body hair and eyelashes as you scratch them and then touch other places on your body.

You can see crabs without a microscope. Look closely. Sometimes even if they are no longer there, you can see the eggs they've left to hatch.

Some people don't itch. They may have crabs without knowing it until they pass them on to someone else.

Tests and Diagnosis. If you aren't sure you have crabs but you itch terribly around the pubic area, go to the clinic for a checkup. The doctor or health worker will be able to see the crabs or their eggs.

Treatment. Soap will not kill crabs. There is a cream treatment called Kwell that can be bought at any drugstore. In the United States you need a prescription for it. It works very quickly and effectively if you follow the instructions on the package exactly. All your clothes must be washed in *hot* water with detergent or dry-cleaned. All your sheets and blankets must be washed or dry-cleaned too. Remember, the crab eggs can live for a week in clothing or bed linen, so if you don't want to or can't wash everything, make sure you don't use them for more than a week.

Follow-up. You may have to repeat the treatment in two weeks. Keep checking yourself for crabs and eggs.

Make sure all your partners are treated too. Otherwise you may keep passing the crabs back and forth.

Complications. The itching will make you want to scratch. The more you scratch, the greater the chance of moving the crabs from one site to another.

Sometimes crabs carry diseases such as typhus.

Prevention

—Keep yourself clean.
—Keep your clothes and bed linen clean.
—*Don't have sex with someone who itches a lot,* unless he/she has some other reason for it. Check for crabs on his or her body.
—*Try not to borrow other people's clothes.*

Facts on Scabies

What Are They? Scabies (*scay*-bees) are microscopic parasites that burrow under people's skin and lay their eggs there.

How Are They Passed? Scabies are passed when a person who has them touches another person. That can be anything from shaking hands to making love. They are *highly* contagious.

What Are the Symptoms? The bug burrows under the skin and causes a red sore or series of sores, or raised reddish tracks along the skin. There is intense itching around the site.

Scabies can appear anywhere on the body.

Tests and Diagnosis. Go to the clinic or doctor's office. The doctor or health worker will prick out some particles from the infected area and examine them under a microscope. He or she will be able to see the scabies if they are present.

Treatment. Same as the treatment for crabs. Use Kwell exactly according to instructions. Use two treatments of Kwell to be sure to get the eggs that the scabies may have left under your skin.

Follow-up. Make sure your sex partners are being treated too. Otherwise you'll pass the bugs back and forth.

If some eggs remain after treatment, you will have to use Kwell another time when the eggs hatch.

Wash clothes and bed linen in *hot* water and detergent; dry in a hot dryer.

Complications. Scabies usually itch terribly, so people scratch. Scratching can cause complications like secondary infections and spreading of the parasite to other parts of the body.

Prevention

—Keep yourself clean.
—*Don't have sex or contact with someone who itches a lot,* unless he/she has some other reason for it.
—Watch for sores and red spots on people's skin.

BUTTERFLY

I am shrouded, here, in my cocoon.
I go through the motions of life, and enjoy it,
as best I can.
I am growing.
Slowly.
I am blossoming into adulthood.
Growing my wings.
Everything seems so confusing now.
My brain is crowded.
Is this a crash course in life and living?
All the chaos shall bust.
Soon.
Too soon, perhaps.
My cocoon will burst.
I will be left open.
Alone.
Vulnerable.
A butterfly at last.

—Janie Leive

INDEX

abdominal pain, lower, as symptom of sexually transmitted disease, 220
abortion, deciding whether to have, 197–206
   advice on, 199
   D-and-C (dilation and curettage) method of having, 204
   emotional aftercare, 205–206
     anger, 205
     depression, 205–206
     fear, 206
     guilt, 205
     sex, feelings about, 206
     strength, 206
   Hyde Amendment, on paying for, 200
   induced method of having, 204
   legal rights, 198–99
   paying for, 200
   physical aftercare, 204–205
   Rh-negative blood and, 201n
   risks and complications associated with, 200–201
     anesthesia, 201
   services, checking out, 199–200
   vacuum suction (vacuum aspiration) method of having, 201–204
     breathing exercises during, 203
   where to get, 199
   See also baby, deciding to have; birth control; pregnancy
adoption choice, after having baby, 214–16
   feelings about, 215
   illegal adoptions, 215
   legal adoptions, 215
   private arrangement, 215
   rights of parent, 214
alcohol
   as blur to deciding on sex with another, 90–91
   erection and, not getting or keeping, 111
   pregnancy and, 191
   See also drugs and alcohol
Alcoholics Anonymous, 49
alveoli of girl's breasts, 21
American Cancer Society, 158n
American Civil Liberties Union, 137, 199
amphetamines (uppers), 149–50
anal sex, 122
anesthesia, abortion and, 201
angel dust (PCP), 150
anger
   as feeling after abortion, 205
   letting out, 135
anus of female, 28
areola of girl's breast, 20–21
aspirin, ease of menstrual cycle and, 35

baby, deciding to have, when pregnant, 206–16
   choices available, 206
   foster care, using, 209–14
     father's rights and, 210n
     legal rights and, 210
     private arrangement, 210–11
     voluntary placement for child, 211–14
   parent, deciding to become, 206–209
   See also abortion, deciding whether to have; birth control
bad trips on drugs, 152
Ballentine, Ralph (*Diet and Nutrition, a Holistic Approach*), 182n
best friends, changing relationships and, 62–64. *See also* friends; oppo-site-sex friendships
birth control, 102, 159–89
   cervical cap, 176–77
   condoms and foam, 166–71
     Consumer Reports on, 167n
     foam, using, 169–70

good and bad points about condoms, 168–69
   good and bad points on foam, 170–71
   how to get condoms, 167
   storing condoms, 167–68
   types of condoms, 166–67
   types of foam, 170
   using condoms, 167–168
diaphragm, 171–76
   checking, 175
   cost of, 172–73
   getting, 172
   good and bad points about, 174–76
   jellies, contraceptive, 172–73
   learning to insert, 173–75
   using, 171, 174
family planning clinics, 164–65
   getting, 162–65
   improving lovemaking by use of, 107
   injectable contraception, 189
IUD (intra-uterine device), 182–86
   antibiotics and, 183
   changing, 185
   checking, 185
   cost of, 185
   getting, 183–84
   good and bad points of, 185–86
   infections, 186
   inserting, 184–85
   perforation and embedding, 186
   pregnancy and, 186–87
   removing, 185
   sexually transmitted diseases and, 186
   using, 183
   who can use, 183
   working of, 182–83
lovemaking without intercourse as, 187
myth about sex, 160–61
natural, 187–89
   calendar method, 187–88
   mucus method, 188
   temperature method, 188
necessity of, 15
pill, 177–82
   cost of, 180
   drugs, working of pill and, 179
   forgetting to take, 178–79
   getting, 180
   good and bad points about, 180–82
   menstrual cycle and, ease of, 35
   nutrition and, 182
   period, missing, 179–80
   if sick, 179
   teenagers and, 35
   types of, 179
   who should not take, 181
   working of, 177–78
respect for oneself and, 161–62
sex, preparing for, 159–60
sexual liberation and, 165
statistics on pregnancy, 159
suppositories and tablets, vaginal, 189
withdrawal as, 188–89
See also abortion, deciding whether to have; baby, deciding to have
bisexuality, 114
bladder infections, in boys, as complication of trichomoniasis, 232
blood
   menstrual cycle and, 31
     fears about, 32

blood, (*continued*)
  test, in physical examination, 155–56
    for pregnancy, 192–93
    for sexually transmitted disease, 221
"blue balls," 81
  relief of, 17
Board of Health, medical treatment for sexually transmitted diseases
    and, 220
body, changes in, 5–40
  of boys, 9–18
    breasts, 17
    effects on self-perception and, 3–4
    erections, 13–14
    genitals, caring for, 17–18
    genitals, inside and outside look of, 12–13
    penis and testicle growth, 13
    proper terms and slang, 11–12
    pubic hair, body hair and whiskers, 16
    semen and ejaculation, 14–16
    voice change, 16–17
  checkup, general, in physical examination and, 156
  of girls, 19–40
    breasts, care of, 22–23
    breasts, developing, 20–22
    breasts, examining, 23–24
    boys' looking at, 19
    feelings about changes in, 19–20
    genitals and reproductive organs, 25–29
    menstruation (period), 29–39
    pubic and body hair, 24–25
    slang terms, 20
    symptoms, unusual, problems related to, 29–40
  self-perception of body, 7–9
    body smells, 8
    comparing self with others, 8
    friends, judgment by, 8
    other sex, judgment by, 8
    parents, judgment by, 8–9
  sexual changes, 5–6
Boston Womens' Health Book Collective (*Our Bodies, Ourselves*), 23n,
    232
boys, body of, 9–18
  breasts, 17
  erections, 13–14
    spontaneous, 14
  genitals, caring for, 17–18
    cancer of testicle, 18
    jock itch or rot, 18
    pain in genital area, 17
    penis discharge, 17
    sexually transmitted diseases (STD), 17
    undescended testicles, 17–18
  genitals, inside and outside look of, 12–13
  penis and testicle growth, 13
  proper terms and slang for, 11–12
  pubic hair, body hair and whiskers, 16
  semen and ejaculation, 14–16
  voice change, 16–17
boys, coping with problems in sex, 109–10
  coming too quickly, 111–12
  erection, not getting or keeping, 111
  pain with lovemaking, 112
  physical examination, 156
bras, wearing of, 22
breasts, of boys, 17
breasts, of girls
  care of, 22–23
  bras, wearing, 22
  hair, 23
  infections, 23
  inverted nipples, 23
  lumps, 23
  secretions, 23
  swelling, monthly, 22–23
  when hit, 23
  development of, 20–22
  examining, 23–24
    self-exam, how to, 24
  milk, flow of, 22
  shape of, 22

size of, 21–22
  slang for, 20

caffeine, pregnancy and, 191
calendar method of natural birth control, 187–88
cancer
  cervical, herpes simplex II and, 225
  in girls, 40
  of testicle, 18
caring, as means of improving lovemaking, 107
cervix, 27
  cap of, birth control and, 176–77
  inflamed, as complication of trichomoniasis, 232
checkups, medical, 153
childbirth techniques, ease of menstrual cycle and, 35
chlamydia, 221, 226
circumcision, 12
clinics, medical help for sexually transmitted diseases and, 220–21
clitoris, 25–26
  slang for, 20
cocaine (coke), 150
coming. *See* ejaculation, semen and
coming out as homosexual, 117–21
  to oneself, 118
  to others, 118–19
  to parents, 119–21
conception, 15, 29
condoms and foams, 166–67
  Consumer Reports on, 167n
  good and bad points about condoms, 168–69
  good and bad points about foam, 170–71
  how to get condoms, 167
  preventing sexually transmitted diseases by using, 218
  storing condoms, 167–68
  types of condoms, 166–67
  types of foam, 170
  using condoms, 167, 168
  using foam, 169–70
consumer's rights, physical health care and, 154
coping with sex, problems in, 108–12
  for boys, 111–12
    coming too quickly, 111–12
    erection, not getting or keeping, 111
    pain with lovemaking, 112
  for girls, 109–10
    orgasm, not reaching, 109–10
    pain with entry of penis, 109
  See also intercourse, sexual; sex
County Department of Public Social Services, 139
crabs. *See* lice, pubic
cramps, menstrual cycle and, 31, 36
"cruising," as technique for homosexuals' meeting each other, 121
culture, as test for sexually transmitted disease, 221
cunnilingus. *See* oral sex
cups, to catch menstrual flow, 38

D-and-C (dilation and curettage) method of having abortion, 204
dating, changing relationships and, 65–66
Depo-Provera, birth control and, 189
depressants (Valium, Quaaludes), 150
depression, as feeling after abortion, 205–206
DES (diethylstilbestrol), 18, 40
  Action Group in New York, 41
  Pap smears and, 158
diaphragm, birth control and, 171–76
  checking, 175
  cost of, 172–73
  getting, 172
  good and bad points about, 174–76
  jellies, contraceptive, 172, 173
  learning to insert, 173–75
  using, 171, 174
discharge, as symptom of sexually transmitted disease, 220
discipline, parents and, 51–52
diseases, sexually transmitted. *See* sexually transmitted diseases
  (STD)
doctor
  going to, 153
  time to talk to, 154–55
"double life," changing relationships and, 54–56

double standard between boys' and girls' behavior, 67–68
  as factor in orgasmic failure, 83
  in refusing sex with another, 93
douching, 231
downers (Valium, Quaaludes). *See* depressants
drugs and alcohol, 149–52
  alcohol, 149
  as blur to deciding on sex with another, 90–91
  depressants, 150
  erection, not getting or keeping and, 111
  hallucinogens, 150
  marijuana and hashish, 149, 150
  narcotics, 150
  precautions against reactions to, 151–52
    legal problems, 152
    overdoses, withdrawal, and bad trips, 152
    physical effects, 151
    psychological effects, 151–52
    quality control, 152
  pregnancy and, 191
  stimulants, 149–50
  See also alcohol

ectopic pregnancy, 39
effleurage, 35
ejaculation, semen and, 14–16
  conception and birth control, 15
  sensation of, 82
emotional health care, 133–52
  drugs and alcohol, 149–52
    alcohol, 149
    depressants, 150
    hallucinogens, 150
    marijuana and hashish, 149, 150
    narcotics, 150
    precautions against reactions to, 151–52
    stimulants, 149–50
  experiences, negative, 137
  family support, 145–46
  feeling bad, feeling better, 133–34
  finding someone to talk to, 141–43
    by friends, 146
  help, trying to ask for, 136
    where to call, 139
  mistakes, dealing with, 136–37
  powerless, feeling, 137–41
    death and suicide, 138–41, 142
  professional helper, 143–45
    obstacles and expectations, 144–45
  resources for help, 148
  self-help, ideas for, 146–48
  talking or not, 134–36, 141
    anger, 135
  See also physical health care
endometriosis, 39
"entrapment" of homosexuals by police, 122
epididymis, 15
Equal Rights Amendment, 49
erections, 13–14
  not getting or keeping, as problem in sex, 111
  spontaneous, 14
estrogen, 5
exercising, ease of menstrual cycle and, 35
extraction, menstrual, menstruation fluid and, 38–39

fallopian tubes, 29
family
  emotional support by, 145–46
  planning clinics, birth control and, 164–65
fantasies, sexual, 77–78
  homosexual, 78
father's rights, using foster care and, 210n
feelings
  bad to better, 133–34
  powerlessness, 137–41
  taking out, 134–36, 141
fellatio. *See* oral sex
fertilization. *See* conception
fibroids and cysts, 39–40
fimbriae of fallopian tubes, 29
Flagyl, as treatment for trichomoniasis, 232

foams. *See* condoms and foams
follicles of ovaries, 29
fooling around (petting), 95–96
foreplay in sexual intercourse, 101
foreskin of penis, 12
foster care, using, 209–14
  father's rights and, 210n
  legal rights and, 210
  private arrangement, 210–11
  voluntary placement for child, 211–14
    agreement, foster care, 212
    alternatives to, 213–14
    feelings about placement, 212–13
    making arrangements, 211–12
    problems with foster care, 213
French kiss, 95
friends
  changing relationships and, 57
  coming out as homosexual to, 118–19
  emotional support from, 146
  as influence in deciding about sex, 88–89
  judging your body, 8
  See also best friends; opposite-ex friendships

Gardner-Loulan, JoAnn (*Period*), 29n
gay men. *See* homosexuality
genderization of fertilized egg in womb, 81n
genitals
  of boys, caring for, 17–18
    cancer of testicle, 18
    external and internal, 12–13
    jock itch or rot, 18
    pain in genital area, 17
    penis discharge, 17
    sexually transmitted diseases (STD), 17
    undescended testicles, 17–18
  of girls. *See* reproductive organs and genitals
  touching each other's, 96
girls' bodies, 19–40
  boys' looking at, 19
  breasts, care of, 22–23
    bras, wearing, 22
    hair, 23
    secretions, 23
    swelling, monthly, 22–23
    when hit, 23
  breasts, developing, 20–22
    age, 21
    shape of, 22
    size, 21–22
  breasts, examining, 23–24
    self-exam, how to, 24
    infections, 23
    inverted nipples, 23
    lumps, 23
  feelings about changes in, 19–20
    sexual harassment, 19–20
  genitals and reproductive organs, 25–29
    internal reproductive organs, 28–29
    outside area, 25–28
  menstruation (having period), 29–39
    cycle, menstrual, 30–31
    difficult moments, 33
    feeling better during, ways of, 34–35
    feelings about, 32
    first period, 31
    history of attitudes toward, 32–33
    menarche, 29
    menstrual fluid, catching, 36–39
    predicting menstrual cycle, 33–35
    problem signs, 39
    readiness for, 31–32
    self-care, 36
    side effects of, knowing, 35–36
  pubic and body hair, 24–25
  slang for, 20
  symptoms, unusual, problems related to, 39–40
    cancer, 40
    DES (diethylstilbestrol), 40
    ectopic pregnancy, 39

girls' bodies, (*continued*)
  endometriosis, 39
    fibroids and cysts, 39–40
    pelvic inflammatory disease (PID), 39
    pregnancy, 39
girls, coping with problems in sex, 109–10
  orgasm, not reaching, 109–10
    pressure, removing, 110
  pain with entry of penis, 109
  physical examination, 156–57
    internal (pelvic) exam, 156–57
    menstruation, 156
    pap smear, 158
    rectal exam, 158
    speculum exam, 157–58
    vaginal exam, bi-annual, 158
glans
  of clitoris, 25
  of penis, 12
globulin injections, for pregnant women with hepatitis, 230
gonorrhea, facts on, 17, 223–24
Gordon, Sol (*You Would If You Loved Me*), 92n
gram-stain test for sexually transmitted disease, 221
groin, pain in, as symptom of sexually transmitted disease, 220
groups, changing relationships and, 57–58
group therapy, emotional health care and, 145
guilt feeling
  after abortion, 205
  over incest, 129
    after rape, 127

hair, pubic and body
  in boys, 16
  in girls, 23, 24–25
HCG hormone, urine and blood test for pregnancy and, 192
head check, in physical examination, 156
health care. *See* emotional health care; physical health care
help, trying to ask for, 136
  professionals and, 143–45
    obstacles and expectations, 144–45
  where to call, 139
hepatitis, facts on, 229–30
herpes, facts on, 224–26
  pap smear and, necessity of, 225
  pregnancy, danger to, 225
homophobia (fear of homosexuals), 97, 113
homosexuality, 112–23
  bisexuality and, 114
  coming out, 117–21
    to oneself, 118
    to others, 118–19
    to parents, 119–21
  discrimination against, 49
  fear of (homophobia), 97, 113
  gay feelings, becoming aware of, 114–17
    denying and hiding feelings, 115–17
    stereotypes, 116–17
  gay-straight line, 112–13
  growing up with, 114
  issues in gay relationships, 122–23
    commitments, 123
    initiating relationships, 122
    roles, 123
  labeling oneself gay, 114
  meeting other gay people, 121–22
    "cruising," 121
    police "entrapment," 122
  misconceptions about, 96
  negative teaching about, 112
  sexual activity and, 122
  sexual fantasies and, 78
  sexually transmitted diseases and, 217
hormones, body changes and, 5
Hyde Amendment, paying for abortions and, 200
hymen, 26–27
  sexual intercourse and, 27
  slang for, 20

incest, 128–29
  as curable sickness, 129
  guilt feelings about, 129

induced method of having abortion, 204
infections
  bladder, in boys, as complication of trichomoniasis, 232
  in girl's breasts, 23
  vaginal. *See* vaginal infections, facts on
influences ("voices") affecting decision to have sex with another, 87–92
  balancing, 90
  blurring, drugs and alcohol and, 90–91
  friends, 88–89
  media, 89
  needs, one's own, 89–90
  parents, 87
  pressure to go further, 91–92
  religious attitudes and beliefs, 89
  standards, one's own, 90
  See also intercourse, sexual, deciding about; sex
initiation, as issue in homosexual relationships, 122
injectable contraception as birth control, 189
inner lips (minor lips) of female genitals, 25
intercourse, sexual, deciding about, 98–104, 187
  having intercourse, 101–104
    first time, 102–104
    pregnancy, 102
    technical aspects of, 101–102
  heterosexual and homosexual, 98
  lovemaking without sex, birth control by, 187
  pregnancy, risk of, 98, 102
  pressures, 99–100
  sexually transmitted disease, risk of, 98, 103
  virginity, opinions about, 99
  waiting, 100–101
  See also sex with another, exploring
intra-uterine device. *See* IUD
itching, as symptom of sexually transmitted disease, 220
IUD (intra-uterine device), 182–86
  antibiotics and, 183
  changing, 185
  checking, 185
  cost of, 185
  getting, 183–84
  good and bad points of, 185–86
  infections from, 186
  inserting, 184–85
  perforation and embedding, 186
  pregnancy and use of, 186–87
  removing, 185
  sexually transmitted diseases and, 186
  using, 183
  who can use, 183
  working nature of, 182–83

jellies and creams, contraceptive, preventing sexually transmitted diseases by using, 171–72, 173, 218
jock itch or rot, 18

kissing, 94–95
  French kiss, 95

labia. *See* outer lips of female genitals
learning about sex with another, 104–105
  sex roles in, 105
legal problems, drugs and, 152
legal rights
  abortion and, 198–99
  foster care and, 210
lesbians. *See* homosexuality
lice, pubic, facts on, 232–33
liver problems, hepatitis and, 230
local VD hot lines, 219–20
loneliness, feeling of, changing relationships and, 60–61
love, falling in, 68–70
lovemaking
  improving, 107
  without intercourse, birth control by, 187
  masturbation and, 81
  talking about, 105
LSD (acid), possible effects after taking, 150
lumps in girl's breasts, 23
Lynch, Peggy (*Sexually Transmitted Diseases (STD) and How to Avoid Them*), 218n

making out, 95
mammary glands, 20, 22
marijuana and hashish, 149, 150
marriage, changing relationships and, 70
masturbation, 17, 79–81
  in boys, care of genitals and, 17
  frequency of, 80
  lovemaking and, 81
  methods of, 79–80
  morality and normality of, 80–81
  privacy and, 79
  See also intercourse, sexual, deciding about; sex with another, problems in
media, as influence in deciding about sex, 88–89
medical examination, 153–55
  complete medical history, 154
  doctor, time to talk to, 154–55
menarche, 29
menstruation (having period), 29–39
  catching, fluid, menstrual 36–39
    cups, 38
    extraction, 38–39
    sanitary napkins, 37–38
    sponges, 38
    tampons, 38
    toxic shock syndrome, 38
  cycle, menstrual, 30–31
    blood, 31
    cramps, 31
    ovulation, 30
  difficult moments, 33
  feelings about, 32
  feeling better during, ways of, 34–35
  first period, 31
  history of attitudes toward, 32–33
  last menstrual period (LMP), determining degree of pregnancy and, 197
  menarche, 29
  myths about, 32
  in physical examination, 156
  predicting menstrual cycle, 33–35
    mucus method, 34–35
  problem signs, 39
  readiness for, 31–32
  self-care and, 36
  side effects, knowing, 35–36
    cramps, 36
miscarriage, hepatitis as possible cause of, 230
mistakes, dealing with, 136–37
mons, 25
moods, changing relationships with parents and, 43
morality of masturbation, 80–81
mucus method
  of natural birth control, 188
  of predicting menstrual cycle, 34–35
mucus of vaginal walls, 27
myths. *See* homosexuality; menstruation; rape

NAACP (National Association for the Advancement of Colored People), 137
narcotics, 150
National Abortion Foundation, 199, 200
National Organization for Women, 199
National Runaway Switchboard, 139
National VD hot line, 219
nipples, inverted, in girls, 23
nocturnal emission. *See* wet dreams
non-gonococcal urethritis (NGU), facts on, 226–27
  caused by chlamydia, 221, 226
non-specific urethritis. *See* non-gonococcal urethritis
normality
  of child, as parents' concern, 46–48
  of masturbation, 80–81
nutrition, good, birth control pill and, 182

opposite-sex friendships, changing relationships and, 64–65. *See also* best friends; friends
oral sex, 96–98
  misconceptions about, 97–98
orgasm
  ease of menstrual cycle and, 35

  in boys, 14–15
    coming too quickly, as problem in sex for, 111–12
  failure of, advice about, 82–83
    anatomical factors, 82
    double standard, 83
    sex education, 83
  girls' not reaching, as problem in sex, 109–10
  by petting/fooling around, 96
  as part of sexual response cycle, 82
  in sexual intercourse, 102
os of cervix, 27–28
others
  accepting in changing relationships, 61–62
  judging one's body by, 8–9
outer lips (major lips), of female genitals, 25
ovaries, 29
overdoses of drugs, 152
ovulation, 30

pain, in genital area of boys, 17
Papanicolaou, Dr. G. N., 158
Pap smear, 158, 158n
  herpes and, 225
parents
  changing relationship with, 41–56
    discipline and, 51–52
    "double life" of child and, 54–56
    normality of child, as concern of parents, 46–48
    seeing parents as people, 48–50
    separating from parents, 41–42
    sex, views on, 52–54
  coming out as homosexual to, 119–21
  as influence in deciding about sex, 87
  judging your body, 8–9
  pregnancy and, 196–97
  sexually transmitted disease, telling about, 222–23
Parents Anonymous, 49
PCP. *See* angel dust
pelvic examination for girls, 156–57
pelvic inflammatory disease (PID), 39
  as complication from gonorrhea, 224
  non-gonococcal urethritis and danger of, 227
pelvic organs
  of female, 27
  of male, 13
penis
  discharge from, 17
  functions of, 12
  growth of, 13
  parts of, 12
  uncircumcised, detail of, 12
perforation and embedding, IUD and, 186–87
period, missing of
  birth control pill and, 179–80
  IUD use and, 187
  as sign of pregnancy, 190
  See also menstruation
petting/fooling around, 95–96
  genitals, touching each others, 96
physical effects of drugs, 151
physical health care, 153–233
  birth control, 159–89
    cervical cap, 176–77
    condoms and foam, 166–71
    diaphragm, 171–76
    family planning clinics, 164–65
    getting, 162–65
    injectable contraception, 189
    IUD (intra-uterine device), 182–86
    lovemaking without intercourse, 187
    myths about sex and, 160–61
    natural, 187–89
    pill, 177–82
    preparing for sex and, 159–60
    respect for oneself and, 161–62
    sexual liberation and, 165
    statistics on pregnancy and, 159–89
    suppositories and tablets, vaginal, 189
    withdrawal as, 188–89
  consumer's rights and, 154

physical health care, (*continued*)
  doctor, going to, 153
  examination, physical, 155–58
    after, 158
    blood test, 155–56
    body check, general, 156
    boy's, 156
    girl's, 156–58
    head check, 156
    measurements, 155
    urine, 155
  medical examination, typical, 153–55
    complete medical history, 154
    doctor, time to talk to, 154–55
  pregnancy, 189–216
    abortion, deciding whether to have, 197–206
    baby, deciding to have, 206–16
    boy's role in, 195–96
    dangers to, 191
    deciding if pregnant, 190
    determining degree of, 197
    feelings about possible, 190–92
    parents, talking with, about, 196–97
    if pregnant, 193–95
    test for, 192–93
  sexually transmitted diseases (STD's), avoiding, 216–33
    birth control as protection from, 223
    body openings and, 217
    gonorrhea, facts on, 223–24
    hepatitis, facts on, 229–30
    herpes, facts on, 224–26
    homosexuality and, 217
    knowing if present, 219
    medical help for, finding, 219–22
    non-gonococcal urethritis (NGU), facts on, 226–27
    pregnancy and, 223
    preventing, 217–19
    pubic lice (crabs), facts on, 232–33
    scabies, facts on, 233
    sex and, feelings about, 217
    symptoms, general, 220
    syphilis, facts on, 227–28
   telling partners about having, 222–23
    vaginal infections, facts on, 230–32
    warts, venereal, facts on, 228–29
  See also emotional health care
PID. *See* pelvic inflammatory disease
pituitary gland, body changes and, 5
Planned Parenthood, 164, 200, 220
police "entrapment" of homosexuals, 122
pregnancy, 39, 189–216
  abortion, deciding whether to have, 197–206
    advice on, 199
    D-and-C (dilation and curettage) method of having, 204
    emotional aftercare, 205–206
    induced method of having, 204
    legal rights, 198–99
    paying for, 200
    physical aftercare, 204–205
    Rh-negative blood and, 201n
    risks and complications associated with, 200–201
    services, checking out, 199–200
    vacuum suction (vacuum aspiration) method of having, 201–204
    where to get, 199
  baby, deciding to have, 206–16
    adoption choice, 214–16
    choices available, 206
    foster care, using, 209–14
    parent, deciding to become, 206–209
  boys' role in, 195–96
  dangers to, 191
  deciding if pregnant, 190
  determining degree of, 197
  feelings about possible, 190–92
  Flagyl, avoidance of, during, 232
  hepatitis infecting fetus during, 230
  herpes, danger of, 225
  IUD use and, 186
  oral sex and, 96, 96n
  parents, talking with, 196–97

petting/fooling around and, 96
  if pregnant, 193–95
    choices to make, 194–95
  process of, 29
  sexual intercourse and, 98, 102
  sexually transmitted diseases and, 223
  tests for, 192–93
    blood test, 192–93
    pelvic exam, 193
    urine test, 192
    where to get, 192
premature ejaculation, 111–12
privacy
  masturbation and, 79
  in sex with another, 106–107
professional help, emotional health care and, 143–45
  obstacles and expectations, 144–45
    group therapy, 145
    prejudging therapist, 144–45
prostaglandins, 36
prostate gland, 12, 15
  infected, as complication of trichomoniasis, 232
psychological effects of drugs, 151–52
puberty, 5, 8, 15
pubic hair
  in boys, 16
  in girls, 24–25
pubic lice. *See* lice, pubic

Quaaludes, 150

rape, 124–28
  by acquaintance, 124
  action to take if raped, 127–28
    after it's over, 128
    guilt feelings, 127
    prosecute, deciding whether to, 128
  knowing if raped, 124–25
  likelihood of, 126–27
  myths about, 125–26
  rapists, 126
rashes, as symptom of sexually transmitted disease, 220
rectal examination
  for boys, 156
  for girls, 158
relationships, changing, 41–70
  accepting others, 61–62
  best friends, 62–64
  dating, 65–66
  double standard, 67–68
  feeling lonely, 60–61
  fitting in, 58–60
  friends and, 57
  groups, 57–58
  love, falling in, 68–70
  marriage, 70
  opposite-sex friendships, 64–65
  parents and, 41–56
    changes in parents, 50–51
    discipline, 51–52
    "double life," 54–56
    moods, 43
    normality of child, as parents' concern, 46–48
    older, trying to look, reaction to, 46–47
    seeing as people, 48–50
    separating from, 41–42
    sex and, 52–54
    style, developing one's own, 43–46
  self-acceptance, 61
  sex-role expectations, 66–67
religion, attitudes and beliefs about, as influence in deciding about sex, 89
reproductive organs and genitals of girls, 25–29
  girls' internal, 28, 29
    conception and, 29
  outside area, 25–28
    anus, 28
    cervix, 27
    clitoris, 25–26
    glans of clitoris, 25
    hymen, 26–27

inner lips (minor lips), 25
mons, 25
mucus of vaginal wall, 27
os of cervix, 27–28
outer lips (major lips, labia), 25
pelvic organs, 27
shaft of clitoris, 25
urethra, 26
vagina, 26–27
vulva, 26
response cycle, sexual, 81–82
  orgasm, 82
  relaxation, 82
  stimulation, 81
  See also intercourse, sexual; sex
Rh blood, positive and negative, abortions and, 201n
Rhogam, abortions on mothers with Rh-negative blood and, 201n
Rome, Esther (*Sexually Transmitted Diseases (STD) and How to Avoid Them*), 218n
Runaway Hot Line, 139

sanitary napkins, menstrual flow and, 37–38
scabies, facts on, 233
scrotum, 12
secretions from girl's breasts, 23
self-acceptance, changing relationships and, 61
self-perception of body, 7–9
  bodily changes and effects on, 3–4
  body smells and, 8
  comparing self with others, 8
  friends, judgment by, 8
  other sex, judgment by, 8
  parents, judgment by, 8–9
semen. *See* ejaculation, semen and
seminal vesicles of testicles, 12
sex with another, exploring, 84–123
  commencing, 85–86
  deciding about, 86–92
    influences, different (or "voices"), 87–92
    relationship, considerations about, 87
  homosexuality, 112–23
    bisexuality and, 114
    coming out, 117–21
    fear of, 113
    gay feelings, becoming aware of, 114–17
    growing up, 114
    issues in gay relationships, 122–23
    labeling oneself gay, 114
    meeting other people, 121–22
    negative teachings about, 112
    sex, 122
  learning about, 104–105
    sex roles in, 105
  lovemaking, improving, 107–108
  making out, 95
  oral sex, 96–98
  petting/fooling around, 95–96
    genitals, touching each other's, 96
  pleasures and pains, 84
  privacy, 106–107
  problems in sex, coping with, 108–109
    for boys, 111–12
    for girls, 109–10
  refusing, 92–93
    double standard, 93
  sexual activity, nature of, 93–95
    kissing, 94–95
  sexual intercourse, 98–104
    having intercourse, techniques of, 101–104
    heterosexual and homosexual, 98
    pressures, 99–100
    sexually transmitted disease, risk of, 98, 103
    virginity, opinions about, 99
  waiting, 100–101
  talking about, 105–106
sex education, 6
  as factor in orgasmic failure, 83
sex-roles
  expectations, changing relationships and, 66–67
  in learning about sex with another, 105

sex with self, exploring, 75–83
  fantasies, sexual, 77–78
    homosexual, 78
  feeling bad about sex, 76–77
    privacy and guilt, 76
    values, 76
  learning about sex, 75–76
  masturbation, 79–81
    frequency of, 80
    lovemaking and, 81
    methods of, 79–80
    morality and normality of, 80–81
    privacy and, 79
  orgasmic failure, advice about, 82–83
    anatomical factors, 82
    double standard, 83
    sex education, 83
  response cycle, sexual, 81–82
    orgasm, 82
    relaxation, 82
    stimulation, 81
sex against will, 124–29
  if raped, action to take, 127–28
  incest, 128–29
  likelihood of rape, 126–27
  myths about rape, 125–26
  rape, 124–25
  who rapes, 126
sexual changes, 5–6
  sex education and, 6
  as mystery, 6
sexual functioning, examination of, for boys, 156
sexual harassment of girls, 19–20
sexual intercourse. *See* intercourse, sexual
sexuality
  being and feeling sexual, understanding of, 73–74
  moving at one's own speed, 74
sexually transmitted diseases (STD's), avoiding, 17, 216–33
  birth control and protection from, 223
  body openings and, 217
  gonorrhea, facts on, 223–24
  hepatitis, facts on, 229–30
  herpes, facts on, 224–26
  homosexuality and, 217
  knowing if present, 219
  medical help for, finding, 219–22
    blood test, 221
    Board of Health, 220
    culture, 221
    free clinics, 220–21
    gram-stain test, 221
    local VD hot lines, 219–20
    National VD hot line, 219
    private doctors, 221
    sexual intercourse, avoiding, 222
    treatment for, 221–22
    women's clinics, 220
  non-gonococcal urethritis (NGU), facts on, 226–27
  pregnancy and, 223
  preventing, 217–19
    techniques of, 218
  pubic lice (crabs), facts on, 232–33
  scabies, facts on, 233
  sex and, feelings about, 217
  symptoms, general, 220
  telling partners about, 222–23
  syphilis, facts on, 227–28
  vaginal infections, facts on, 230–32
    trichomoniasis, 231–32
    yeast infections, 230–31
  warts, venereal, facts on, 228–29
shaft of clitoris, 25
shaft of penis, 12
"simultaneous orgasm," 102
smegma, 12
smells, body, self-perception and, 8
sores, as symptom of sexually transmitted disease, 220
sore throat, as symptom of sexually transmitted disease, 220
speculum examination for girls, 157–58
sperm, 12

sperm, *(continued)*
ejaculation, conception and birth control, 15
spermicidal cream, applying, 173
sponges, menstrual flow and, 38
spontaneous erection, 14
standards, one's own, as influence in deciding about sex, 90
stereotypes, homosexuals as, 116–17, 119
stimulants (uppers, amphetamines), 149–50
stimulation
in sexual intercourse, direct and indirect, 101–102
during sexual response cycle, 81
straights (heterosexuals), 112. *See also* homosexuality
strength, feeling of, after abortion, 206
style, developing one's own, changing relationships with parents and, 43–46
suicide, feelings about, 138–41
myths and facts about, 142
suppositories and tablets, vaginal, birth control and, 189
syphilis, facts on, 227–28
death from, 227

talking
emotional health care and, 141–43
about sex with another, 105–106
pretending, 106
tampons
inserting, 26, 27
for menstrual flow, 38
toxic shock syndrome from, 38
temperature method of natural birth control, 188
testicles, 12
cancer of, 18
examining, 18
growth of, 13
inside of, 15
undescended, 17–18
testosterone, 5, 16
therapy. *See* professional help, emotional health care and
timing, as means of improving lovemaking, 107–108
toxic shock syndrome, tampons and, 38
trichomoniasis, as infection of vagina, facts on, 231–32
Flagyl, danger of, as treatment for, 232

undescended testicles, 17–18
United Way Information and Referral Services, 139
uppers (amphetamines). *See* stimulants
urethra
of female genitals, 26
inflamed, as complication of trichomoniasis, 232
in penis, 12–13
urethritis. *See* non-gonococcal urethritis
urination, burning, as symptom of sexually transmitted disease, 220
urine test, in physical examination, 155
for pregnancy, 192
uterus (womb), 29

vacuum suction (vacuum aspiration) method of having abortion, 201–204
breathing exercises during, 203
vagina, 27
examination of, bi-manual, 158
infections of, facts on, 230–32
slang for, 20
trichomoniasis, 231–32
yeast infections, 230–31
douche for curing, 231
Valium, 150
vas deferens (sperm duct), 12, 15
vasectomy, 15
VD Handbook, The, 222n
venereal diseases (VD). *See* sexually transmitted diseases (STD's)
virginity, opinions about, 99
vitamin B, 148n
vitamins B and C, ease of menstrual cycle and, 34
voice change, in boys, 16–17
vulva, slang for, 20

warts, venereal, facts on, 220, 228–29
wet dreams, 16
whiskers, in boys, 16
withdrawal from drugs, 152
womb of woman. *See* uterus

yeast infection of vagina, facts on, 230–31